RC

D1447432

PICK'S DISEASE AND PICK COMPLEX

PICK'S DISEASE
AND PICK COMPLEX

Edited by

Andrew Kertesz, M.D.
Department of Clinical Neurological Sciences
Lawson Research Institute
St. Joseph's Health Centre
The University of Western Ontario

David G. Munoz, M.D.
Department of Pathology
The University of Western Ontario

⊛ WILEY-LISS

A JOHN WILEY & SONS, INC., PUBLICATION

New York • Chichester • Weinheim • Brisbane • Singapore • Toronto

5/98

#37410534

Copyright © 1998 by Wiley-Liss, Inc. All rights reserved.

Published simultaneously in Canada.

Library of Congress Cataloging-in-Publication Data:
Pick's disease and Pick complex / edited by Andrew Kertesz, David G. Munoz.
    p. cm.
   Includes bibliographical references and index.
   ISBN 0-471-17792-X (cloth : alk. paper)
   1. Presenile dementia.   I. Munoz, David G.
   [DNLM: 1. Dementia, Presenile. WM 220 P597 1998]
  RC522.P53   1998
  616.8′3–dc21
  DNLM/DLC
  for Library of Congress   97-34191

Printed in the United States of America.

10 9 8 7 6 5 4 3 2 1

CONTENTS

▬▬▬ FOREWORD

Few areas of brain disease are as bewildering to the uninitiated as those of localized brain degeneration. The editors and authors of this book face a formidable dilemma: unjudicious lumping may obscure important differences, while unjustified splitting may withdraw a key piece in an emerging pattern. The editors have chosen an approach both comprehensive and reflective of the state-of-the-art. They begin with a nosological and historical introduction, followed by the contributions of all the major investigators in the field and end with chapters on inflammation, genetics and the editors' clinico-pathological summing up.

The fact that the editors were able to secure the contributions of most of the active international community in this area speaks to the editors' standing and the eagerness of the authors to have one book where all current knowledge can be assessed and the remaining questions formulated. Having one volume that summarizes where we are and where we should be going marks a milestone and offers a platform for further progress. Science can wait, but medicine must act. While knowledge remains incomplete, decisions have to be made in regard to diagnosis, prognosis and potential treatment of patients. This necessitates adopting schemes of classification and clinical and pathological criteria in the absence of sufficient data.

Kertesz and Munoz propose the term "Pick's complex" to interpret the syndromes with common pathologies and clinical features. They provide considerable clinical and pathological evidence that corticobasal degeneration is also part of Pick's complex and they show that some discoveries are rediscoveries. The extrapyramidal variety of Pick's disease was described in the 1930's and later rediscovered as corticonigral and then corticobasal degeneration. Similarly, Pick and his contemporaries described frontotemporal lobar degeneration mainly manifesting as a frontal type of personality and behavioural alternations and progressive aphasia. These have been "rediscovered" as separate entities because they did not contain the typical inclusions or Pick bodies. Kertesz and Munoz provide compelling evidence for the convergence of these clinical entities and spectrum of pathologies.

Their interpretive concept has been boosted by the recent discovery of chromosome 17 localization of some families with frontal temporal degeneration or Pick complex, with Pick variant pathology, which may be only a superficial spongiosis of the cortex. (also a feature of Pick's disease)

This book brings together behavioural neurologists, neuropsychologists, pathologists, neurobiologists, neurochemists and neurogeneticists to present a wealth of information and compelling evidence of the integration of various neurodegenerative disorders and clinical, pathological, biological and genetic commonalities. This volume will become the standard text of its time.

Vladimir Hachinski, M.D., FRCP(C), DSc(Med)
Richard & Beryl Ivey Professor and Chair
Department of Clinical Neurological Sciences
The University of Western Ontario

ACKNOWLEDGMENTS

The idea of this book came to us when we discovered the substantial number of patients with Pick complex and the bewildering profusion of terminology at various levels of description that have appeared in the literature, which to us seemed to be dealing with closely related entities. We hope to restore Pick's disease to its original importance and have the unifying concept of Pick complex to bridge the gap between the clinical and pathological descriptions. We also attempted to provide a forum for most recent ideas and advances in this field. Although not all the contributors to this volume subscribe to the concept of the unitary nature of the clinical or the pathological variants, there is agreement that these represent a relatively common form of degenerative dementia.

Special acknowledgments are due to our collaborators, who helped us with some of the material in the book technically and in a clerical fashion. We thank Wilda Davidson and Patricia McCabe for testing the patients and maintaining the data base, Ian McKenzie and John Wolf who helped to review the pathological material, Roy Taylor for technical assistance, and Bonita Caddel for typing, organizing, proof-reading the manuscripts. We are grateful to many members of the Department of Clinical Neurological Sciences and Psychiatry in London, as well as from other centres in Ontario and nationally, who contributed by referring patients knowing our interest in progressive aphasia and frontal lobe dementia. We appreciate their generosity, clinical insights and interest.

Andrew Kertesz, M.D.
David G. Munoz, M.D.
London, Ontario
February 1998

Dr. Kyle Boone, Department of Psychiatry, Harbor-UCLA Medical Center, 1000 W. Carson Street, Torrance, CA 90509

Dr. Arne Brun, Department of Pathology, Lund University Hospital, Box 638, 220 09 Lund, Sweden

Dr. Lorraine N. Clark, UCSF, Department of Neurology, 1001 Potrero Avenue, San Francisco, CA 94110

Dr. André Delacourte, Department of Research, Unite INSERM 422, Place de Verdun, 59045 Lille, Cedex, France

Dr. Peter Garrard, University of Cambridge Neurology Unit, Addenbrooke's Hospital, Hills Road, Cambridge, CB2 2QQ, United Kingdom

Dr. Phillipe Gasque, Department of Medical Biochemistry, University of Wales, College of Medicine, Heath Park, Cardiff, CF4 4XN, United Kingdom

Dr. Gloria M. Grace, Department of Psychology, London Health Sciences Centre, University Campus, 339 Windermere Rd., London, Ontario N6A 5A5, Canada

Dr. Lars Gustafson, Department of Psychogeriatrics, Lund University Hospital, Box 638, 220 09 Lund, Sweden

Dr. John R. Hodges, University of Cambridge, Neurology Unit, Addenbrooke's Hospital, Hills Road, Cambridge, CB2 2QQ, United Kingdom

Dr. Andrew Kertesz, Department of Clinical Neurological Sciences, St. Joseph's Health Centre, University of Western Ontario, London, Ontario N6A 4V2, Canada

Dr. David S. Knopman, Department of Neurology, University of Minnesota Hospitals, Box 295, Minneapolis, MN 55455

Ms. Nancy Koras, Department of Neurology, Harbor-UCLA Medical Center, 1000 W. Carson Street, Torrance, CA 90509

Jonathan Kushii, Department of Neurology, Harbor-UCLA Medical Center, 1000 W. Carson Street, Torrance, CA 90509

Dr. Ramón Leiguarda, Instituto de Investigaciones Neurologicas, Raúl Carrea, Montañeses 2325, 1428 Buenos Aires, Argentina

Dr. Peter A. LeWitt, Clinical Neuroscience Center, Wayne State University School of Medicine, 5821 West Maple Road, #192, West Bloomfield, MI 48322

Dr. Timothy Lynch, Department of Neurology, Columbia University, 650 West 168th Street, Room BB-307, New York, NY 10032

Dr. David M. A. Mann, Department of Pathological Sciences, University of Manchester, M13 9PT, United Kingdom

Dr. Pablo Martinez-Lage, University of Navarra, c/Santa Cruz 31-8B, Azur Mayor (Navarra) 31180, Spain

Dr. Bruce L. Miller, Department of Neurology, Harbor-UCLA Medical Center, 1000 W. Carson Street, Bldg. F9, Torrance, CA 90509

Dr. Fred Mishkin, Department of Radiology, Harbor-UCLA Medical Center, 1000 W. Carson Street, Torrance, CA 90509

Dr. David G. Munoz, Department of Pathology, University of Western Ontario, London, Ontario, N6A 5C1, Canada

Dr. James W. Neal, Department of Histopathology, Neuropathology Laboratory, University of Wales, College of Medicine, Heath Park, Cardiff, CF4 4XN, United Kingdom

Dr. David Neary, Department of Neurology, Manchester Royal Infirmary, Manchester, M13 9WL, United Kingdom

Dr. Geoff R. Newman, Medical Electron Microscopy Unit, University of Wales, College of Medicine, Heath Park, Cardiff, CF4 4XN, United Kingdom

Dr. Karalyn Patterson, MRC Applied Psychology Unit, 15 Chaucer Rd, Cambridge, United Kingdom

Dr. Yves Robitaille, Hôpital Côte des neiges, 4565 chemin de la Reine Marie, Montréal, H3W 1W5, Canada

Nicolas Sergeant, Department of Research, Unite INSERM 422, Place de Verdun, 59045 Lille, Cedex, France

Sim K. Singhrao, Departments of Medical Electron Microscopy and Medical Biochemistry, University of Wales, College of Medicine, Heath Park, Cardiff, CF4 4XN, United Kingdom

Dr. Julie S. Snowden, Department of Neurology, Manchester Royal Infirmary, Manchester, M13 9WL, United Kingdom

Dr. Sergio E. Starkstein, Instituto de Investigaciones Neurologicas, Raúl Carrea - Montañeses 2325, 1428 Buenos Aires, Argentina

Dr. Michael J. Strong, Department of Clinical Neurological Sciences, London Health Sciences Centre, Room 7OF10, University Campus, 339 Windermere Rd., London, Ontario, N6A 5A5, Canada

Dr. J. Randolph Swartz, Department of Psychiatry, Harbor-UCLA Medical Center, 1000 W. Carson Street, Torrance, CA 90509

Annick Wattez, Department of Research, Unite INSERM 422, Place de Verdun, 59045 Lille, Cedex, France

Dr. Kirk Wilhelmsen, UCSF, Department of Neurology, Bldg. 1, Room 101, 1001 Potrero Avenue, San Francisco, CA 94110

PICK'S DISEASE AND PICK COMPLEX

CHAPTER 1

Pick's Disease and Pick Complex: Introductory Nosology

ANDREW KERTESZ

Department of Clinical Neurological Sciences, St. Joseph's Health Centre, University of Western Ontario, London, Ontario N6A 4V2, Canada

INTRODUCTION

Pick's disease (PiD) is like the proverbial elephant. When blind men are asked to define it, one feeling a leg calls it a tree; another touching the trunk, a snake; and a third encountering the body, a wall. The term means different things to different people. The term *Pick's disease* is used to designate either clinically defined cases of progressive frontal and temporal degeneration or a pathological entity defined histologically by the presence of argyrophilic globular inclusions (Pick bodies) and swollen, achromatic neurons (Pick cells). Arnold Pick described the clinical picture of focal atrophies, particularly in the frontal and temporal lobes, around the turn of the century (Pick 1892, 1904, 1905, 1906). Pick's initial description of a progressively aphasic patient with behavioral disturbances and cases of frontal lobe dementia was based on gross examination alone, without any microscopic data, but the clinical descriptions and their relationship to focal atrophy are the basis of the syndrome. Gans (1922) suggested the eponymic term and considered a predilection for the phylogenetically younger frontal and temporal lobes in the etiology. Subsequently, PiD was defined on the basis of histology, initially described by Alzheimer (1911). Onari and Spatz (1926) and Stertz (1926) reexamined a series of cases of Pick and others, emphasizing this histological picture associated with focal atrophy. A dichotomy of nosology arose because some people use the term *Pick's disease* on the basis of histological criteria, while others describe the clinical picture of focal atrophies, as Pick did originally. Most series of PiD were based on postmortem examination, and often the clinical features were incompletely described because of the retrospective nature of these studies. This gave rise to the notion that PiD is difficult to diagnose *in vivo*. It also became apparent that cases of clinical PiD with frontal lobe and temporal lobe symptomatology may not show the typical histological picture at autopsy (Malamud and Boyd, 1940; Winkelman and Book, 1944; Constantinidis et al., 1974; case records of the Massachusetts General Hospital, 1986). Fur-

Pick's Disease and Pick Complex, Edited by Andrew Kertesz and David G. Munoz
ISBN 0-471-17792-X   ©1998 Wiley-Liss, Inc.

TABLE 1.1   Glossary of PC

Circumscribed cerebral atrophy	Dementia lacking distinctive histology (DLDH)
Pick's disease (PiD)	Semantic dementia
Lobar atrophy	Frontal lobe dementia with motor neuron disease
Progressive subcortical gliosis (PSG)	Frontotemporal dementia (FTD)
Corticodentatonigral degeneration	Primary progressive apraxia
Generalized Pick's disease	Nonspecific familial dementia
Frontal lobe dementia (FLD)	Atypical presenile dementia
Primary progressive aphasia (PPA)	Spongiform encephalopathy of long duration
Corticobasal degeneration (CBD)	Hereditary dysphasic dementia
Corticobasal degeneration syndrome (CBDS)	Disinhibition-dementia-parkinsonism-amyotrophy

thermore, various clinical and pathological manifestations of PiD were described under different labels, at times as distinct entities (Table 1.1). In order to alleviate the nosological dichotomy while retaining the well-established eponym, we suggested the term *Pick complex* (*PC*) to encompass all the related entities both clinically and pathologically (Kertesz et al., 1994). In this chapter, I will summarize the clinical concepts concerning this family of syndromes.

PICK'S DISEASE: EVOLUTION OF A SYNDROME

After the initial descriptions of PiD, which were concerned mostly with the extent and location of the atrophy and some with the unique histology, mainly clinicopathological papers appeared. Most of the patients described in these papers had dramatic frontal lobe deficits (Schneider, 1927, 1929; Thorpe, 1932; Löewenberg, 1935; Ferraro and Jervis, 1936, Nichols and Weigner, 1938). Schneider (1927, 1929) described several stages of PiD: first, a "disturbance of judgement and asocial behavior" followed by aphasia and later by more generalized dementia. He also distinguished rapid and slow forms. The aphasic variety of PiD was described quite early (Pick, 1892; Rosenfeld, 1909; Malamud and Boyd, 1940, Akelaitis, 1944; Wechsler et al., 1982; Holland et al., 1985), and the cases resemble reports of primary progressive aphasia, appearing later (see below). Caron (1934), in his review of PiD, stated that the most common form is characterized by early development of aphasia, and other investigators also emphasized early speech disturbance or aphasia in PiD (Lüers, 1947; Kosaka, 1976; Ohashi, 1983).

It was recognized that at times the disease occurred in families (Malamud and Waggoner, 1943). A report of a large family with PiD, in which 25 of 51 examined members were affected (Schenk, 1958–1959) with a mostly frontal presentation, was published. Subsequently, a study of this family was republished, with a genetic linkage to chromosome 17 (Heutink et al., 1997). Descriptions of what could be classified clinically as familial PiD continue to be published, but there is a tendency to reclassify these because of the pathological variations (Lynch et al., 1994; Brown et al., 1996; Bird et al., 1997) (see Chapters 14 and 18 in this volume).

Several series of PiD were described in the European literature in the early 1950s (Sjogren et al., 1952; van Mansvelt, 1954; Lüers and Spatz, 1957; Delay and Brion, 1962). Frontotemporal atrophy was the most common form of the disease (54%). Frontal atrophy occurred in only 25% and temporal atrophy in only 17%. The brunt of the atrophy was found most often in the medial orbital and the inferior frontal gyri and the anterior third of the superior temporal gyrus. More than half the cases showed atrophy on the left side more than on the right, and in 20% of the cases right frontal atrophy was more prominent than on the left. Constantinidis et al. (1974) classified PiD as: A—with Pick bodies, B—only with swollen neurons, and C—only gliosis. They believed that "in spite of the dissimilarities between these forms, considering the absence of sufficient knowledge about pathogenesis, it seems prudent at present to maintain the uniqueness of Pick's entity." They thought that the clinical differences between these forms were not related to the nature of histological alterations but rather to the temporal lobe or frontal predominance of the abnormality.

The predominantly behavioral changes due to the frontal lobe syndrome often begin with apathy and disinterest, which may be mistaken for depression. On the other hand, the symptoms of disinhibition may suggest a manic psychosis or a personality disorder (Gregory and Hodges, 1996). Cases of PiD with frontal lobe manifestations therefore are more likely to be presented to a psychiatrist than to a neurologist. Those who are more interested in behavioral disorders are less likely to report the language disorder in great detail, often describing the progressive, nonfluent aphasia as mutism (Gustafson et al., 1990). Neurologists, on the other hand, may see the primarily aphasic disorder more often and may underreport the multifacted behavioral syndrome often accompanying the language disturbance or appearing somewhat later.

Behavioral terminology is undergoing constant change; in early reports, it was less standardized or defined than in more recent ones. Disinterest, apathy, and what is now called "executive deficit," for instance, were often misinterpreted as memory loss. The psychiatric descriptions from the French-Swiss literature (Tissot et al., 1985) bear little resemblance to those of the Swedish (Gustafson et al., 1990), English (Neary et al., 1988), or American papers (Knopman et al., 1990). Sometimes the symptoms resembled those of the so-called Kluver-Bucy syndrome, which is produced in monkeys by bilateral ablation of the temporal neocortex, the amygdala, or the orbitofrontal cortex. This syndrome consisting of hyperorality, hypersexuality, and compulsive touching can be seen in humans after encephalitis, and PiD (Cummings and Duchen, 1981). Since frontal lobe symptomatology is highly complex and requires special training to recognize, early cases often remain puzzling for first-time observers. Even authorities on dementia claimed at various times that Alzheimer's disease (AD) and PiD are similar clinically and cannot be distinguished reliably by neuropsychological methods (Katzman, 1986; American Psychiatric Association, 1987; Kamo et al., 1987; Knopman et al., 1989).

There have been several case descriptions of PiD in which the patients had prominent extrapyramidal features (von Braunmühl, 1930; Löwenberg, 1936; Akelaitis, 1944; Winkelman and Book, 1944). Ferraro and Jervis (1936) stated that extrapyramidal symptoms were common in PiD. Sometimes unilateral rigidity and parkinsonism were the first symptoms to attract attention. It was recognized that subcortical changes occur in PiD, even without extrapyramidal symptomatology (Winkelman and Book, 1944). Constantinidis et al. (1974) described extrapyramidal involvement particularly in "group B" patients and Mann et al. (1993) in 8/12 of patients with frontal lobe dementia. Changes in the basal ganglia, especially in the striatum and the substantia nigra, in addition to cortical pathology occurred in the majority of 30 cases in one review (von Bagh, 1941).

Munoz-Garcia and Ludwin (1984) distinguished the "generalized" variety of PiD from the cortical variety because of the subcortical extension of the pathological findings. The clinical description of these patients is quite similar to that of patients with the cortical variety of PiD. They may have been distinguished in the paper by Munoz-Garcia and Ludwin by the young age at disease onset. One patient had incontinence and hyperorality, restlessness, and echolaia, another patient had progressive logopenia and hyperorality and still another had irrational behavior, poor judgment, and loss of speech. None of these patients had prominent extrapyramidal symptoms, but some had features of the Kluver-Bucy syndrome. Many of the subcortical varieties of PiD are very similar to corticonigral and corticobasal degeneration (CBD) clinically and pathologically (see below). Some cases with published pathology have CBD, others only superficial vacuolation or spongiosis, cell loss, and gliosis in the subcortical and cortical structures (Brown et al., 1996). The relatively early age of disease onset has been observed by authors describing the subcortical or generalized varieties of PiD (Winkelman and Book, 1944; Neumann, 1949; Munoz-Garcia and Ludwin, 1984).

Progressive subcortical gliosis (Neumann, 1949; Neumann and Cohn, 1967) is clinically similar to PiD and remains so far only a pathological diagnosis. More than 30 cases have been described in the literature, the largest series by Verity and Wechsler (1987) and Bergeron et al. (1996). In one family with this pathology, not only a linkage to chromosome 17 was found (see Chapter 18 in this book) but also prion proteins, which leaves the nosology in doubt (Petersen et al. 1995).

With the development of neuroimaging, frontal lobe atrophy was demonstrated with increasing frequency *in vivo,* first with air studies, then with computed tomography (CT) scans in the 1970s, and with magnetic resonance imaging (MRI) and single photon emission computed tomography (SPECT) more recently. The clinical diagnosis of PiD continued to be made sporadically on the basis of frontal and temporal symptomatology supported by the focal atrophy on imaging and a normal electroencephalogram. However, instead of shifting the diagnosis of PiD back to the clinic, the *in vivo* studies applied new labels such as *frontal lobe dementia (FLD), primary progressive aphasia (PPA)* and *frontotemporal degeneration* as distinct entities, reserving the diagnosis of PiD for increasingly restricted histological criteria. Further development of histochemistry contributed to the fractionation of the pathological variations labeled with an astonishing variety of terms (see Table 1.1) while often underemphasizing the commonalities clinically and pathologically.

FRONTAL LOBE DEMENTIA OR FRONTOTEMPORAL DEGENERATION

In the second half of the 1980s, two European groups described frontal lobe dementia (FLD) as a distinct entity and contrasted its clinical features with those of AD (Neary et al., 1986, 1988; Brun, 1987; Gustafson, 1987). They estimated its relative incidence to be 15–20% of degenerative dementias. Both groups recognized that even thought some of the cases had Pick bodies and the majority did not, the clinical syndrome was the same. They called the pathology without Pick bodies "frontal lobe dementia type," consisting of neuronal loss and gliosis in the frontal cortex, with or without spongiform changes or ballooned neurons (Brun, 1987). At the same time, Knopman et al. (1990) described a similar clinicopathological picture as "dementia lacking distinctive histology (DLDH)." More recently, an association with motor neuron disease (MND) has been increasingly recognized (Neary et al. 1990; Chapter 12, this volume).

The groups who described dementia of the frontal lobe type changed the term to *frontotemporal degeneration (FTD)* and summarized the consensus criteria for diagnosis (The Lund and Manchester Groups, 1994). The term *frontotemporal degeneration* or *frontotemporal dementia* (Kumar and Gottlieb, 1993) does not include frequent subcortical involvement, parietal pathology, and extrapyramidal symptomatology. Furthermore, it does not distinguish between the clear-cut behavioral presentation of FLD and the aphasic presentation of PPA, which is one of the most valuable contributions of the recent descriptions of the clinical picture in these conditions.

Further distinctions have been made between clinical subtypes of FTD, such as the "apathetic, disinhibited, and stereotypic" (Snowden et al., 1996). The disinhibited type mainly involves the orbitofrontal region. In the apathetic type, the dorsal lateral convexity appears to be affected more, and in the stereotypic type appears to have more extra pyramidal involvement and striatal pathology. These distinctions tend to become blurred as the disease progresses and not all patients can be easily categorized into these subtypes. Several families with FTD have been described with linkage to chromosome 17 q21. (Basun et al., Foster et al., 1997 also see Chapter 18.) Despite the phenotypic variability that emphasized personality changes in some patients, aphasia and extrapyramidal features in others, these families were characterized by early age of disease onset and at times rapid progression. Furthermore, they showed a pheno-type combination suggesting the relatedness of the various clinical manifestations. These cas-es are very similar to those described in familial PiD, but because of the pathological varia-tions, they were called *familial FTD* (Basun et al., 1997).

PRIMARY PROGRESSIVE APHASIA

A similar instance of relabeling PiD occurred with the description of primary progressive apha-sia (PPA) as a separate entity. In the original series by Mesulam (1982), only one patient had a biopsy, which showed nonspecific pathology with lipofuscinosis. However, many subsequent (and preceding) cases of PPA were described with classical PiD (Rosenfeld, 1909; Wechsler et al., 1982; Holland et al., 1985; Graff-Radford et al., 1990; Kertesz et al., 1994). Other cases had histology characterized by gliosis, neuronal loss, spongiosis of layers II and III in the cor-tex (Kirshner et al., 1987) identical to that described in FLD, and subcortical involvement with neuronal achromasia similar to CBD (Lippa et al., 1990; Kertesz et al., 1994). Although much has been made of the heterogeneity of the underlying pathology, Mesalum and Weintraub (1992), in a review, found the majority of the cases have PiD or a Pick variant pathology.

PPA is defined as a progressive language impairment without dementia existing for at least 2 years (Mesulam, 1987), although it is recognized that other modalities are affected subse-quently, particularly behavior changes suggesting a frontal deficit. Several varieties of PPA have been described, the more common nonfluent variety leading to mutism (the majority of published cases), the aphemic variety with verbal apraxia and stuttering initially, and seman-tic aphasia (dementia) in which speech output is preserved but the naming and comprehension of objects appear to be lost (Snowden et al., 1989). At times, extrapyramidal complications (Morris et al., 1984; Goulding et al., 1989; Kertesz et al., 1994) and even MND supervenes (Caselli et al., 1993). The variety associated with MND tends to be more rapidly progressive (Caselli et al., 1993, Kertesz et al., 1994). PPA has been frequently described with progressive apraxia and frontal dementia. FLD and CBD, in turn, also have a progressive language distur-bance (see Chapters 6 and 9 this volume). Therefore, not only the pathology but also the symp-tomatology of PPA overlaps among the entities belonging to the Pick complex.

CORTICONIGRAL, OR CORTICOBASAL DEGENERATION

When Rebeiz et al. (1968) described corticodentatonigral degeneration, they recognized the similarity of the pathology to PiD. This was subsequently confirmed by several investigators who contributed further clinical details, including the prominent apraxia, gaze palsy, reflex my-oclonus, and alien hand syndrome to the condition and relabeled it *corticobasal* or *corticobasal ganglionic degeneration* (Gibb et al., 1989; Lang et al., 1992). Including the original descrip-tion, most of the literature concerning this condition acknowledges the clinical and pathologi-cal overlap between CBD and PiD (Clark et al., 1986; Luthert et al., 1992; Jendroska et al., 1995; Brown et al., 1996).

CBD suffers from a dichotomy similar to that of PiD in that the pathological and clinical descriptions do not fully overlap. There are some case reports describing patients with the clinical presentation of CBD, defined by unilateral rigidity, apraxia, and alien hand syndrome, but the pathological findings of PiD with Pick bodies (von Braunmühl, 1930; Hassin and Levitin, 1941). Other cases pathologically typical of CBD have a frontal type of dementia without the presenting extrapyramidal features (Clark et al., 1986; Paulus and Selim, 1990; Frisoni et al., 1995; Rey et al., 1995). Typical pathology of CBD can be seen with a clinical picture of PPA (Lippa et al., 1990, 1991; Dobato et al., 1993; Kertesz et al., 1994; Martí-Massó et al., 1994; Brown et al., 1996; Sakurai et al., 1996). In a recent study, we suggested that the clinical syndrome of prominent apraxia, unilateral extrapyramidal syndrome, and alien hand phenomenon should be designated the *corticobasal degeneration syndrome* (*CBDS*) (Kertesz and Munoz, 1997). Further evidence of the neuropathological overlap between PiD and CBD will be commented on in Chapters 8 and 9 of this volume, as well as in the pathological summary (see chapter 15). The evidence is overwhelming that CBD is also part of the Pick complex and that subcortical involvement is much too frequent to allow us to restrict the complex to frontotemporal degeneration.

THE PICK COMPLEX

Conditions combining several features of the Pick complex (PC) continue to be reported under different names, such as *dementia with nonspecific pathology* (Kim et al., 1981), *dementia lacking distinctive histology* (Knopman et al., 1990), *hereditary dysphasic dementia* (Morris et al., 1984), and *disinhibition dementia-parkinsonism-amyotrophy complex* (Lynch et al., 1994). Table 1.1 summarizes the terms used to describe conditions similar to a clinicopathological entity that was originally called *Pick's disease* (some obvious duplications or idiosyncratic variations were omitted). However, the use of *Pick's disease* has been restricted by some to designate at this time a specific histopathology. We suggested the term *Pick complex* to avoid the confusion which continues to surround the term *Pick's disease* (Kertesz et al., 1994). *Pick complex* designates both the pathological and the clinical overlap between the variations. It has an advantage over *frontotemporal degeneration* because it avoids the restriction of pathology and clinical symptomatology to the frontotemporal cortex and acknowledges the relationship to PiD. *Pick complex* is a unifying concept of overlapping clinical syndromes and neuropathological findings (see Chapter 15, this volume) emphasizing the commonalities rather than the differences between them (Figure 1.1).

If one considers all the cases of FLD, PPA with and without MND, and CBD as part of PC, the entity becomes much less rare. According to some estimates including all pathological variants, the incidence of FLD may be as high as 20% of degenerative dementias (Neary et al., 1988; Gustafson et al., 1990), and PPA reports may represent another 10%, even considering the substantial overlap with FLD (Kertesz, 1996). We have now examined over 80 cases of PC in our clinic and continue to see a suspected case almost weekly. The numbers match those of patients with vascular dementia. The ratio of PC to AD may be 1:4, or about 25% of degenerative dementias, rather than the estimates of PiD based on autopsy material using restrictive histological criteria. Admittedly, epidemiological studies are lacking and selection bias is playing a role in centers with an interest in the disease.

An increasing number of clinicians believe that many, if not all the labels mentioned above describe a similar disease entity that clinically and probably biologically is related to PiD. However, as new immunohistological techniques are applied to varieties of PiD, fractionation of the entity continues (see Chapter 15, this volume). The "elephant" is being defined by smaller and

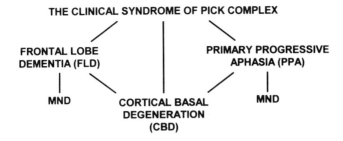

THE CLINICAL SYNDROME OF PICK COMPLEX

FRONTAL LOBE
DEMENTIA (FLD)

PRIMARY PROGRESSIVE
APHASIA (PPA)

MND

CORTICAL BASAL
DEGENERATION
(CBD)

MND

MND = motor neuron disease (may occur with any of the
components of the complex)

FIGURE 1.1. The major clinical components of PC. For other histological and pathological entities included in PC, see Table 1.1.

smaller details, and the differences rather than the similarities are being emphasized. One of the purposes of this chapter, and indeed of this book, is to remove the blindfold and recognize the cohesion of the syndrome which is large enough to deserve the metaphor.

REFERENCES

Akelaitis AJ (1944): Atrophy of basal ganglia in Pick's disease. Arch Neurol Psychiatry 51:27–34.

Alzheimer A (1907): Über eine eigenartige Erkrankung der Hirnrinde. Allgem Z Psychiatrie 64:146–148.

Alzheimer A (1911): Über eigenartige Krankheitsfälle des späteren Alters. Z Gesamte Neurol Psychiatr 4:356–385.

American Psychiatric Association (1987): Diagnostic and Statistical Manual of Mental Disorders (DSM-III-R). Washington, DC: American Psychiatric Association.

Basun H, Almkvist O, Axelman K, Brun A, Campbell TA, Collinge J, Forsell C, Froelich S, Wahlund LO, Wetterberg L, Lannfelt L (1997): Clinical characteristics of a chromosome 17-linked rapidly progressive familial frontotemporal dementia. Arch Neurol 54:539–544.

Bergeron C, Pollanen MS, Weyer L, Black SE, Lang AE (1996): Unusual clinical presentations of cortical-basal ganglionic degeneration. Ann Neurol 40:893–900.

Bird TD, Wijsman EM, Nochlin D, Leehey M, Sumi SM, Payami H, Poorkaj P, Nemens E, Rafkind M, Schellenberg GD (1997): Chromosome 17 and hereditary dementia: Linkage studies in three non-Alzheimer families and kindreds with late-onset FAD. Neurology 48:949–954.

Brown J, Lantos P, Roques P, Fidani L, Rossor MN (1996): Familial dementia with swollen achromatic neurons and corticobasal inclusion bodies: A clinical and pathological study. J Neurol Sci 135:21–30.

Brun A (1987): Frontal lobe degeneration of non-Alzheimer type. I. Neuropathol. Arch Gerontol Geriatr 6:193–208.

Caron M (1934): Etude clinique de la maladie Pick. Paris: Vigot.

Case records of the Massachusetts General Hospital (Case 16–1986): N Engl J Med 314:1101–1111.

Caselli RJ, Windebank AJ, Petersen RC, Komori R, Parisi JE, Okazake H, Kokmen E, Iverson R, Dinapol R, Graf-Radford NR (1993): Rapidly progressive aphasic dementia and motor neuron disease. Ann Neurol 33:200–207.

Clark AW, Manz HJ, White CL III, Lehmann J, Miller D, Coyle JT (1986): Cortical degeneration with swollen chromatolytic neurons: Its relationship to Pick's disease. J Neuropathol Exp Neurol 45:268–284.

Constantinidis J, Richard J, Tissot R (1974): Pick's disease. Histological and clinical correlations. Eur Neurol 11:208–217.

Cooper PN, Jackson M, Lennox G, Lowe J, Mann DMA (1995): τ-Ubiquitin and αß-crystallin—immunohistochemistry defines the principal causes of degenerative frontotemporal dementia. Arch Neurol 52:1011–1015.

Cummings JL, Duchen LW (1981): Kluver-Bucy syndrome in Pick's disease: Clinical and pathological correlations. Neurology 31:1415–1422.

Delay J, Brion S (1952): Les Démences Tardives. Paris: Masson, p 234.

Dickson DW, Yen S-H, Suzkui KI, Davies P, Garcia JH, Hirano A (1986): Ballooned neurons in select neurodegenerative diseases contain phosphorylated neurofilament epitopes. Acta Neuropathol (Berl) 71:216–223.

Dobato JL, Mateo D, de Andrés C, Gimenez-Roldán S (1993): Degeneración gangliónica corticobasal presentándose como un síndrome de afasia progresiva primaria. Neurologia 8:141.

Ferraro A, Jervis GA (1936): Pick's disease. Arch Neurol Psychiatry 36:739–767.

Frisoni GB, Pizzolato G, Zanetti O, Bianchetti A, Chierichetti F, Trabucchi M (1995): Corticobasal degeneration: Neuropsychological assessment and dopamine D2 receptor SPECT analysis. Eur Neurol 35:50–54.

Gans A (1922): Betrachtungen über Art und Ausbreitung des krankhaften Prozesses in einem Fall von Pickscher Atrophie des Stirnhirns. Ztschr. f. d. ges. Neurol. u. Psychiatr. 80:10–28.

Gibb WRG, Luthert PJ, Marsden CD (1989): Corticobasal degeneration. Brain 112:1171–1192.

Goulding PJ, Northen B, Snowden JS, MacDermott N, Neary D (1989): Progressive aphasia with right-sided extrapyramidal signs: Another manifestation of localised cerebral atrophy. J Neurol Neurosurg Psychiatry 52:128–130.

Graff-Radford NR, Damasio AR, Hyman BT, Hart MN, Tranel D, Damasio H, van Hoesen GW, Rezai K (1990): Progressive aphasia in a patient with Pick's disease: A neuropsychological, radiologic, and anatomic study. Neurology 40:620–626.

Gregory CA, Hodges JR (1996): Frontotemporal dementia: Use of consensus criteria and prevalence of psychiatric features. Neuropsychiatr Neuropsychol Behav Neurol 9:145–153.

Gustafson L (1987): Frontal lobe degeneration of non-Alzheimer type. II. Clinical picture and differential diagnosis. Arch Gerontol Geriatr 6:209–223.

Gustafson L, Brun A, Risberg J (1990): Frontal lobe dementia of non-Alzheimer type. In Wurtman RJ, Corkin S, Growdon J, Ritter-Walker E (eds): Advances in Neurology, Volume 51: Alzheimer's Disease. New York: Raven Press, pp. 65–71.

Hassin GB, Levitin D (1941): Pick's disease, clinicopathologic study and report of a case. Arch Neurol Psychiatr 45:814.

Heutink P, Stevens M, Rizzu P, Bakker E, Kros JM, Tibben A, Niermeijer MF, van Duijn CM, Oostra BA, van Swieten JC (1997): Hereditary frontotemporal dementia is linked to chromosome 17q21–q22: A genetic and clinicopathological study of three Dutch families. Ann Neurol 41:150–159.

Holland AL, McBurney DH, Moossy J, Reinmuth OM (1985): The dissolution of language in Pick's disease with neurofibrillary tangles: A case study. Brain Lang 24:36–58.

Jackson M, Lowe J (1996): The new neuropathology of degenerative frontotemporal dementias. Acta Neuropathol 91:127–134.

Jendroska K, Rossor MN, Mathias CJ, Daniel SE (1995): Morphological overlap between corticobasal degeneration and Pick's disease: A clinicopathological report. Mov Disord 10:111–114.

Kamo H, McGeer PL, Harrop R, McGeer EG, Calne DB, Martin WRW, Pate BD (1987): Positron emission tomography and histopathology in Pick's disease. Neurology 37:439–445.

Kaplan HI, Freedman AM, Sadock BJ (1980): Comprehensive Textbook of Psychiatry, Volume III. Baltimore: Williams and Wilkins.

Katzman R (1986): Differential diagnosis of dementing illness. Neurol Clin North Am 4:329–340.

Kertesz A (1996): Pick complex and Pick's disease. Eur J Neurol 3:280–282.

Kertesz A, Hudson L, Mackenzie IRA, Munoz DG (1994): The pathology and nosology of primary progressive aphasia. Neurology 44:2065–2072.

Kertesz A, Munoz D (1997): Clinical and pathological overlap between frontal dementia, progressive aphasia and corticobasal degeneration—the Pick complex. Neurology 48:A293.

Kim RC, Collins GH, Parisi JE, Wright AW, Chu YB (1981): Familial dementia of adult onset with pathologic findings of a "non-specific" nature. Brain 104:61–78.

Kirshner HS, Tanridag O, Thurman L, Whetsell WO Jr (1987): Progressive aphasia without dementia: Two cases with focal spongiform degeneration. Ann Neurol 22:527–532.

Knopman DS, Christensen KJ, Schut LJ, Harbaugh RE, Reeder T, Ngo L, Frey W II (1989): The spectrum of imaging and neuropsychological findings in Pick's disease. Neurology 39:362–368.

Knopman DS, Mastri AR, Frey WH, Sung JH, Rustan T (1990): Dementia lacking distinctive histologic features: A common non-Alzheimer degenerative dementia. Neurology 40:251–256.

Kosaka K (1976): On aphasia of Pick's disease—a review of our own 3 cases and 49 autopsy cases in Japan (in Japanese). Seishin Igaku 18:1181–1189, as quoted by Ohashi (1983).

Kumar A, Gottlieb G (1993): Frontotemporal dementia—a new clinical syndrome? Am J Geriatr Psychiatry 1:95–107.

Lang AE, Bergeron C, Pollanen MS, Ashby P (1992): Parietal Pick's disease mimicking cortical-basal ganglionic degeneration. Neurology 44:1436–1440.

Lippa CF, Smith TW, Fontneau N (1990): Corticonigral degeneration with neuronal achromasia. A clinicopathological study of two cases. J Neurol Sci 98:301–120.

Lippa CF, Cohen R, Smith TW, Drachman DA (1991): Primary progressive aphasia with focal neuronal achromasia. Neurology 41:882–886.

Löwenberg K (1935): Pick's disease. Arch Neurol Psychiatry 36:768–789.

Löwenberg K (1936): Pick's disease: A clinicopathologic contribution. Arch Neurol Psychiatrie 36:768–789.

Lüers T (1947): Ueber den Verfall der Sprache bei der Pickschen Krankheiten. (umschriebene Atrophie der Grosshirnrinde). Z Gesamte Neurol Psychiatr 179:94–131.

Lüers T, Spatz H (1957): Picksche Krankheit (Progressive umschriebene Grosshirnatrophie). In Lubarsch O, Henke F, Roessle R (eds): Handbuch der Speziellen Pathologischen Anatomie und Histologie. Bd 13, Nervensystem, Teil 1. Berlin: Springer-Verlag, pp 614–715.

Luthert PJ, Wightman G, Leigh PN, Marsden CD (1992): Corticobasal degeneration: Immunohistochemical study. Neuropathol Appl Neurobiol 18:293.

Lynch T, Sarno M, Marder KS, Bell KL, Foster NL, Defendini RF, Sima AAF, Keohane C, Nygaard TG, Fahn S, Mayeux R, Rowland LP, Wilhelmsen KC, (1994): Clinical characteristics of a family with chromosome 17-linked disinhibition-dementia-parkinsonism-amyotrophy complex. Neurology 44:1878–1884.

Malamud N, Boyd DA (1940): Pick's disease with atrophy of the temporal lobes—a clinicopathologic study. Arch Neurol Psychiatry 43:210–222.

Malamud N, Waggoner RW (1943): Genealogic and clinicopathologic study of Pick's disease. Arch Neurol Psychiatry 40:288–303.

Mann DMA, South PW, Snowden JS, Neary D (1993): Dementia of frontal lobe type: Neuropathology and immunohistochemistry. J Neurol Neurosurg Psychiatry 56:605–614.

Mansvelt J van (1954): Pick's Disease. A Syndrome of Lobar Cerebral Atrophy, Its Clinico-anatomical and Histopathological Types. Utrecht: These.

Martí-Massó JF, López de Muniain A, Poza JJ, Urtasun M, Carrera N (1994): Degeneración corticobasal gangliónica: A propósito de siete observaciones diagnosticadas clínicamente. Neurologia 9:115–120.

Mesulam MM (1982): Slowly progressive aphasia without dementia. Ann Neurol 11:592–598.

Mesulam MM (1987): Primary progressive aphasia—differentiation from Alzheimer's disease. Ann Neurol 22:533–534.

Mesulam MM, Weintraub S (1992): Primary progressive aphasia: Sharpening the focus on a clinical syndrome. In Boller F, Forette F, Khachaturian Z, Poncet M, Christen Y (eds): Heterogeneity of Alzheimer's Disease. Berlin: Springer-Verlag, pp 43–66.

Morris JC, Cole M, Banker BQ, Wright D (1984): Hereditary dysphasic dementia and the Pick-Alzheimer spectrum. An Neurol 16:455–466.

Munoz-Garcia D, Ludwin SK (1984): Classic and generalized variants of Pick's disease: A clinicopathological, ultrastructural and immunocytochemical study. Ann Neurol 16:467–480.

Neary D, Snowden JS, Bowen DM, Sims NR, Mann DMA, Benton JS, Northen B, Yates DO, Davison AN (1986): Neuropsychological syndromes in presenile dementia due to cerebral atrophy. J Neurol Neurosurg Psychiatry 49:163–174.

Neary D, Snowden JS, Mann DMA, Northen B, Goulding PJ, Macdermott N (1990): Frontal lobe dementia and motor neurone disease. J Neurol Neurosurg Psychiatry 53:23–32.

Neary D, Snowden JS, Northen B, Goulding PJ (1988): Dementia of the frontal lobe type. J Neurol Neurosurg Psychiatry 51:353–361.

Neumann MA (1949): Pick's disease. J Neuropathol Exp Neurol 8:255–282.

Neumann MA, Cohn R (1967): Progressive subcortical gliosis: A rare form of presenile dementia. Brain 90:405–418.

Nichols IC, Weigner WC (1938): Pick's disease—a specific type of dementia. Brain 61:237–249.

Ohashi H (1983): An aphasiologic approach to Pick's disease. In Hirano A, Miyoshi K (eds): Neuropsychiatric Disorders in the Elderly. Tokyo: Igaku-Shoin, pp 132–135.

Onari K, Spatz H (1926): Anatomische Beitrage zur Lehre von der Pickschen umschriebenen Grosshirnrindenatrophie (Piscksche Krankheit). Z Gesamte Neurol Psychiatr 101:470–511.

Paulus W, Selim M (1990): Corticonigral degeneration with neuronal achromasia and basal neurofibrillary tangles. Acta Neuropathol 81:89–94.

Petersen RB, Tabaton M, Chen SG, Monari L, Richardson SL, Manetto V, Lanska D, Markesberry W, Lynch T (1995): Familial progressive subcortical gliosis: Presence of prions and linkage to chromosome 17. Neurology 45:1062–1067.

Pick A (1892): Über die Beziehungen der senilen Hirnatrophie zur Aphasie. Prag Med Wochenschr 17:165–167.

Pick A (1904): Über primäre progressive Demenz bei Erwachsenen. Prag Med Wochenschr 29:417–420.

Pick A (1905): Zur Symptomatologie der linksseitigen Schläfenlappenatrophie. Monatsschr Psychiatr (Berl) 16:378–388.

Pick A (1906): Über einen weiteren Symptomenkomplex im Rahmen der Dementia senilis, bedingt durch umschriebene stärkere Hirnatrophie (gemischte Apraxie). Vortrag, gehalten im Wiener Vereine für Psychiatrie und Neurologie. Monatsschr Psychiatr (Berl) 19:97–108.

Rebeiz JJ, Kolodny EH, Richardson EP Jr (1968): Corticodentatonigral degeneration with neuronal achromasia. Arch Neurol 18:20–33.

Rey GJ, Tomer R, Levin BE, Sanchez-Ramos J, Bowen B, Bruce JH (1995): Psychiatric symptoms, atypical dementia, and left visual field inattention in corticobasal degeneration. Mov Disord 10:106–110.

Rosenfeld M (1909): Die partielle Grosshirnatrophie. J Psychol Neurol 14:115–130.

Sakurai Y, Hashida H, Uesugi H, Arima K, Murayama S, Bando M, Iwata M, Momose T, Sakuta M (1996): A clinical profile of corticobasal degeneration presenting as primary progressive aphasia. Eur Neurol 36:134–137.

Schenk VWD (1958–1959): Re-examination of a family with Pick's disease. Ann Hum Genet 23:325–333.

Schneider C (1927): Uber Picksche Krankheit. Monatsschr Psychiatr Neurol 65:230–275.

Schneider C (1929): Weitere Beitrage zur Lehre von der Pickschen Krankheit. Z Gesamte Neurol Psychiatr 120:340–384.

Sjogren T, Sjogren H, Lindgren AGH (1952): Morbus Alzheimer and Morbus Pick. Acta Psychiatr Neurol Scand 82(Suppl):1–152.

Snowden JS, Goulding PJ, Neary D (1989): Semantic dementia: a form of circumscribed cerebral atrophy. Behav Neurol 2:167–182.

Snowden JS, Neary D, Mann DMA (1996): Frontotemporal Lobar Degeneration: Frontotemporal Dementia, Progressive Aphasia, Semantic Dementia. London: Churchill Livingston.

Stertz G (1926): Ueber die Picksche Atrophie. Z Gesamte Neurol Psychiatr 101:729–747.

The Lund and Manchester Groups (1994): Clinical and neuropathological criteria for frontotemporal dementia. J Neurol Neurosurg Psychiatry 57:416–418.

Thorpe FT (1932): Pick's disease (circumscribed senile atrophy) and Alzheimer's disease. J Ment Sci 78:302–314.

Tissot R, Constantinidis J, Richard J (1985): Pick's disease. In Frederiks JAM (ed): Handbook of Clinical Neurology, Vol 2 (46): Neurobehavioural Disorders. Amsterdam: Elsevier, pp 233–246.

van Bogaert L (1934): Syndrome extrapyramidal au cours d'une maladie de Pick. J Belge Neurol Psychiatrie 34:315.

Verity MA, Wechsler AF (1987): Progressive subcortical gliosis of Neumann: A clinicopathologic study of two cases with review. Arch Gerontol Geriatr 6:245–261.

von Bagh K (1941): Anatomic findings in 30 cases of systematic atrophy of cortex (Pick's disease) with special consideration of basal ganglia and long descending nerve tracts, preliminary report. Arch Psychiatrie 114:68.

von Branmühl A (1930a): Ueber Stammganglienveränderungen bei Pickscher Krankheit. Z Gesamte Neurol Psychiatr 124:214.

von Branmühl A (1930b): In Bumke O (ed): Handbuch der Geisteskrankheiten, Vol XI, pt 7. Berlin: Julius Springer, p 673.

Wechsler AF, Verity A, Rosenschein S, Freid I, Scheibel AB (1982): Pick's disease. A clinical, computed tomographic, and histologic study with Golgi impregnation observations. Arch Neurol 39:287–290.

Winkelman NW, Book MH (1944): Asymptomatic extrapyramidal involvement in Pick's disease. Arch Neurol Psychiatry 8:30–42.

CHAPTER 2

Arnold Pick: A Historical Introduction

ANDREW KERTESZ

Department of Clinical Neurological Sciences, St. Joseph's Health Centre, University of Western Ontario, London, Ontario N6A 4V2, Canada

Arnold Pick (Figure 2.1) was born in 1851 in Gross Messeritsch (now Velke-Meziříčí), a small town in Moravia, then a province of the Hapsburg Empire. His secondary school education in the gymnasium of Iglau (now Jihlava) emphasized a must for future physician at that time in the classics, language and history. As far as education was concerned, Moravia at that time was one of the most bilingually integrated provinces in the empire. As the official business of law, commerce, and government were carried out in German, there were few with a high school diploma who did not speak German. Most educated Austrians in Moravia and Bohemia were fluent in Czech, the language used by the majority for day-to-day activities. Pick graduated from the Medical School in Vienna in 1875 at the age of 24. He did an elective at the Landesirrenanstalt (state mental institution) in Vienna in 1872 as a student, and between 1872 and 1874 became an assistant to Theodore Meynert, the chairman of neurology and psychiatry in Vienna. At about that time, Carl Wernicke, who was a few years senior to Pick, also spent 6 months with Meynert, whose main interest was neuroanatomy. Meynert influenced both young men considerably, as evidenced by their subsequent work. After his graduation, it was Pick's turn to pursue a 6-month elective in Westphal's department of neuropsychiatry in the Charité hospital in Berlin, while Wernicke was there as Westphal's assistant. Pick did several projects on the anatomy and pathology of the brainstem and the spinal cord there. Pick was an Austrian, trained in the Austro-Hungarian Empire, while Wernicke trained in Prussia, but there was a great deal of movement across the borders in German-speaking academia, a tradition that goes back to the Middle Ages and, apart from a few interruptions by war, continues to this day.

For his residency, Pick worked in a state mental hospital in Wehnen from 1875 to 1877 and in the Prague asylum (Irrenanstalt) from 1877 to 1880. Here he met Otto Kahler, which was the beginning of a fruitful collaboration and friendship. He received his Habilitation (a teaching qualification) in neurology and psychiatry from the faculty of medicine in Prague in July 1878. The Prague asylum was in the old quarters of the medieval St. Catherine monastery, the tower of which still stands. It became the first academic department of neuropsychiatry, established in 1841 under the direction of von Riedel, who, following Pinel's example, intro-

Pick's Disease and Pick Complex, Edited by Andrew Kertesz and David G. Munoz
ISBN 0-471-17792-X ©1998 Wiley-Liss, Inc.

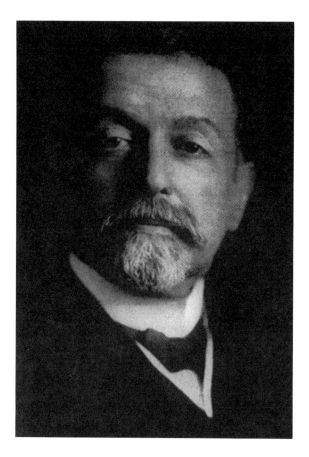

FIGURE 2.1. Arnold Pick - Unattributed photograph reproduced from History of Neurology with permission of Little Brown.

duced progressive steps such as occupational and music therapy in caring for mental patients and founded the first German journal of psychiatry. To this day, the No. 1 Department of Neurology of Charles University is located on Katerinská Street in Prague, named after the ancient monastery with its baroque additions from 1790 (Figure 2.2). The name of the building was once synonymous with mental illness in Prague (similar to Bedlam in England). To say that "one belongs to Katerinky" in Czech is to doubt one's sanity.

Prague achieved greatness during the Middle Ages under foreign kings. Charles IV, who became Holy Roman Emperor and placed the seat of the empire in Prague, was from Luxembourg and had a French cultural background but loved Bohemia and the Czechs. He invited the best architects, such as Peter Parler, to build medieval Prague, St. Vitus Cathedral, the famous stone bridge with the gate tower named after him, and many other monuments that still exist. Prague became the seat of the Hapsburg Empire again under Rudolph II in the sixteenth century, and it remained a principal Hapsburg city until the dissolution of the empire at the end of World War I. During the time of Pick, Prague flourished peacefully under the Emperor Franz

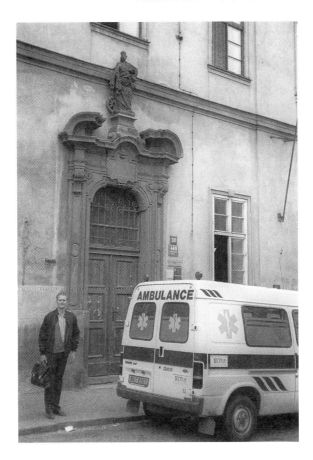

FIGURE 2.2. The entrance to Pick's department on Katerinska St. in Prague, today it is the first Department of Neurology.

Joseph. This is when Wenceslas Square was built and the famous horse statue of King Wenceslas was erected, heralding the rise of Czech nationalism.

In 1880 Pick was first appointed assistant director of the new psychiatric institute in Dobrzan (Dobrany), about 110 km from Prague, and then became director of the institute from 1882 to 1886. In 1886 he was promoted to full professor and a few months later, at the age of 35, he took over the chair of the neuropsychiatry department in Prague from Jakob Fischel. The selection committee records (Figure 2.3) obtained from the Archives of the Carolinum in Prague show that von Krafft-Ebbing from Graz was the first choice, but Krafft-Ebbing held out for the chair in Vienna, which he obtained a few years later. Pick reorganized the department based on research and patient care. He was considered an excellent clinician and teacher. He took a keen interest in neuroanatomy, neuropathology, and the organic diseases of the nervous system. In one of his letters to the Ministry of Education, he asks to be identified as a professor of neuropathology, in addition to psychiatry, similarly to his counterparts in Vienna and Graz (Figure 2.4). The official language of instruction at the University of Prague was German, just as

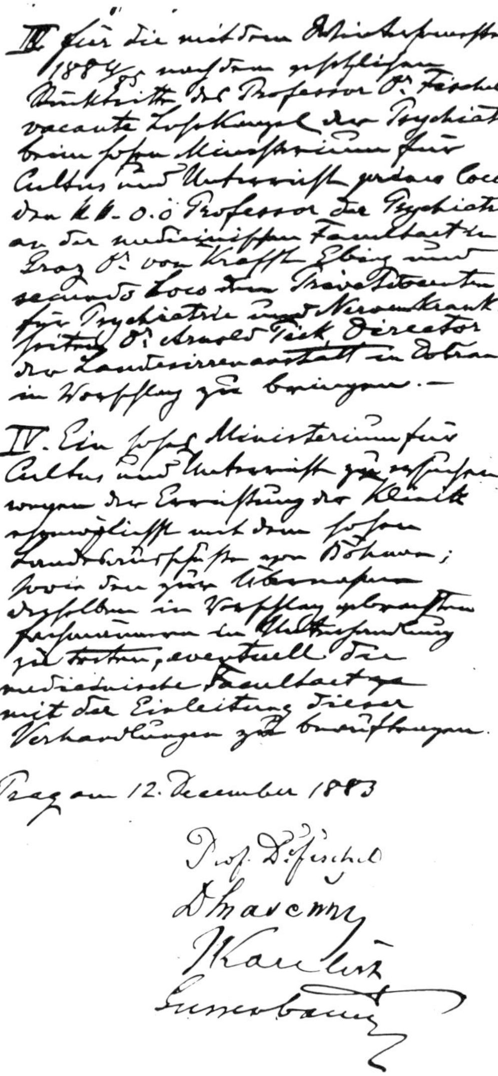

FIGURE 2.3. The recommendation of the Selection Committee naming von Krafft-Ebbing as 1st (line 9) and Arnold Pick as 2nd candidate to succeed Dr. Fischel (top signature).

it was in all aspects of administration in the nineteenth century. The end of the century saw the rise of Czech nationalism, and on the instigation of the Czech deputies in the Imperial Council in Vienna, a bill was passed in 1882 to establish a Czech university in Prague. Thomas Masaryk was appointed as professor of philosophy in 1882. After the faculties of law and philosophy, the faculty of medicine duplicated all its departments and began to provide Czech instruction (Vencovský, 1987). A parallel Czech department of neuropsychiatry was established

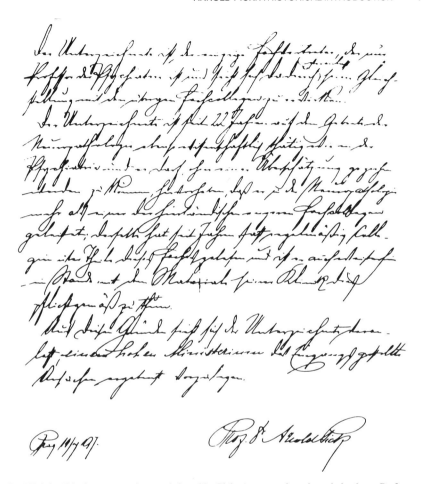

FIGURE 2.4. This document written and signed by Pick requests to be acknowledged as a Professor of Neuropathology, dated in Prague 1897.

in the same building under the leadership of Dr. Cumpelik and later by Kuffner, who was Pick's counterpart for the most part of his tenure.

Neurology and psychiatry were not yet separated in Austro-Hungary at the time of Pick. The split of these specialities came later in German universities than in England and France, even though Romberg, chief physician at the University Hospital in Berlin, had already written the first clinical neurology textbook in 1840 and could be considered the father of neurology. The situation was different in England and France, where neurological institutes and departments were established in the 1860s. Because German neuropsychiatry remained integrated, most physicians in the speciality had widely ranging interests. As they described the basic psychiatric entities, they also dealt with the effects of alcohol and syphilis on the nervous system, and the topics of their publications ranged from the spinal cord to behavior. Dementia and schizophrenia were defined at around that time; until then, dementia had encompassed all forms of insanity. Not until Alzheimer and Pick championed neuropathology in their study of mental illness were these conditions clearly defined.

Pick remained chairman of his department for 35 years and became one of the leaders in neurology and neuropsychiatry, with 280 publications to his name, an extraordinary number at that time. The majority of them deal with aphasia, apraxia, agnosia, memory, consciousness, and other topics belonging to what is now called *behavioral neurology*. His overall output in this field exceeds that of Wernicke, in part because he lived longer (Wernicke died in a bicycle accident in 1905 at the age of 45). Pick became interested in aphasia, probably following Wernicke's inspiration, "Der Aphasische symptomencomplex" was published in 1874, and Pick was one of the first to validate Wernicke's observations. He initially followed Wernicke's classification of the aphasias but later became interested in a linguistic approach to speech disorders. He began a series of articles on agrammatism because he considered it a central problem in aphasia, but the work remained unfinished (Pick, 1902, 1909a, 1913, 1973). In the first volume of "Die Agrammatischen Sprachstörungen," Pick reviewed the psychological and linguistic knowledge pertaining to aphasia. His concept of agrammatism included not only the deficit of syntax, but also other disturbances in language use. He considered the sentence not just a conglomeration of words but a psychological entity. Pick distinguished two forms of agrammatism. The temporal variety is characterized by defective syntax with a quickened pace of speech but wrong inflexions, prefixes, and suffixes. In the frontal variety, on the other hand, only substantive words are juxtaposed, as in a telegram without syntactic elements. Since Pick's introduction, agrammatism has become a popular and fertile area among modern linguists interested in aphasia.

Some interpreted Pick's emphasis on the linguistic explanations of aphasic phenomena as turning away from Wernicke's concepts and considered Pick one of the "holists" unwilling to divide aphasic phenomena (Geschwind, 1963; Vondráček, 1977). His ideas on aphasia were undoubtedly influenced by Hughlings Jackson's concepts of the hierarchical organization of the brain. An example is his model of language comprehension (Pick, 1909b), which to a considerable degree resembles the models in modern cognitive science. Pick described stages of cognition that included the formulation of thought, preliminary to the use of language, as distinct from the formulation of words, presaging modern linguistic concepts of preword processes. He even went further back to what he called the "mental attitude," where thought is still undifferentiated. Subsequent stages of comprehension would represent differentiated ideas and the scheme of the phrase. Only after these processes would words be chosen. Pick also thought of the cortical acoustic area as a monitor of other speech mechanisms. He cautioned against oversimplification in observing aphasic phenomena and interpreting deficits: "the abnormal responses do not reveal the elements out of which speech is built," which is often reiterated in arguments today.

The breadth of Pick's publications is remarkable, ranging from microscopic study of the central canal in the spinal cord to hysterical psychosis. He did experimental work on the visual systems of dogs and wrote about counseling the relatives of psychiatric patients. He coauthored a text on the pathological anatomy of the central nervous system with his friend Otto Kahler. He described reduplicative paramnesia, subsequently a commonly recognized delusional misidentification syndrome in degenerative dementia (Pick, 1903). His patient not only had reduplication of location but also mistook a relative for a "double," a delusion that was subsequently named *Capgras syndrome*. Several of his works became eponymous, such as *Pick's visual hallucinations* (Pick, 1904a), *Pick's bundle* (in the medulla), and *Pick's disease* (Pick, 1892, 1901d, 1904a, 1905a, 1906).

Arnold Pick is best known for the description of a distinct form of presenile dementia presenting with behavioral syndromes due to circumscribed lobar atrophy. The original articles by

Pick dealing with this entity do not contain any histological description. Pick's first patient had progressive aphasia and a concomitant behavioral disorder (Pick, 1892). His second patient also had fluent progressive aphasia with temporal lobe atrophy (Pick, 1901a). His third patient, a 41-year-old housewife, developed apathy; neglect of her household, children, and hygiene; and logopenia. She also overate, was irritable and aggressive, and had significant personality changes (Pick, 1904b). The fourth publication covered a series of three patients under the title "The Symptomatology of Left-Sided Temporal Lobe Atrophy" (Pick, 1905a). All three patients were fluent aphasics with anomia and word deafness, and appear to some extent to correspond to modern descriptions of progressive fluent or semantic aphasia. The third patient in this series had a cystic lesion in the temporal lobe that may have contributed to the symptoms, although this may have been an asymmetrically enlarged temporal horn. The fifth publication in 1906 presented a patient who began with apathy followed by disinhibition, personal neglect, anomic aphasia, logopenia, and severe ideational apraxia described at length in the article (Pick, 1906).

The use of the term *Pick's disease* has been shifted to mean the pathological entity with silver staining globular inclusions (Pick bodies), first described by Alzheimer (Alzheimer, 1911), ballooned neurons, and circumscribed atrophy (Onari and Spatz, 1926). Restricted to this pathological definition, it is considered relatively rare compared to Alzheimer's disease (a ratio of 1:10). Recently, frontal dementia, primary progressive aphasia, dementia with amyotrophic lateral sclerosis (ALS), and corticobasal degeneration have been recognized as having a high degree of clinical and pathological similarity to Pick's disease (Kertesz et al., 1994). If one considers these clinical conditions with *Pick variant pathology* as a continuum or *Pick complex,* Pick's disease may be second in incidence only to Alzheimer's disease, particularly in the presenile age group. Arnold Pick's contribution to behavioral neurology and neuropsychiatry may be appreciated even further since the ratio of Pick complex to Alzheimer's disease is closer to 1:4, as converging evidence indicates.

Pick's fame has spread far beyond the German-speaking medical and scientific community. He and Hughlings Jackson held each other in high esteem. Pick had Jackson's portrait on his desk and wrote several articles in the English literature (Pick, 1901b, 1901d, 1903, 1905b, 1909a). Jackson wrote about Pick and popularized his work in England. Pick counted among his friends several members of the intellectual elite in Prague, such as Ernst Mach, the physicist; Friedrich Jodl, a philosopher; Steinach, a biologist and physiologist; and Sauer, a linguist, and corresponded with many of the leading neurologists of his time, such as Dejerine, Marie, Head, Jolly, and Raymond (Brown, 1952). He lived in central Prague at 6 Krakauergasse, as attested to by a letter written on his personal stationery. The elegant apartment house there now houses the Bulgarian Embassy. Our efforts to find his descendants were unsuccessful.

Pick became dean of medicine in Prague for 1 year (1891–1892), which is standard practice in German universities. A dean was only *primus inter pares,* a rotating chair of the body of professors that constituted the executive committee of the faculty. He was said to prefer clinical activities to administration. In 1907 he was honored with the title of *Hofrat* (court councillor). After writing several articles about the cognitive effects of war injuries, he retired in 1921. Pick's last years were marred by illness; he lost his sight due to a cataract and retinal detachment, and one of his eyes had to be enucleated. A renal stone was removed, with many complications, and in 1924, at the age of 73, he died of urinary sepsis following another operation. His many pupils carried on his work. Otto Sittig, another behavioral neurologist, is well known for his significant work on apraxia, among other achievements. He edited Pick's work on aphasia posthumously, available in an English translation by Jason Brown (Pick, 1973), and wrote Pick's obituary. Sittig died in a concentration camp during World War II. Oscar Fischer, who did significant work on senile plaques in the neuropathology laboratory in Pick's department at around the same time as Alzheimer, also perished in a concentration camp. Other well-known pupils included Bruno Fischer, Max Löwy, and Alexander Margulis.

After Pick's retirement, Otto Poetzl from Vienna, whose main interest was in cortical visual disturbances such as visual agnosia, continued the emphasis on neurology in the German department of neuropsychiatry in Prague. The Czech Republic maintained the German university even after the breakup of the Austro-Hungarian Empire in 1918. This is astonishing considering the intense nationalism and anti-Austrian feeling that brought about the creation of Czechoslovakia. However, about a quarter of the population of the new republic was German-speaking, and a large number of academics and intellectuals were bilingual. Although Masaryk, the president of this new nation, led the struggle against Austrian and Hungarian domination, he was also a product of German academic institutions and culture, very much like his contemporary, Arnold Pick (Newman, 1960). The German and Czech departments were located above each other in the same building, but they apparently had minimal scientific contact (Vencovský, 1987). Only during the lectures by outstanding visitors would they attend each other's meetings. This situation, of course, did not exclude personal friendships between individual members of both clinics.

Arnold Pick's work represented the integration of neurology, psychiatry, and neuropathology at the turn of the century in German neurology. His professorship survived a major historical upheaval, the breakup of one of the longest-lasting empires, and the birth of a new country. A comparison of his original articles with the recent literature on focal atrophies suggests that his contribution to neurology, particularly to neurodegenerative disorders, is substantial and needs to be recognized. Frontotemporal circumscribed atrophy, as described originally by Pick, is more common than has been recognized although it has been recently rediscovered and relabeled. Although the term *Pick's disease* is now often used to denote a specific histological picture characterized by globular argyrophilic inclusions and swollen neurons, the more recently described frontal lobe dementia and primary progressive aphasia have pathological features which overlap with the histology of Pick's disease, and they are clinically indistinguishable from Pick's original descriptions. Arnold Pick is a major intellectual ancestor of modern behavioral neurology, and hopefully this book will contribute to a well-deserved acknowledgment of his work.

REFERENCES

Alzheimer A (1911): Über eigenartige Krankheitsfälle des späteren Alters. Z Gesamte Neurol Psychiatr 4:356–385.

Brown MR (1952): Arnold Pick (1851–1924). In Haymaker W (ed): The Founders of Neurology. Springfield, IL: Charles C Thomas.

Geschwind N (1963): Carl Wernicke, the Breslau School and the history of aphasia. In Carterette EC (ed): Brain Function, Volume III: Speech, Language and Communication. Berkeley: University of California Press, pp 1–16.

Kertesz A, Hudson L, Mackenzie IRA, Munoz DG (1994): The pathology and nosology of primary progressive aphasia. Neurology 44:2065–2072.

Newman EP (1960): Masaryk. London: Campion Press.

Onari K, Spatz H (1926): Anatomische Beiträge zur Lehre von der Pickschen umschriebenen Grosshirn-rinden-Atrophie ("Picksche Krankheit"). Z Gesamte Neurol Psychiatr 101:470–511.

Pick A (1892): Ueber die Beziehungen der senilen Hirnatrophie zur Aphasia. Prag Med Wochenschr 17:165–167.

Pick A (1901a): Senile Hirnatrophie als Gundlage von Hernderscheinunger. Wien Klin Wochenschr Monatsschr Psychiatr Neurol 14:403–404.

Pick A (1901b): Clinical studies in pathological dreaming. J Ment Sci 485–499.

Pick A (1901c): On the study of the true tumours of the optic nerve. Brain 502–508.

Pick A (1901d): The deleterious results following operations in hypochondriasis, performed for the sake of mental impression. Philadelphia Med J 482–484.

Pick A (1902): Ueber Agrammatismus als Folge von Herderkrankung. Z Heilk (Prag) 23:82–90.

Pick A (1903): Clinical studies—I. On "dreamy mental states" as a permanent condition in epileptics; II. On the pathologically protracted duration of impressions on the senses as a cause of various disturbances of the sensory perception and especially of the sight; III. On reduplicative paramnesia. Brain 26:242–251, 251–260, 260–267.

Pick A (1904a): Über primäre progressive Demenz bei Erwachsenen. Prag Med Wochenschr 29:417–420.

Pick A (1904b): The localizing diagnostic significance of so-called hemianopic hallucinations with remarks on bitemporal scintillating scotomata. Am J Med Sci 77:82–92.

Pick A (1905a): Zur Symptomatologie der linksseitigen Schläfenlappenatrophie. Monatsschr Psychiatr (Berl) 16:378–388.

Pick A (1905b): The psychology of a particular form of pathological intoxication. J Ment Sci 51:62–70.

Pick A (1906): Über einen weiteren Symptomenkomplex im Rahmen der Dementia senilis, bedingt durch umschriebene stärkere Hirnatrophie (gemischte Apraxie). Vortrag, gehalten im Wiener Vereine für Psychiatrie und Neurologie. Monatsschr Psychiatr (Berl) 19:97–108.

Pick A (1909a): On the localisation of agrammatismus. Rev Neurol Psychiatry 7:757–762.

Pick A (1909b): Über das Sprachverständnis. Drei Vorträge. Leipzig: Barth.

Pick A (1913): Die agrammatischen Sprachstörungen. Studien zur psychologischen Grundlegung der Aphasielehre. Berlin: J. Springer.

Pick A (1973): Aphasia (trans by Brown JW). Springfield, IL: Charles C Thomas.

Vencovskỳ E (1987): "Stolet České psychiatrické kliniky v. Praze 1886–1986 (One Hundred Years of the Czech Psychiatric Clinic in Prague). Praha: Univerzita Karlova Praha.

Vondráček V (1977): Lékař Dále Vzpoíná (A Physician Recollects) (1920–1938). Praha: Avicenum.

CHAPTER 3

Clinical and Neuropsychological Features of Frontotemporal Dementia

BRUCE L. MILLER, KYLE BOONE, FRED MISHKIN, J. RANDOLPH SWARTZ, NANCY KORAS, and JONATHAN KUSHII

Departments of Neurology (B.L.M., N.K., J.K.), Psychiatry (K.B., J.R.S.), and Radiology (F.M.), Harbor-UCLA Medical Center, UCLA School of Medicine, Los Angeles, CA

INTRODUCTION AND NOMENCLATURE

This chapter focuses on a clinically and anatomically heterogeneous dementing disorder associated with selective degeneration of the anterior frontal and temporal lobes for which we will use the term *frontotemporal dementia* (*FTD*) (Gustafson et al., 1987; Neary et al., 1988; Miller et al., 1991). The nomenclature for this group of disorders is reviewed. Additionally, we describe the epidemiology, as well as the neuropsychological, diagnostic, neuropsychiatric, and imaging features of FTD and review the UCLA experience with FTD in these areas.

Arnold Pick offered the first clinical description of patients with selective lobar degeneration in 1892, and 15 years later Alois Alzheimer described cytoplasmic inclusions within ballooned cortical neurons in Pick's original two patients. Although Pick himself did not describe these cytoplasmic inclusions, they were subsequently called *Pick bodies,* and *Pick's disease* became synonymous with frontal lobe dementias. Ironically, neuropathologists require neuronal cytoplasmic inclusions never described by Pick in order to make a diagnosis of Pick's disease.

Later, other subtypes of frontal lobe dementia were defined, such as progressive subcortical gliosis (Neumann and Cohn, 1967), in which pathology was localized primarily to subcortical regions. Similarly, the coassociation of motor neuron disease with frontal lobe dementia (Mitsuyama, 1993) was described. Most of these patients did not have classical Pick bodies (Mitsuyama, 1993). A similar association has been found between primary progressive aphasia and motor neuron disease (Caselli et al., 1993). Further complicating the issue of what constitutes Pick's disease are patients with selective frontotemporal atrophy and Pick-like inclusions without the classical features of a Pick body (Chang et al., 1995). Some investigators include the pale, achromatic inclusions in parietal neurons in cortico-basal-ganglionic degeneration as an FTD subtype (Jackson and Lowe, 1996).

Pick's Disease and Pick Complex, Edited by Andrew Kertesz and David G. Munoz
ISBN 0-471-17792-X   ©1998 Wiley-Liss, Inc.

In the late 1980s, Brun (1987), Gustafson (Gustafson et al., 1987), and Neary and colleagues (Neary et al., 1987) reported on dementia patients with a progressive frontal lobe disorder. These patients had neuronal loss, gliosis, and macrovacuolization of frontal tissue, but the plaques and tangles typically found in Alzheimer's disease (AD) were absent. However, in Brun's series (1987), only 20% of the frontally predominant subjects had classical Pick bodies within cortical neurons. Brun (1987) suggested the name *frontal dementia of the non-Alzheimer type* for these patients, while Neary coined the term *dementia of the frontal type* (Neary et al., 1988). More recently, the Lund-Manchester groups collectively suggested the term *frontotemporal dementia* (*FTD*), which acknowledged that along with the frontal lobes, the anterior temporal lobes are also involved in many patients with this disorder (Brun et al., 1994).

Another nomenclature relates to patients in whom frontotemporal degeneration is selective and involves primarily the left or right hemisphere. Mesulam (1982) and Morris et al. (1984) described patients with unilateral left frontal or temporal degeneration in whom aphasia was the presenting feature. Ten years later, patients with selective right-sided predominant degeneration with primarily behavioral defects were described (Miller et al., 1993). Like patients with bilateral frontotemporal degeneration, most unilateral subjects show either classical Pick's disease or frontal gliosis and neuronal loss without Pick bodies. Brun (1993) suggested separating patients with Pick bodies (Pick's disease) from those with frontal gliosis and neuronal loss but no Pick bodies. In contrast, Kertesz et al. (1994) noted the clinical and pathologic overlap of these conditions and coined the term *Pick complex*.

Genetic studies are likely to settle many nomenclature controversies related to FTD. Gustafson (1993) noted that approximately 50% of patients with FTD have a family history of dementia. Similarly, in the UCLA population, approximately 20% of the subjects had a first-degree relative with either dementia or motor neuron disease (Miller et al., 1995). Wilhelmsen and colleagues (1994) reported a linkage to the short arm of chromosome 17 in a family with dementia, parkinsonism, and motor neuron disease. Subsequently, at least seven families have shown a linkage to this region.

In addition to Lynch and Wilhelmsen's original family with dementia, parkinsonism, and motor neuron disease (Lynch et al., 1994), the diverse syndromes now linked to chromosome 17 include progressive subcortical gliosis (Petersen et al., 1995), familial parkinsonism (Wilhelmsen et al., 1996), and hereditary dysphasic dementia (J.C. Morris, personal communication). The clinical evaluation of different patient groups has not been standardized, so it is still unknown whether there is greater overlap between these seemingly separate clinical disorders. Because progress in mapping the genetics of the various dementing conditions has occurred at such a rapid pace, rigid adherence to a nomenclature system based on clinical or pathological characteristics seems premature.

EPIDEMIOLOGY

Overview

Except for a family history, little is known about the risk factors for FTD. Until recently, neurology textbooks stated that FTD is a rare condition that cannot be differentiated from AD prior to death (Adams and Victor, 1993). However, others suggest that FTD is not rare (Knopman et al., 1990), and Snowden and colleagues (1996) estimate that 25% of subjects with presenile dementia suffer from FTD. Misdiagnosis continues to be a serious impediment to determining the true prevalence of FTD, and many investigators tend to classify FTD patients as having AD. In 1993 Mendez and colleagues reported that 18/21 patients with Pick's disease at post mortem were diagnosed as having AD during life.

At UCLA, FTD is a common disorder, although we see more FTD patients than most centers due to our special interest in this condition. Using strict clinical and functional neuroimaging parameters, we have diagnosed more than 60 patients with FTD. Most were seen over the past few years, and currently we evaluate one new FTD patient weekly. Community-based studies will be necessary to determine the true prevalence of FTD, but based on our experience, we concur with Knopman et al. (1990) and Snowden et al. (1996) that FTD is a common dementia.

In addition to the problem that many FTD patients are misdiagnosed as having AD, we suspect that some patients with FTD are never seen in dementia clinics. In studies on patients with late-life onset of psychosis, we encountered three patients in whom the first clinical manifestation of a degenerative disorder was a bizarre psychosis. In two, FTD was the likely etiology for the dementia, while the third was thought to have AD (Lesser et al., 1989). Two of the three patients had predominantly right-sided functional deficits with single photon emission computed tomography (SPECT).

Previous studies found that 50% of patients with Pick's disease had asymmetric left-sided involvement, while only 20% showed asymmetric right-sided disease. The lower percentage of right-sided subjects may reflect the fact that patients with right-sided disease were more likely to present with psychiatric problems, and we suspect that some FTD patients with predominantly right-sided involvement were chronically institutionalized in psychiatric facilities without ever receiving a neurological evaluation. In contrast, because left-sided patients had aphasia, they were more likely to be seen by neurologists (and neuropathologists).

UCLA Population

We have analyzed the epidemiological features of our first 54 subjects. Fifty percent (27) were male and 50% (27) were female. Right handers presented 93%, and left handers accounted for 7%. The socioeconomic status was high, with a mean educational level of more than 14 years. They were slightly younger than typical AD patients; the mean age at presentation for FTD was 56 years. We found a strong association between motor neuron disease in our patients with suspected FTD, and 14% of these patients had findings of motor neuron disease or a first-degree relative with a history of this disease. This underestimates the true prevalence of motor neuron disease in FTD, as many subjects develop motor findings only late in the disease, and others show motor neuron disease at pathology yet are free of clinical manifestations. In one small study of 10 subjects, we found no association with apolipoprotein E4 and FTD, although larger studies are planned (Miller et al., 1995).

These findings are congruent with reports from others (Gustafson, 1993) and suggest that FTD is typically a presenile dementia which affects males as often as females. If often has a familial basis, and there is a strong association with motor neuron disease. Apolipoprotein E4 does not appear to be a risk factor for FTD. Similarly, there are no known treatable risk factors associated with FTD. Perhaps with pooling of clinical populations from different sites, better understanding of the nongenetic risk factors in FTD will become possible.

DIAGNOSIS: FUNCTIONAL NEUROIMAGING

Despite the currently high misdiagnosis rate for FTD, several groups have demonstrated that recognition of the clinical and neuroimaging features of this condition allows accurate diagnosis during life. Recently, the UCLA group (Read et al., 1995) and the Lund group in Sweden (Risberg et al., 1993) reported greater than 90% diagnostic accuracy for patients with FTD

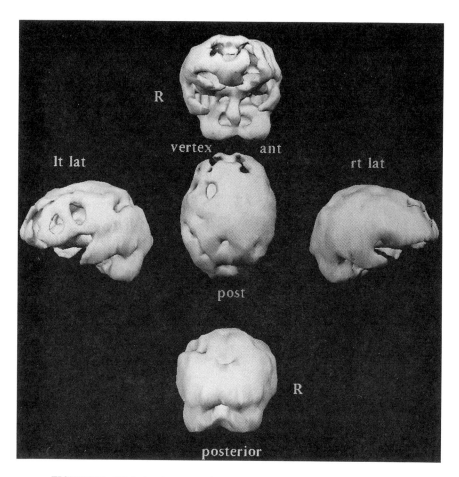

FIGURE 3.1. Clinical and neuropsychological features of frontotemporal dementia.

using SPECT combined with clinical diagnosis. Both groups found that FTD patients had bifrontal and bitemporal hypoperfusion, while AD patients had temporal-parietal hypoperfusion. Figure 3.1 shows typical SPECT findings in a patient with FTD. There are marked deficits in anterior frontal and temporal perfusion, while posterior temporal-parietal perfusion is relatively normal.

Many FTD patients with functional deficits on SPECT also show structural deficits with computed tomography (CT) or magnetic resonance imaging (MRI), but the value of SPECT over structural imaging is still unknown. Although functional imaging studies like SPECT seem to differentiate patients with FTD from most patients with AD, the sensitivity and specificity of SPECT need to be more extensively studied. Importantly, there have been no systematic evaluations of SPECT in patients with FTD compared to healthy or psychiatrically ill elderly patients. Many elderly depressed and psychotic individuals show frontal and anterior temporal hypoperfusion on SPECT (Miller et al., 1992). Therefore, the specificity of frontal hypoperfusion for differentiating depression or psychosis from FTD is likely to be low.

One group of patients in whom SPECT can be misleading are AD patients in whom frontal hypoperfusion occurs early in the illness. Unlike patients with FTD, these AD patients typically show more temporal-parietal than frontal hypoperfusion on SPECT, although in some FTD patients prominent temporal-parietal hypoperfusion also occurs. Similarly, even though most patients with predominantly frontal or anterior hypoperfusion will eventually turn out to have FTD pathology, purely frontal and anterior temporal presentations of AD probably do exist. Therefore, even though SPECT will differentiate most patients with FTD from those with AD, neuroimaging is neither 100% sensitive nor 100% specific. Perhaps the additional imaging of neurotransmitter systems such as the serotonin or dopamine system will improve diagnosis in the future.

CLINICAL/NEUROLOGICAL DIAGNOSIS: OVERVIEW AND UCLA EXPERIENCE

The Lund-Manchester groups have devised research criteria for FTD based on the clinical features of FTD (Brun et al., 1994). These research criteria include 29 items within the categories of behavior, speech, affect, spatial orientation/praxis, physical signs, investigations, and supportive findings. There are also 14 exclusion items which exclude other dementias. Although many of the items are highly sensitive and specific for FTD, others seem to have less value for diagnosis.

In a comparison of 30 FTD subjects and 30 AD subjects, we discovered that the behavioral items were most sensitive and specific for FTD (Miller et al., 1996a). In particular the behavioral items of early behavioral disinhibition, apathy, loss of personal awareness, loss of social awareness, stereotyped motor behaviors, and hyperoality strongly differentiated FTD from AD subjects. There were some subjects with predominantly left-sided hypoperfusion on SPECT in whom none of the behavioral items were rated as positive in the FTD group. However, this asymmetric left-sided group of FTD subjects was captured by the progressive loss of speech items.

This study suggests that the constellation of symptoms found in an individual FTD patient is due to the separate and additive effects of right and left frontal and temporal pathology. In patients with selective left frontal hypoperfusion on SPECT, nonfluent aphasia is an early and prominent symptom. Most subjects with selective left frontal hypoperfusion show intact social graces and exhibit no behavioral disinhibition. Self-deprecation, depression, and social withdrawal are common. With predominantly right frontal dysfunction, a picture of marked behavioral alteration with poor impulse control and childish, silly, poorly modulated affect emerges. Some subjects with selective right frontal degeneration become highly critical of others, and their appeal to others diminishes.

Among the most interesting subjects we have seen are those in whom SPECT demonstrates anterior temporal hypoperfusion in conjunction with relative sparing of the anterior frontal lobes. This subgroup represents approximately 20% of our FTD population. In all of the temporally predominant patients we have seen, both temporal lobes were abnormal on SPECT, although in most, either the right or left side was more severely affected.

We suggested the term *temporal lobe variant* (*TLV*) of FTD for these individuals (Edwards-Lee et al., 1996), while Snowden and colleagues (1992) and Hodges and colleagues (1992) have emphasized the linguistic deficits in left-sided-predominant patients and use the term *semantic dementia* to describe them. Although *semantic dementia* captures the aphasic features found in many of the left temporally predominant subjects, it does not describe many TLV patients with predominantly right-sided temporal pathology.

Left TLV subjects typically show semantic anomia and semantic alexia. The anomia is characterized by the loss of word meaning; clueing with the first syllable, or even the whole word, does not improve the anomia. With semantic alexia there is trouble in moving from the phoneme to meaning, and atypical phonetic phrases are handled poorly. Recently, we saw a subject who could read the word *not* but not *knot* due to the *kn* phoneme and could not read the word *right* due to inability to pronounce *ght*. In addition, the subject could not give the meaning of *knot* or *right*.

In patients with right temporally predominant hypoperfusion, the clinical manifestations are often psychiatric. Bizarre, remote affect is a common feature of these patients, and many are disinhibited. This constellation of bizarre/remote affect and disinhibition can sometimes suggest schizophrenia, although unlike many patients with schizophrenia, auditory hallucinations in these patients are uncommon. Also, the aphasia and dementia in these patients differentiate them from classical psychiatric patients. Right TLV patients develop eccentric, sometimes stereotyped behaviors. One of our patients waved goodbye to all of the pictures in his house before going to bed, and another wore only lavender shirts and yellow pants. Bizarre hyperoral behaviors also occur; repetitive spitting and eating only a single food item are also common.

In patients with both left and right temporal degeneration, we have seen unexpected talents develop. The subject described above with semantic anomia became an accomplished "whistler" and, despite her aphasia, created interesting songs regarding her dog. Several patients who showed no previous interest in art became accomplished artists in the setting of the dementia (Miller et al., 1996b). In two subjects, an obsessive interest in written words occurred. This led to the copying of phrases from books and the playing of "search and circle" word games for may hours every day. There is striking sparing of visuospatial skills in patients with TLV. For some, the only item correctly answered on the Mini-Mental State Examination is copying intersecting pentagons.

NEUROPSYCHOLOGICAL DIAGNOSIS: OVERVIEW AND UCLA EXPERIENCE

Several studies have shown that FTD subjects show deficits in executive skills, with variable performance on memory and attentional tasks and normal or only mild difficulties in constructions and word retrieval (Neary et al., 1986; Jagust et al., 1989; Johanson and Hagberg, 1989; Miller et al., 1991; Boone et al., 1993). However, surprisingly few systematic evaluations of neuropsychological function in subjects with FTD have been published.

We recently analyzed archival neuropsychological data on 15 FTD patients, 16 AD patients, and 16 normal controls (Pachana et al., 1996). Both patient groups scored significantly below the controls on measures of verbal and nonverbal free recall, executive functions, and complex constructional ability, although the AD patients had more widespread memory impairment. The three groups did not differ in confrontation naming, recognition memory, or basic attention. The only neuropsychological measure on which the two patient groups differed was visual recall, with the FTD patients outperforming the AD group.

Analysis of the relative patterns of test scores between the two patient groups allowed better differentiation of the FTD and AD subjects. AD patients exhibited greater impairment on memory than on executive measures, while FTD subjects performed mostly poorly on executive functions compared to memory. Specifically, all of the AD patients demonstrated standardized scores (i.e., z scores based on control means and standard deviations) that were higher for verbal fluency (FAS) than visual recall (Rey-Osterrieth percent retention), while only four (29%) of the FTD patients showed this pattern. This study showed that neuropsychological batteries differentiate both FTD and AD patients from healthy controls. However, the neuropsychological scores in FTD and AD patients are sufficiently similar to make differential diagnosis between these two conditions difficult. It is not possible to point to a single test that will differentiate FTD from AD, although the relative rankings of test scores do offer some guidance.

One of the problems with approaching FTD patients as a homogeneous neuropsychological group is the fact that they are often asymmetric with regard to anatomical involvement. Recently we observed a unique constellation of cognitive abnormalities in five patients with predominantly right-sided frontotemporal degeneration (Paul et al., 1996). These patients had a performance IQ lower than the verbal IQ. Additionally, design fluency was lower than verbal fluency. Both verbal and nonverbal memory were impaired, although recognition was relatively intact. Even though these patients had predominantly right-sided involvement, basic visuconstructional abilities were relatively normal, which probably reflects the sparing of parietal function in FTD. Of interest, all four FTD patients in the study by Pachana and colleagues (1996) who did not have visual memory scores that were superior to verbal fluency scores had a predominantly right frontotemporal pattern of hypoperfusion on SPECT.

Additional research is needed to corroborate the initial indications that cognitive profiles in FTD differ, depending on whether the cerebral dysfunction is primarily right-sided or left-sided. Also, it may be possible to further delineate unique cognitive patterns in FTD, depending on whether the dysfunction within a hemisphere is more frontal or temporal. To this end, experimental paradigms such as working memory tasks should be explored in this population. In the future, with the development of genetic markers for FTD, it may become possible to study neuropsychological function in patients in the very earliest stages of this disorder.

NEUROPSYCHIATRY/NEUROCHEMISTRY: OVERVIEW AND CLINICAL IMPLICATIONS

The spectrum of behavioral disorders associated with FTD is daunting, and many symptoms may be secondary to the neurochemical deficits that occur with this disorder. Although the effect of FTD on caregivers has not been formally studied, the psychiatric burden associated with FTD is extremely high. In a recent study (Levy et al., 1996), we found that apathy, disinhibition, aberrant motor behaviors, irritability, and euphoria all occurred with a significantly higher frequency in FTD than in AD. We have found antisocial behavior in nearly 50% of subjects with FTD (Miller et al., 1997).

Delusions occurred in approximately 10% of FTD subjects, and Lesser and colleagues (1989) have shown that psychosis is sometimes the presenting feature of FTD. The cause of delusions in FTD is unknown, although it has been our experience that FTD individuals with disabling delusions are usually treated with neuroleptics, with profound parkinsonian side effects. This is unfortunate because parkinsonian features occur with FTD (Knopman et al., 1990).

Additionally, FTD is associated with profound presynaptic and postsynaptic serotonergic defects (Sparks and Markesbery, 1991; Neary et al., 1993). This serotonergic defect is found with cortical, brainstem and hypothalamic structures. Unlike AD, FTD is not associated with cholinergic loss in the nucleus basalis of Meynert (Wood et al., 1983). Therefore, there is no rational for using medications that increase brain acetylcholine in FTD patients, and in our experience, cholinergic boosting compounds exacerbate psychiatric symptoms in these patients.

We suggested (Miller et al., 1995) that some of the symptoms associated with FTD are related to serotonergic dysfunction. Weight gain exceeding 10 lb occurred in 64% of FTD patients, and a change in food preference to carbohydrates occurred in 75%. Also, severe, disabling compulsions were found in 64% of individuals with FTD. In contrast, in AD patients, eating disorders and compulsions were rare. The eating disorders and compulsions could all be attributed to central losses of brain serotonin. If this hypothesis is correct, then one might be able to treat behavioral components of FTD with serotonin-boosting antidepressants.

In fact, Swartz (1997) has demonstrated in preliminary studies that it is possible to ameliorate specific symptoms in many FTD patients by using serotonin-boosting compounds. Swartz and colleagues have found that many of the symptoms associated with FTD, including impulsivity, depression, carbohydrate craving, and compulsions, are improved with serotonin-selective reuptake inhibitors. Mild improvements in eating disorders have also been noted. However, no significant changes in neuropsychological function have been found.

Many questions still remain regarding potential therapies for FTD. In particular, the best serotonin-boosting antidepressant for FTD is unknown. Similarly, newer antipsychotics should be evaluated as potential therapies for FTD. Without a better understanding of the mechanism of brain degeneration in FTD, preventive therapies have not been attempted. However, further studies in this areas are needed.

FUTURE DIRECTIONS IN FTD

FTD is finally getting the attention that it warrants and is no longer considered to be a rare or undiagnosable condition. In the near future, genetic mapping studies are likely to be successful and should lead to a better understanding of the molecular mechanisms resulting in frontal and anterior temporal lobe degeneration. As with AD, more than one gene is likely to predispose to this disorder. Genetic studies should also help to clarify the complex nomenclature issues that currently impair the systematic diagnosis and study of FTD. For example, whether Pick's disease should be considered as separate from FTD without Pick bodies will require a better understanding of the pathogenesis of both conditions.

Clinical diagnosis is already improving, and the combination of better clinical, neuroimaging, and genetic testing will become available in the near future. However, the currently used clinical criteria, along with SPECT alone, are unlikely to yield 100% sensitivity or specificity. Receptor imaging, particularly of the cortical serotonin system, may eventually offer a significant diagnostic improvement.

What is clear is that FTD offers a relatively untapped clinical, neuropsychological, and psychiatric model for understanding what happens to individuals who slowly lose function within selective frontal and anterior temporal brain regions. When clinically asymptomatic patients can be diagnosed with genetic testing, the earliest manifestations of dysfunction in these areas may become possible. The prevention and/or ultimately the cure of FTD seems possible in the coming decades.

ACKNOWLEDGMENTS

This work was supported by the UCLA Alzheimer Disease Center AG-10123, the Christine Risse Award, and the Sidell-Kagan Research Foundation through the UCLA Medical School.

REFERENCES

Adams RD, Victor M (1993): Principles of Neurology, 5th ed. New York: McGraw-Hill.

Boone KB, Miller BL, Lesser IM (1993): Frontal lobe cognitive functions in aging: Methodologic considerations. Dementia 3:232–236.

Brun A (1987): Frontal lobe degeneration of non-Alzheimer type. I. Neuropathology. Arch Gerontol Geriatr 6:193–208.

Brun A (1993): Frontal lobe dementia of the non-Alzheimer type revisited. Dementia 4:126–131.

Brun A, Englund B, Gustafson L, Passant U, Mann DMA, Neary D, Snowden JS (1994): Clinical and neuropathological criteria for frontotemporal dementia. J Neurol Neurosurg Psychiatry 57:416–418.

Caselli RJ, Windebank AJ, Petersen RC, Komori R, Parisi JE, Okazake H, Kokmen E, Iverson R, Dinapol R, Graff-Radford NR (1993): Rapidly progressive aphasic dementia and motor neuron disease. Ann Neurol 33:200–207.

Chang L, Cornford M, Miller BL, Itabashi H, Mena I (1995): Neuronal ultrastructural abnormalities in a patient with frontotemporal dementia and motor neuron disease. Dementia 6:1–8.

Edwards-Lee T, Miller BL, Benson DF, Cummings JL, Russell G, Mena I (1997): The temporal lobe variant of frontotemporal dementia. Brain 120:1027–1040.

Gustafson L (1993): Clinical picture of frontal lobe degeneration of non-Alzheimer type. Dementia 4:143–148.

Gustafson L, Brun A, Risberg J. (1987): Frontal lobe degeneration of non-Alzheimer type. II. Clinical picture and differential diagnosis. Arch Gerontol Geriatr 6:209–223.

Hodges JR, Patterson K, Oxbury S, Funnell F (1992): Semantic dementia. Progressive fluent aphasia with temporal lobe atrophy. Brain 115:1783–1806.

Jackson M, Lowe J (1996): The new neuropathology of degenerative frontotemporal dementias. Acta Neuorpathol 91:127–134.

Jagust WL, Reed BR, Scab JP, Kramer JN, Budinger TF (1989): Clinical-physiologic correlates of Alzheimer's disease and frontal lobe dementia. Am J Physiol Imag 4:89–96.

Johanson A, Hagberg B (1989): Psychometric characteristics in patients with frontal lobe degeneration of non-Alzheimer type. Arch Gerontol Geriatr 8:129–137.

Johnson K, Davis DR, Buonanno FS, Brady T, Rose TJ, Growdon JD (1987): Comparison of magnetic resonance imaging and roentgen ray computerized tomography in dementia. Arch Neurol 144:1075–1080.

Kertesz A, Hudson L, Mackenzie I, Munoz D (1994): The pathology and nosology of primary progressive aphasia. Neurology 44:2065–2072.

Knopman DS, Mastri AR, Frey WH, Sung JH, Ruston T (1990): Dementia lacking distinctive histologic features: A common non-Alzheimer degenerative dementia. Neurology 40:251–256.

Lesser IM, Miller BL, Boone K, Hill E, Mena I (1989): Psychosis as the first manifestation of degenerative dementia. Bull Clin Neurosci 4:59–64.

Levy M, Miller BL, Cummings, JL, Fairbanks, LA, Craig A (1996): Alzheimer's disease and frontotemporal dementia: Behavioral distinctions. Arch Neurol 53:687–690.

Lynch T, Sano M, Marder KS, Bell K, Foster N, Defendini R, Sima A, Keonane C, Nygaard TG, Fahn S (1994): Clinical characteristics of a family with chromosome 17-linked disinhibition-dementia-parkinsonism-amyotrophy complex. Neurology 44:1878–1884.

Mendez MF, Selwood A, Mastri AR, Frey WH (1993): Pick's disease versus Alzheimer's disease: A comparison of clinical characteristics. Neurology 43:289–292.

Mesulam MM (1982): Slowly progressive aphasia without generalized dementia. Ann Neurol 11:592–598.

Miller BL, Chang L, Mena I, Boone KB, Lesser I. (1993): Clinical and imaging features of right focal frontal lobe degenerations. Dementia 4:204–213.

Miller BL, Cummings JL, Boone K, Chang L, Schuman S, Pahan N, Darby AL (1995a): Clinical and neurobehavioral characteristics of fronto-temporal dementia and Alzheimer disease. Neurology 45:A318.

Miller BL, Cummings JL, Villanueva-Meyer J, Boone K, Mehringer CM, Lesser IM, Mena I (1991): Frontal lobe degeneration: Clinical, neuropsychological and SPECT characteristics. Neurology 41:1374–1382.

Miller BL, Darby A, Benson DF, Cummings JL, Miller MH (1997): Antisocial behavior in frontotemporal dementia. Br J Psychiatry 170:1–6.

Miller BL, Darby AL, Swartz JR, Yener GG, Mena I (1995b): Dietary changes, compulsions and sexual behavior in fronto-temporal degeneration. Dementia 6:195–199.

Miller BL, Ikonte C, Cummings JL, Levy M, Darby A, Schuman S (1996a): Evaluation of the Lund Manchester criteria for frontotemporal dementia. Neurology 46:A185.

Miller B, Lesser I, Mena I, Villanueva-Meyer J, Hill E (1992): Regional cerebral blood flow in late-life-onset psychosis. Neuropsychiatry Neuropsychol Behav Neurol 5:132–137.

Miller BL, Ponton M, Benson DF, Cummings JL, Mena I (1996b): Enhanced artistic creativity with temporal lobe degeneration. Lancet 348:1744–1755.

Mitsuyama Y. (1993): Presenile dementia with motor neuron disease. Dementia 4:137–142.

Morris JC, Cole M, Banker BQ, Wright D (1984): Hereditary dysphasic dementia and the Pick-Alzheimer spectrum. Ann Neurol 16:455–466.

Neary D, Snowden JS, Bowen DM, Sims NR, Mann DMA, Benton JS, Northen B, Yates DO, Davison AN (1986): Neuropsychological syndromes in presenile dementia due to cerebral atrophy. J Neurol Neurosurg Psychiatry 49:163–174.

Neary D, Snowden JS, Mann DMA (1993): The clinical pathological correlates of lobar atrophy. Dementia 4:154–160.

Neary D, Snowden JS, Northen B, Goulding PJ (1988): Dementia of frontal lobe type. J Neurol Neurosurg Psychiatry 51:353–361.

Neary D, Snowden JS, Shields RA (1987): Single photon emission tomography using ^{99m}Tc-HM-PAO in the investigation of dementia. J Neurol Neurosurg Psychiatry 50:1101–1109.

Neumann MA, Cohn R. (1967): Progressive subcortical gliosis, a rare form of presenile dementia. Brain 90:405–418.

Pachana N, Boone KB, Miller BL, Cummings JL (1996): Comparison of neuropsychological functioning in Alzheimer's disease and frontotemporal dementia. JINS 2:505–510.

Paul LK, Boone KB, Miller BL, Mena I (1996): Cognitive deficits in right frontotemporal dementia. Int Congress Neuropsychiatry, Seville, Spain.

Petersen RB, Tabaton M, Chen SG, Monari L, Richardson SL, Manetto V, Lanska D, Markesberry W, Lynch T (1995): Familial progressive subcortical gliosis: Presence of prions and linkage to chromosome 17. Neurology 45(6):1062–1067.

Pick A (1977): On the relationship between aphasia and senile atrophy of the brain. In Rottenberg D, Hochberg FH (eds): Neurological Classics in Modern Translation. New York: Hafner Press, pp 35–40.

Read SL, Miller BL, Mena I, Kim R, Darby A (1995): SPECT in dementia: Clinical and pathological correlations. J Am Geriatr Soc 43:1243–1247.

Risberg J, Passant U, Warkentin S, Gustafson L (1993): Regional cerebral blood flow in frontal lobe dementia of non-Alzheimer type. Dementia 14:186–187.

Snowden JS, Neary D, Mann DMA (eds) (1996): Fronto-temporal Lobar Degeneration. New York: Churchill-Livingstone.

Snowden JS, Neary D, Mann DMA, Goulding PJ, Testa HJ (1992): Progressive language disorder due to lobar atrophy. Ann Neurol 31:174–183.

Sparks DL, Markesbery WR (1991): Altered serotonergic and cholinergic synaptic markers in Pick's disease. Arch Neurol 48:796–99.

Swartz R, Miller BL, Darby A, Schuman S (1997): Frontotemporal dementia: treatment response to serotonin selective reuptake inhibitors. J Clin Psychiatry 58(5):212–216.

Wilhelmsen K, Lynch T, Pavlou E, Nygaard TG (1994): Localization of disinhibition-dementia-parkinsonism-amyotrophy complex to 17q21–22. Am J Hum Genet 55:1150–1165.

Wilhelmsen K, Wszolek ZK, Currier RC, Lanska DJ (1996): The clinical spectrums of chromosome 17q21–22-linked degenerative syndromes. Neurology 46(2):A188.

Wood PL, Etienne P, Lal S, Nair NPV, Finaltson MH, Gauthier S, Palo J, Haltia M, Paetau A, Bird ED (1983): A post-mortem comparison of the cortical cholinergic system in Alzheimer's disease and Pick's disease. J Neurol Sci 62:211–217.

Frontal Lobe Degeneration of Non-Alzheimer Type and Its Relation to Other Frontotemporal Dementias and Alzheimer's Disease

LARS GUSTAFSON and ARNE BRUN

Departments of Psychogeriatrics (L.G.) and Pathology (A.B.), Lund University Hospital, S-220 09, Lund, Sweden

INTRODUCTION

A 30-year clinicopathological prospective study of dementia has resulted in a topographically based classification of dementias headed by a group of degenerative frontotemporal dementias (FTD), presented in greater detail in a consensus between the Lund and Manchester research groups (Brun et al., 1994). During the first years of our longitudinal study, we soon recognized a group of patients with a predominant frontal lobe clinical pathology and frontotemporal regional cerebral blood flow (rCBF) pathology. The tentative clinical diagnosis usually became Pick's disease. Later, however, the detailed postmortem examination revealed a cortical degeneration that was neither Alzheimer's disease (AD) nor typical Pick's disease (Brun and Gustafson, 1978). We tried to find a suitable descriptive designation, and *frontal lobe degeneration of non-Alzheimer type* (*FLD*) was suggested (Brun, 1987; Gustafson, 1987), not primarily as a demarcation against Pick's disease but rather to stress the possibility of a clinical differentiation from AD. AD has often been described erroneously as having a marked frontal lobe character.

Our most recent survey of neuropathological diagnoses (Brun and Gustafson, 1993) showed that the majority of severe dementias are caused by AD (42%), cerebrovascular disease (26%), or a combination of these two conditions (12%). A surprisingly high proportion (9%) was diagnosed as FTD. Here FLD is the dominating disorder (8%) and thus is more prevalent than Pick's disease, diagnosed in 1%. One reason why we have found such a large number of FLD patients is probably that our longitudinal dementia study, from its start 30 years ago, also included early-onset cases (Gustafson, 1975). Other research groups have been presenting sim-

Pick's Disease and Pick Complex, Edited by Andrew Kertesz and David G. Munoz
ISBN 0-471-17792-X ©1998 Wiley-Liss, Inc.

ilar clinical materials, some with even higher proportions of FTD cases, although with somewhat different designations. Neary and his colleagues in Manchester described *dementia of frontal lobe type* (Neary et al., 1988), Knopman et al. (1990) introduced the term *dementia lacking distinctive histological features,* and Clark et al. (1986) described cases with *primary degenerative dementia without Alzheimer pathology.* There are striking similarities between the clinical pictures described in these different studies and our own findings. Other studies in France, Germany, Italy, the United States, and the Netherlands have added important information on clinical, neuropsychological, brain imaging, and genetic findings in FTD (Miller et al., 1993; Förstl et al., 1994; Pasquier et al., 1995; Heutink et al., 1997; Frisoni et al., 1996). The group of FTD originally consisting of FLD, Pick's disease, and motor neuron disease (MND) with dementia (MNDD) will probably expand to include several other diseases, many of which have the basic clinical and pathological features of the FTD group. Original and additional disorders are presented elsewhere in this book, such as Pick's disease, MNDD, progressive aphasia, and chromosome 17-related disorders (Lynch et al., 1994). The position of FLD in this context is discussed here, as well as its relation to AD, the main clinical differential diagnostic problem. Our view of FLD is based on repeated clinical observations including rCBF measurements of patients with the diagnosis confirmed postmortem.

PATHOLOGICAL CONSIDERATIONS

Frontal Lobe Degeneration of Non-Alzheimer Type (FLD)

On gross inspection of the brain, either no atrophy, mild atrophy, or in a few cases moderate atrophy of the frontal cortex is noted, and in about 30% of the cases there is also mild atrophy of the anterior third of the temporal cortex. Circumscribed atrophy, as in Pick's disease, is never seen, although preservation of the adjoining central, sensory, and motor gyri may create a situation slightly reminiscent of a circumscription. On cut brain slices, slight widening of the frontal part of the ventricular system is seen. The amygdala and hippocampal formation, as well as the striatum and thalamus, are of normal size. The substantia nigra in some cases shows a mild loss of pigment.

Microscopically, the same picture is noted in all cases, showing in the cortical areas mentioned, including the anterior cingulate cortex, a degenerative process that in advanced cases may also though in a mild form be present in postcentral parietal areas. In between, the central gyri are remarkably well preserved. This degenerative process is marked by a microvacuolation of supragranular layers, at the same time showing atrophy, some loss of neurons, and gliosis, most easily detected in the molecular layer (Brun, 1993). In these cortical layers there is also a loss of synapses amounting to about 40–50% compared to age-matched controls (Liu and Brun, 1996). In the infragranular layers no changes are usually noted, and in the immediately adjoining white matter there is mild to moderate gliosis with only slight loss of myelin (Englund and Brun, 1987). On microscopical examination in about 30% of the cases, the grossly unchanged striatum and amygdala show a mild to moderate change of the type reported above. In the substantia nigra there is a loss of pigmented neurons, but never as severe as in Parkinson's disease.

Neuronal inclusions, Lewy bodies, and tau immunopositivity are absent, and the methods used to detect prions give a negative result (Collinge et al., 1994). Alzheimer-type changes such as plaques, tangles, and amyloid are not seen or are present in only the oldest patients, and then in an amount expected for the age. In a few cases mild loss of anterior horn spinal neurons may be seen, but without other MND-type changes such as demyelination of ventral or lateral pyramidal tracts.

This histopathological picture has also been reported in some cases under the designation *dementia lacking distinctive histology* (Knopman et al., 1990). Other cases included under this heading differ with respect to localization of changes and also show additional features not observed in FLD. Histologically similar changes have also been seen as nonspecific dementia in cases of progressive aphasia and were thought to be forerunners of a more global dementia (Green et al., 1990). Such changes were also found by Clark et al. (1986) and were interpreted as primary degenerative dementia without Alzheimer pathology.

Motor neuron disease with dementia (MNDD) is also included in the FTD group in view of its great similarities to FLD, showing the same cortical histological changes, though MNDD by definition also includes spinal and bulbar motor system degeneration and neuronal inclusions, especially in the hippocampal formation neurons (Mitsuyama, 1993). A relationship between the two disorders might be indicated by the relatively frequent frontal clinical involvement in MNDD noted by Ludolph et al. (1993), Lopez et al. (1994), and others.

Progressive nonfluent aphasia and semantic dementia are also related histopathologically to the FTD group. These conditions show the cortical changes seen in FLD, though with a slightly different frontotemporal pattern and without neuronal inclusions and ballooned cells (Snowden et al. 1996).

Frontotemporal dementia linked to chromosome 17, recently summarized by Sima et al. (1996) and Foster et al. (1997), constitutes another group of relatively rare familial disorders with changes in common with those of FLD but with additional features varying from family to family, most often a parkinsonism, giving rise to the designation *frontotemporal dementia and Parkinsonism linked to chromosome 17.* The parkinsonian symptomatology correlates with a degeneration of the substantia nigra. It might here be of interest to note that FLD also shows such degeneration, though less intense that in the chromosome 17-linked group and not giving rise to marked parkinsonian symptoms. One further link to FLD is a family in this group presented by Basun et al. (1997) showing changes generally identical to those in FLD.

In *Pick's disease* the degeneration involves the same areas as in FLD, including the anterior portion of the cingulate gyrus, though with much greater severity within well-defined cortical areas, resulting in a circumscription of the atrophic regions. In keeping herewith both supra- and intragranular layers are involved, (Gustafson and Brun 1997). Central and basal gray structures such as the striatum and limbic areas also participate consistently in the degenerative process; in particular, the frontal white matter shows obvious atrophy and demyelination, with pronounced and often asymmetric ventricular widening. In all these respects, then, Pick's disease differs from FLD, a difference further underscored by the presence of Pick bodies and inflated neurons. In our opinion, these features define Pick's disease, an opinion shared, for example, by Verity and Wechsler (1987) and Baldwin and Förstl (1993). Such features, especially the neuronal changes, have not been observed either in our most advanced and long-standing cases of FLD or in further examples of the disease in the affected families. Other authors are of a different opinion. For example, Kertesz et al. (1994), based on the finding of Pick cells and inflated neurons in cases of primary progressive aphasia but with other features of FLD, suggest lumping other disorders such as FLD, Pick's disease, and progressive aphasia into a larger group called the *Pick complex.* Here it should be recalled that Snowden et al. (1996) described a Pick type of frontal lobe degeneration in which some cases showed neuronal inclusions and, on the other hand, Constantinides et al.'s variety of Pick's disease without such cellular changes (1974). The latter may, however, represent a variety of what is now called FLD.

AD is a common diagnostic alternative to FLD, particularly in the early stages. It should, however, be noted that the two disorders are almost diametrically opposite in terms of pathological changes (Brun and Gustafson, 1978; Brun, 1987). FLD entirely lacks plaques, tangles, and amyloid deposits save for the nonspecific, diffuse deposits and a few plaques and tangles in elderly FLD patients. Of particular importance for the difference in clinical expression of these disorders is the difference in the topographical distribution of changes. In FLD, these changes selectively involve the frontal lobes and the anterior temporal cortex, whereas in AD the postcentral temporoparietal areas and the hippocampus bear the brunt of the pathology. A more pronounced frontal involvement in AD is seen in a minority of presenile patients. In the senile variety of AD, frontal changes are more common than in the presenile form, though still less intense than the postcentral alterations. Furthermore, hippocampal changes are compulsory and severe in AD and rare or absent in FLD.

CLINICAL PICTURE

Changes in Personality and Behavior

The clinical onset of FLD is insidious, and its progression is slow and gradual. The first clinical manifestations usually appear in the presenium and seldom after 70 years of age. The mean age at onset in our 30 postmortem-verified cases was 56 ± 7.6 years (range, 45–70 years), with a total duration of the illness of 3–17 years (mean, 8.1 ± 3.4 years). The duration was somewhat shorter than in the eight cases with pure Pick's disease, 11.0 ± 4.1 years (range 4–17 years), and in presenile AD it was 10.6 ± 3 years (range, 5–16 years) in the longitudinal study. This is in accordance with the age characteristics reported in other studies (Neary et al., 1988; Knopman et al., 1990).

Due to the distribution of degenerative changes, the clinical picture in the early stage of FLD is characterized by changes and deterioration of personality and behavior, affective symptoms, and a progressive dynamic aphasia. The most common clinical features are presented in Table 4.1. Cognitive dysfunction, mostly seen as memory failure and increased distractibility, is almost always present, although often overshadowed by other, more obvious and dramatic manifestations of the brain lesions. Changes in personality traits with levelling of emotions, social neglect, lack of judgment, and apathy are typical findings. The appearance of such symptoms without indications of cognitive failure may easily lead to diagnostic considerations of nonorganic mental disorders such as mood disorder, schizophrenia, delusional disorder, and adult personality deviations of nonorganic origin. Such diagnostic misinterpretation probably becomes less common at a later stage of the disease, although a number of FLD cases may remain clinically unrecognized and may be revealed only if there is postmortem follow-up.

Signs of disinhibition and lack of insight into the present condition and its consequences are early manifestations in FLD. Impaired control of emotions is manifested as irritability, tearfulness, inadequate smiling, and spells of crying and laughing. There may be an initial period of unrestrained behavior with restlessness, irritability, hypersexuality, and increased talkativeness, but more often the changes are toward stereotypy, aspontaneity, and, at a later stage, severe apathy and emotional unconcern. The patient's habitual personality traits may, however, deteriorate slowly, which makes it difficult even for a close relative to decide when the signs of FLD started. Therefore, alternative explanations of the patient's strange behavior may be offered, such as problems at work or in the family. Most FLD patients are judged to have a fairly normal premorbid personality, although restlessness and anxiety are sometimes reported (Gustafson, 1987). Moreover, the emotional features of FLD do not seem strongly related to premorbid personality traits but rather to the metabolic pattern, as shown by single photon emission computed tomography (SPECT) (Lebert et al., 1995). This relationship between emotional symptoms and SPECT findings is not disease specific but is also found in other types of organic dementia (Miller et al., 1993; Luauté et al., 1994; Lebert et al., 1995).

TABLE 4.1   Clinical Findings in FLD

Insidious onset and slow progression

Changes in personality
  Disinhibition—social neglect
  Levelling of emotions
  Lack of insight and judgment
  Restlessness, agitation
  Irritability, euphoria
  Apathy

Dissolution of language
  Progressively reduced speech
  Stereotyped phrases
  Echolalia
  Mutism, amimia

Depressive episodes
Anxiety
Hypochondriasis, symptoms of pain
Stereotyped behavior
Deceptions, delusions

Changes in oral/dietary behavior
Utilization behavior
Hypersexuality

Memory, receptive speech, and spatial functions
  comparatively spared
Dyscalculia
Intermittent dyspraxia

Normal EEG despite evident dementia
Epileptic seizures less common
Low, labile blood pressure
Incontinence, early appearance

As pointed out, the emotional changes in FLD may be difficult to differentiate from those of affective disorders. The emotional tuning may be that of euphoria, sometimes combined with increased verbal output and confabulation. This clinical picture may be misinterpreted as a hypomanic or manic stage, at least in a short time perspective. Stereotyped smiling and giggling, when present, seem less related to elated mood than to dysregulation of emotional expression. Differentiation from nonorganic depressive disorders may also be difficult since many FLD patients display episodes of depressed mood with suicidal ideation. The slowly developing emotional shallowness, apathy, social withdrawal, reduced speech, and lack of mimical movements may be misinterpreted as signs of a major depression. The majority of our FLD and Pick patients had received antidepressant medication at an early stage of the disease. Suicide was suspected in one postmortem verified FLD case and in one additional case lacking autopsy. In spite of the fact that FLD patients lose their insight early, many of them complain of anxiety and various somatic symptoms, sometimes in combination with fixed hypochondriacal ideas.

These features, in combination with the changes in personality and language, may lead to the diagnosis of schizophrenia. The severity of anxiety is, however, difficult to evaluate, both in FLD and in Pick's disease, due to the patient's restlessness and the limited and stereotyped verbal communication. The strategies used to handle anxiety in FLD patients have been studied with psychological techniques which are used for differentiation from AD (Johanson et al., 1990).

The early personality changes in FLD with social and personal neglect, lack of judgment, and unpredictable behavior may easily lead to conflicts with family and society, especially as long as there is no reasonable explanation for the patient's strange, antisocial behavior. The severe strain on the family will easily cause mental ill health, economic and legal problems, and even divorce and suicide. Complications of this type are uncommon in families with an AD patient. In AD the habitual personality traits are usually well preserved. The typical AD patient may therefore, under optimal conditions, appear friendly, socially cooperative, and more or less aware of his or her constant need of support from other people. By contrast, the FLD patient becomes self-centered, less concerned about family and friends, and often described as uninterested, emotionally cold, and even hostile. Another possible consequence of the frontal lobe dysfunction is traffic accidents. The FLD patient often continues to drive after clinical onset of the disease. Practical and spatial abilities are comparatively spared, but the patient becomes careless and inattentive and therefore a constant risk factor on the road. By contrast, the typical AD patient is self-critically and anxiously aware of his or her practical difficulties, impaired sense of locality, and left-right insecurity and is therefore ready to give up driving.

Psychotic Features

Hallucinations and illusions were observed in about 20% of FLD and early-onset AD patients, as well as in 50% of the late-onset AD group in our longitudinal dementia study (Gustafson and Risberg, 1993). Such symptoms will probably be reported even more often when the patients are followed closely from the early stage of the disease (Johansson and Gustafson, 1996). The clinical analysis of psychotic features has to consider the access ability of ideas and emotions in FLD patients due to lack of communication. The psychotic traits easily give the impression of functional psychosis with schizophrenia as an early tentative diagnosis (Gustafson, 1987; Neary et al., 1988; Knopman et al., 1990), especially when they appear in combination with lack of insight, stereotypy, and language dysfunction of the frontal lobe type. About one-third of our FLD patients had psychotic episodes, mostly of a paranoid aggressive type, occasionally with acts of easily provoked violence.

The psychotic features in AD seem more directly related to the cognitive failure with dysmnesia, dysgnosia, and disorientation, while the psychotic symptoms and ideation in FLD show important clinical variability without such a connection. Moreover, hallucinations and delusions in AD can often be influenced and diverted by psychological methods and treated with psychotropic medication, while in FLD these symptoms are less liable to respond favorably in these respects (Gustafson and Risberg, 1993). An association between psychosis and frontal lobe damage has also been described in AD and vascular dementia with lesions in the frontal lobes (Brun and Gustafson, 1991; Miller et al., 1991). Sensory distortions, especially hyperestesia, were found in about 30% of the FLD group and in 10% of the AD cases. Stereotyped and preservative behavior, seen as a preoccupation with daily routines such as washing, dressing, locking of doors, physical training, and wandering, is common in FLD. Such ritualistic behavior, which at times may reach psychotic dimensions, has also been reported in other clinical studies of patients with frontal and caudate frontal lesions (Luria, 1973; Seibyl et al., 1989; Tonkonogy and Barreira, 1989).

Klüver-Bucy Syndrome

Several components of the human Klüver-Bucy syndrome, such as hyperorality, hypersexuality, and bulimia, as well as other changes in oral/dietary behavior are prevalent in FLD and Pick's disease (Brun and Gustafson, 1978; Cummings and Duchen, 1981; Gustafson, 1987). Excessive smoking, drinking, and eating, with a preference for special foods, were observed in 50% and 80% of our FLD and Pick patients, respectively. Some of these patients were first misdiagnosed as alcoholics due to their excessive drinking and its social consequences. The changes in alcohol consumption may sometimes be controlled by firmness on the part of relatives. Craving for affection and sexual contacts were reported in more than 50% of FLD patients but were uncommon in early-onset AD patients (Gustafson, 1993); surprisingly, they were seldom reported in our eight patients with pure Pick's disease. FLD patients may also show the "utilization behavior" described in patients with various frontal lobe lesions (Lhermitte et al., 1986) and easily revealed by neuropsychological testing (Snowden et al., 1996). This lack of impulse control shows important similarities to the "hypermetamorphosis" and distractibility of the Klüver-Bucy syndrome. Traits of the Klüver-Bucy syndrome, such as hyperorality, may also be observed in AD, although seldom with the productivity and complexity reported in FLD and Pick's disease.

Speech Disorder

The speech disorder in FLD and Pick's disease is described as progressive reduction of verbal output, usually starting as verbal aspontaneity with stereotyped comments and perseveration of a limited number of set phrases. There may be an initial period of increased unrestrained talking and singing, which, especially in Pick's disease, may appear in combination with confabulation. Imitating behavior such as echolalia was found in about 50% of postmortem-verified FLD and Pick cases. Echophenomena and utilization behavior belong to the *environmental dependency syndrome* in patients with frontal lobe lesions (Lhermitte et al., 1986). Sometimes the normal pitch of voice is changed in FLD, which in combination with stereotypy leads to a similarity to verbal mannerisms associated with schizophrenic processes. The handwriting may also change in various ways, such as changes in the size of letters, misspellings, and stereotypes. The language dysfunction is thus dominated by a dynamic expressive failure rather than by a receptive one. In the end state, the patient may become mute but still capable of understanding verbal communication. These speech disturbances are different from the global dysphasia with paraphasia and dysgraphia of the postcentral type in AD. The dissolution of language in FLD and Pick's disease, as well as the disappearance of nonverbal communication, makes it extremely difficult to evaluate to what extent the patients understand what is said. Probably, however, even at an advanced stage, these patients are capable of some understanding and recognition. The symptom constellation of palilalia, echolalia, mutism, and amimia (PEMA syndrome of Guiraud) is typical of FLD and Pick's disease but rare in AD. The stuttering-like phenomenon logoclonia, which is prevalent in AD, is extremely uncommon in FLD and Pick's disease.

Cognitive Impairment

Memory impairment, mainly reduced recent memory and lack of concentration, appear early in FLD, although they are less predominant and disturbing than in early-onset AD. Temporal and spatial orientation and practical ability are usually preserved even at a late stage of the disease, although they are difficult to evaluate by traditional methods. Memory impairment, like confabulation, is more prominent in Pick's disease, probably due to the more severe hippocampal degeneration (Johanson and Hagberg, 1989). FLD patients with the best preserved memory function also show the best preserved hippocampal structures at autopsy (Johanson and Hagberg, 1989). FLD patients who are testable are usually able to copy simple geometric figures, in contrast to the more general failure among AD patients. Surprisingly often, dyscalculia is mentioned as an early problem in FLD.

In our experience, neuropsychological testing can be used for the early recognition of FLD and to distinguish it from other dementias, normal aging, and nonorganic mental disease. Dyspraxia, right-left disorientation, and spatial disorientation develop comparatively late in FLD and Pick's disease, in consequence with the relative sparing of temporoparietal cortical areas in FLD. FLD patients may, however, describe a transitory type of dyspraxia similar to that previously described in Pick's disease (Mallison, 1947). This temporary dysfunction of sequential behavior may be connected to the frontal (especially prefrontal) degeneration (Luria, 1973) and differs from the dyspraxia of pure AD, which is stable, with only small variations over time.

The early test profile in FLD is characterized by reduced vocabulary, slow verbal production, and relatively intact reasoning and memory. By contrast, early AD is characterized by relatively intact verbal production and simultaneous impairment of reasoning ability, verbal and spatial memory dysfunction, dysphasia, and dyspraxia. AD with a later onset shows a less consistent test profile and more marked verbal memory dysfunction. Systematic evaluation of behavior qualities such as cooperation, self-criticism, distractibility, flight reactions, and strategy in the test situation strongly contributed to the differentiation of FLD from AD (Johanson and Hagberg, 1989; Pachana et al., 1996). There are significant correlations between cognitive performance and rCBF pathology in FTD. Elfgren and coworkers (1993, 1996) have shown significant correlations between global impairment and verbal fluency scores and left frontal lateral, frontal medial, and left temporal anterior inferior rCBF, as measured with SPECT.

Physical Signs

There are few pathological somatic findings, including neurological findings, in FLD. Primitive reflexes appear, however, comparatively early, while rigidity, tremor, and akinisia are late phenomena. Increased muscular tension is significantly more common in AD than in FLD and Pick's disease. Generalized epileptic seizures may appear in FLD, but they are less prevalent than in AD, and myoclonic twitchings, which are present in 50% of early-onset AD patients, are extremely uncommon in FLD. The electroencephalogram (EEG) is usually normal at an early stage of FLD (Johannesson et al., 1977; Rosén et al., 1993). However, in FLD there is an increase in EEG pathology with longer duration of the disease. This has also been shown in Pick's disease, MNDD, and other dementias of the frontal lobe type. By contrast, the EEG in AD is almost always pathological, even at an early stage. Quantitative EEG analysis will probably improve the differential diagnosis between FTD, AD, and vascular dementia (Rosén et al., 1993).

Surprisingly often, FLD patients have a low and labile blood pressure, with a high prevalence of orthostatic blood pressure drops and syncopal attacks (Gustafson, 1987). Low and labile blood pressure is, however, also prevalent in early-onset AD and vascular dementia (Passant et al., 1996). The relationship between blood pressure changes and the brain disease in FLD is still unclear, except that FLD is unlikely to be of ischemic origin. Urinary incontinence, which is reported early in about 50% of our FTD cases, is a comparatively late feature in uncomplicated AD. These symptoms, which are also common in vascular dementia and in AD, are probably caused by the frontobasal and anterior cingulate damage (Andrew and Nathan, 1964; Wilson and Chang, 1974).

Differential Diagnosis

The clinical diagnosis of FLD, especially at an early stage, and differentiation from other organic brain diseases with frontal features and functional mental diseases with similar changes in personality, mood, and behavior, may be difficult. FLD as a constituent of FTD can, however, be recognized by systematic evaluation of the patient's history and clinical picture, supported by neuropsychological testing, brain imaging (Gustafson et al., 1977; Neary et al., 1988; Pasquier et al., 1995; Risberg and Gustafson, 1997), and other diagnostic techniques. The Lund-Manchester consensus is recommended as a basis for clinical recognition. In our daily clinical work we use a combination of three diagnostic rating scales: one scale for recognition of dementia of the Alzheimer type (DAT score), one scale for diagnosis of FTD (FTD score) (Gustafson and Nilsson, 1982; Brun and Gustafson, 1993), and the original ischemic score suggested by Hachinski et al. (1975) to estimate the probability of a vascular etiology of the disease. Diagnoses based on the scoring profile in the three rating scales have been validated against rCBF findings and neuropathological diagnoses (Risberg and Gustafson, 1988).

There are important clinical similarities between FLD and Pick's disease. Differentiation based purely on clinical grounds is still very difficult in spite of the described neuropathological distinction. Similar personality changes, expressive speech disorder, and gradual loss of mimical expressions are found in both diseases, as are a normal EEG, early incontinence, and low, labile blood pressure. However, affective symptoms, especially depression, are more often reported in FLD, while severe memory failure and confabulation are more frequent in Pick's disease. Moreover, positive heredity for dementia of a similar type is reported to the same extent in the two diseases (Groen and Endtz, 1982; Passant et al., 1993). Hopefully, the use of functional brain imaging will improve the differentiation by showing the more severe cortical involvement with sharp demarcation from better-preserved tissue in Pick's disease. The guidelines for diagnosis of other types of dementia such as the NINCDS-ADRDA criteria (McKhann et al., 1984), although focusing on AD, may easily include cases of FLD and Pick's disease in that group. DSM-III-R (APA, 1987) offers few diagnostic guidelines for Pick's disease, while DSM-IV (APA, 1994) describes Pick's disease as a pathologically distinct etiology of frontotemporal brain atrophy. According to ICD-10 (1992), *dementia in Pick's disease* is a slowly progressive dementia with frontal lobe features and selective frontal and temporal lobe atrophy but without the pathological changes of AD. Thus these guidelines give little information on the growing knowledge of heterogeneity in FTD.

There are several significant clinical differences between FLD and Pick's disease, on the one hand, and AD, on the other hand (Gustafson, 1987). These differences, which are evident even at an early stage, may remain distinguishable even at the fully developed stage of the diseases. Memory failure, spatial disorientation, and dyspraxia are more prevalent in AD, while lack of insight, disinhibition, and hyperorality are more common in FTD. AD is characterized by global dysphasia, logoclonia, increased muscular tension, and epileptic seizures, especially myoclonia, while expressive dynamic aphasia and components of the PEMA syndrome are typical of FLD and Pick's disease. However, an important minority of AD patients, about 5%, have early involvement of the frontal lobes and therefore manifest frontal lobe symptoms at an early stage. Differential diagnosis is, however, still possible, considering the total clinical picture in the two types of dementia (Brun and Gustafson, 1991).

Clinical onset of dementia in MMND usually occurs in the sixth decade of life, as in other types of FTD (Mitsuyama, 1984, 1993; Morita et al., 1987; Neary et al., 1990). The clinical picture is similar to that of FLD, with early changes in personality and behavior, loss of insight, and signs of disinhibition such as restlessness, irritability, unrestrained sexuality, and hyperorality. Differential diagnosis from FLD and Pick's disease may be difficult when these symptoms precede the signs of anterior horn cell involvement. Speech may become stereotyped and perseverative, developing into mutism, while receptive speech function, orientation, and practical abilities remain comparatively spared. The emotional changes are often toward euphoria. The diagnosis is based on recognition of a rapidly aggressive dementia of the frontal lobe type and the presence of the physical signs of anterior horn involvement. The EEG may remain normal, as in FLD, and functional brain imaging often shows predominant frontal or frontotemporal pathology (Ludoph et al., 1993). It may be difficult to differentiate FLD from Creutzfeldt Jacob disease with a frontal emphasis and from Huntington's disease when personality changes and psychotic features dominate. The clinical diagnosis of FLD may also be considered in cases with frontal cortical and subcortical vascular lesions (Brun and Gustafson, 1991).

There are important similarities between FLD at an early stage and the clinical spectrum of progressive aphasia, as described by Mesulam (1982) and Neary et al., (1993). The progressive aphasia is dominated by language disturbances, and memory impairment and dyspraxia are less pronounced. Later in the course, however, many of these patients seem to develop global dementia (Green et al., 1990; Snowden et al., 1992). SPECT studies of progressive aphasia often show asymmetric pathology with predominant left hemispheric involvement (Neary et al., 1993). Whether progressive aphasia and FLD represent two distinct disorders or different clinical profiles of the same degenerative process with different topographic distribution remains undetermined. The syndrome of semantic dementia in which the brain pathology is mainly restricted to the middle and inferior temporal gyri (Snowden et al., 1996) is accompanied by behavioral changes, although these are less severe than those in FLD and Pick's disease. Dynamic aphasia similar to that in FLD and Pick's disease has also been described in progressive supranuclear palsy (Esmonde et al., 1996).

The changes in personality and cognition in frontotemporal dementia linked to chromosome 17 usually start between the ages of 30 and 60 (Wilhelmsen et al., 1994; Sima et al., 1996; Foster et al., 1997). Average duration of the condition in the families described has been less than 10 years. Age at onset is difficult to determine due to the type of deterioration and the slow progression. The spectrum of personality changes is similar to that in FLD, but the type and severity of memory impairment, dyspraxia and dysgnosia are more similar to those of AD. As in FLD, most patients become mute, but the extrapyramidal features with bradykinesia, rigidity, and postural instability are more pronounced than in FLD. Functional brain imaging shows focal, usually frontotemporal, hypoperfusion and hypometabolism in chromosome 17-linked dementia, which is uncommon in AD (Brun and Gustafson, 1991; Gustafson and Risberg, 1993; Waldemar et al., 1994).

In summary, during the last 10 years we have seen the emergence of a new group of frontal dementias, different from AD, the largest single member of which is FLD. The group is characterized by a common basic pathology structurally and topographically, but with some variations in form-specific features clinically and pathologically, the differential weight of which is still difficult to determine. Hopefully, future research will provide answers to the question of whether these conditions are fundamentally different or represent the spectrum of one disorder, may be based on mutations primarily on chromosome 17.

REFERENCES

American Psychiatric Association (APA) (1987): Diagnostic and Statistical Manual of Mental Disorders (DSM-III-R), 3rd ed, rev. Washington, DC: APA.

American Psychiatric Association (APA) (1994): Diagnostic and Statistical Manual of Mental Disorders (DSM-IV). Washington, DC: APA.

Andrew J, Nathan PW (1964): Lesions of anterior frontal lobes and disturbances of micturition and defecation. Brain 87:232–262.

Baldwin B, Förstl H (1993): Pick's disease—101 years on Still there; but in need of reform. Br J Psychiatry 163:100–104.

Basun H, Almqvist O, Axelman K, Brun A, Campbell TA, Collinge J, Forsell C, Froelich S, Wahlund L-O, Wetterberg L, Lannfelt L (1997): Clinical characteristics of a family with chromosome 17-linked rapidly progressive frontotemporal dementia. Arch Neurol 54:539–544.

Brun A (1987): Frontal lobe degeneration of non-Alzheimer type. I. Neuropathology. Arch Gerontol Geriatr 6:193–208.

Brun A. (1993): Frontal lobe degeneration of non-Alzheimer type, revisited. I. Neuropathology. Arch Gerontol Geriatr 4:126–131.

Brun A, Englund B, Gustafson L, Passant U, Mann DMA, Neary D, Snowden JS (1994): Clinical and neuropathological criteria for frontotemporal dementia. J Neurol Neurosurg Psychiatr 57:416–418.

Brun A, Gustafson L (1978): Limbic lobe involvement in presenile dementia. Arch Psychiatrie Nervenkrankh 226:79–93.

Brun A, Gustafson L (1991): Psychopathology and frontal lobe involvement in organic dementia. In Iqbal K, McLachlan DRC, Winbald B, Wisenewski HM (eds): Alzheimer's Disease: Basic Mechanisms, Diagnosis and Therapeutic Strategies London: Wiley, pp 27–33.

Brun A, Gustafson L (1993): I. The Lund longitudinal dementia study: A 25-year perspective on neuropathology, differential diagnosis and treatment. In Corain B, Nicolini M, Winblad B, Wisniewski H, Zatta P (eds): Alzheimer's Disease. Advances in Clinical and Basic Research. Chichester, New York, Bristone, Toronto, Singapore, Wiley, pp 4–18.

Clark AW, White CL III, Manz JH, Parhad JM, Curry B, Whitehouse PJ, Lehman L, Cole JT (1986): Primary degenerative dementia without Alzheimer pathology. Can J Neurol Sci 13:462–470.

Collinge J, Hardy J, Brown J, Brun A (1994): Familial Pick's disease and dementia in frontal lobe degeneration of non-Alzheimer type are no variants of prion disease. J Neurol Neurosurg Psychiatry 57: 762.

Constantinidis J, Richard J, Tissot R (1974): Pick's disease. Histological and clinical correlations. Eur Neurol 11:208–217.

Cummings JL, Duchen LW (1981): Klüver-Bucy syndrome in Pick's disease: Clinical and pathological correlations. Neurology 31:1415–1422.

Elfgren C, Passant U, Risberg J (1993): Neuropsychological findings in frontal lobe dementia. Dementia 4:214–219.

Elfgren C, Ryding E, Passant U (1996): Performance on neuropsychological tests related to single photon emission computerised tomography findings in frontotemporal dementia. Br J. Psychiatry 169:416–422.

Englund E, Brun A (1987): Frontal lobe degeneration of non-Alzheimer type. II. White matter changes. Arch Gerontol Geriatr 6:235–243.

Esmonde T, Giles E, Xuereb J, Hodges J (1996): Progressive supranuclear palsy presenting with dynamic aphasia. J Neurol Neurosurg Psychiatry 60:403–410.

Foster NL, Wilhelmsen K, Sima AAF, Jones MZ, D'Amato C, Gildman S (1997): Frontotemporal dementia and Parkinsonism linked to chromosome 17: A consensus. Ann Neurol 41:706–715.

Förstl H, Hentschel F, Besthorn C, Geiger-Kabisch C, Sattel H, Schreiter-Gasser U, Bayerl JR, Schmitz F, Schmitt HP (1994): Frontal und temporal beginnende Hirnatrophie. Nervenarzt 65:611–618.

Frisoni GB, Beltramello A, Geroldi C, Weiss C, Bianchetti A, Trabucchi M (1996): Brain atrophy in frontotemporal dementia. J Neurol Neurosurg Psychiatry 61:157–165.

Green J, Morris JC, Sandson J, McKeel DW, Miller JW (1990): Progressive aphasia: A precursor of global dementia? Neurology 40:423–429.

Groen JJ, Endtz LJ (1982): hereditary Pick's disease: Second re-examination of a large family and discussion of other heredity cases, with particular reference to electroencephalography and computerized tomography. Brain 105:442–459.

Gustafson L (1975): Psychiatric symptoms in dementia with onset in the presenile period. Acta Psychiatrica Scandinavica, Suppl 257. Copenhagen: Munksgaard, pp 9–35.

Gustafson L (1987): Frontal lobe degeneration of non-Alzheimer type. II. Clinical picture and differential diagnosis. Arch Gerontol Geriatr 6:209–233.

Gustafson L, Brun A. (1997): Fokal beginnende Hirnatorphie, "Morbus Pick". In: Förstl H (ed): Lehrbuch der Gerontopsychiatrie. Stuttgart: Ferdinand Enke Verlag, pp. 278–290.

Gustafson L, Brun A, Ingvar DH (1977): Presenile dementia: Clinical symptoms, pathoana-tomical findings and cerebral blood flow. In Meyer JS, Lechner H, Reivich (eds): Cerebral Vascular Disease. Amsterdam: Excerpta Medica, pp 5–9.

Gustafson L, Nilsson L (1982): Differential diagnosis of presenile dementia on clinical grounds. Acta Psychiatr Scand 65:194–209.

Gustafson L, Risberg J (1993): Deceptions and delusions in Alzheimer's disease and frontal lobe dementia. In Katona C, Levy R (eds): Delusions and Hallucinations in Old Age. Gaskell, UK: Royal College of Psychiatrist, pp 216–225.

Hachinski VC, Iliff LD, Zilhka E, du Boulay GH, McAllister VL, Marshall J, Ross Russel RW, Symon L (1975): Cerebral blood flow in dementia. Arch Neurol 32:632–637.

The ICD-10 Classification of Mental and Behavioural Disorders. Clinical Descriptions and Diagnostic Guidelines (1992). Geneva: World Health Organization.

Johannesson G, Brun A, Gustafson L, Ingvar DH (1977): EEG in presenile dementia related to cerebral blood flow and autopsy findings. Acta Neurol Scand 56:89–103.

Johansson A, Gustafson L (1996): Psychiatric symptoms in patients with dementia treated in a psychogeriatric day hospital. Int Psychogeriatrics 8:645–658.

Johanson A, Gustafson L, Smith GJW, Risberg J, Hagberg B, Nilsson B (1990): Adaptation in different types of dementia and in normal elderly subjects. Dementia 1:95–101.

Johanson A, Hagberg B (1989): Psychometric characteristics in patients with frontal lobe degeneration of non-Alzheimer type. Arch Gerontol Geriatr 8:129–137.

Kertesz A, Hudson L, Mackenzie IRA, Munoz DG (1994): The pathology and nosology of primary progressive aphasia. Neurology 44:2066–2072.

Knopman DS, Mastri AR, Frey WH, Sung JH, Rustan T (1990): Dementia lacking distinctive histologic features. A common non-Alzheimer degenerative dementia. Neurology 40:251–256.

Lebert F, Pasquier F, Petit H (1995): Personality traits and frontal lobe dementia. Int J Geriatr Psychiatry 10:1046–1049.

Lhermitte F, Pillon B, Serdaru M (1986): Human autonomy and the frontal lobes. Part I: Imitation and utilization behaviour: A neuropsychological study of 75 patients. Ann Neurol 19:326–334.

Liu X, Brun A (1996): Regional and laminar synaptic pathology in frontal lobe degeneration of non-Alzheimer type. Int J Geriatr Psychiatry 2:47–55.

Lopez OL, Becker JT, De Kosky ST (1994): Dementia accompanying motor neuron disease. Dementia 5:42–47.

Luauté JP, Favel P, Rémy C, Sanabria E, Bidault E (1994): Troubles de l'humeur et démence de type frontal. Hypothèse d'un rapport pathologénique. L'Encéphale 20:27–36.

Ludolph AC, Langen KJ, Regard M, Herzog H, Kemper B, Kuwert T, Böttger IG, Feinendegen L (1993): Frontal lobe function in amyotrophic lateral sclerosis: A neuropsychologic and positron emission tomography study. Acta Neurol Scand 85:81–89.

Luria AR (1973): The Working Brain. London: Penguin Books.

Lynch T, Sano M, Marder KS, Bell KL, Foster NI, Defendini RF, Sima AAF, Keohande C, Nygaard TG, Fahn S, Mayeux R, Rowland LP, Wilhelmsen KC (1994): Clinical characteristics of a family with chromosome 17-linked disinhibition-dementia-parkinsonism-amyotrophy complex. Neurology 44:1878–1884.

Mallison R (1947): Zur Klinik der Pickschen Atrophie. Nervenarzt 6:247–256.

McKhann G, Drachman D, Folstein M, Katzman R, Price D, Stadlan EM (1984): Clinical diagnosis of Alzheimer's disease: Report of the NINCDS-ADRDA Work Group under the auspices of the Department of Health and Human Services Task Force on Alzheimer's Disease. Neurology 34:939–944.

Mesulam MM (1982): Slowly progressive aphasia without generalized dementia. Ann Neurol 11:592–598.

Miller BL, Chang L, Mena I, Boone K, Lesser IM (1993): Progressive right frontotemporal degeneration: Clinical, Neuropsychological and SPECT characteristics. Dementia 4:204–213.

Miller BL, Cummings JL, Villanueva-Meyer J, Boone K, Mehringer CM, Lesser IM, Mena I (1991): Frontal lobe degeneration: Clinical, neuropsychological and SPECT characteristics. Neurology 42:1374–1382.

Mitsuyama Y (1984): Presenile dementia with motor neuron disease in Japan: Clinico-pathological review of 26 cases. J Neurol Neurosurg Psychiatry 47:953–959.

Mitsuyama Y (1993): Presenile dementia with motoneuron disease. Dementia 4:137–142.

Morita K, Kaiya H, Ikeda T, Namba M (1987): Presenile dementia combined with amyotrophy. A review of 34 Japanese cases. Arch Gerontol Geriatr 6:263–277.

Neary D, Snowden JS, Mann DMA (1990): Frontal lobe dementia and motoneuron disease. J Neurol Neurosurg Psychiatry 53:23–32.

Neary D, Snowden JS, Mann DMA (1993): The clinical pathological correlates of lobar atrophy. Dementia 4:154–159.

Neary D, Snowden JS, Northen B, Goulding PJ (1988): Dementia of frontal lobe type. J Neurol Neurosurg Psychiatry 51:353–361.

Pachana NA, Brauer-Boone K, Miller BL, Cummings JL, Berman N (1996): Comparison of neuropsychological functioning in Alzheimer's disease and frontotemporal dementia. J Int Neuropsychol Soc 2:505–510.

Pasquier F, Lebert F, Grymonprez L, Petit H (1995): Verbal fluency in dementia of frontal lobe type and dementia of Alzheimer type. J Neurol Neurosurg Psychiatry 58:81–84.

Passant U, Gustafson L, Brun A (1993): Spectrum of frontal lobe dementia in a Swedish family. Dementia 4:160–162.

Passant U, Warkentin S, Karlson S, Nilsson K, Edvinsson L, Gustafson L (1996): Orthostatic hypotension in organic dementia: Relationship between blood pressure, cortical blood flow and symptoms. Clin Autonom Res 6:29–36.

Risberg J, Gustafson L (1988): Regional cerebral blood flow in psychiatric disorders. In Knezevic S, Maximilian VA, Mubrin Z, Prohovnik I, Wade J (eds): Handbook of Regional Cerebral Blood Flow. Hillsdale, NJ: Lawrence Erlbaum, pp 219–240.

Risberg J, Gustafson L (1997): Regional cerebral blood flow measurements in the clinical evaluation of demented patients. Dementia 8:92–97.

Rosén I, Gustafson L, Risberg J (1993): Multichannel EEG frequency analysis and somatosensory-evoked potentials in patients with different types of organic dementia. Dementia 4:43–49.

Seibyl PJ, Krystal JH, Goodman WK, Lawrence HP (1989): Obsessive-compulsive symptoms in a patient with a right frontal lobe lesion—response to lithium augmentation of tranylcypromine. Neuropsychiatry Neuropsychol Behav Neurol 1:295–299.

Sima AAF, Defendini RD, Keohande D, D'Amato C, Foster NL, Parchi P, Gambetti P, Lynch T, Wilhelmsen KC (1996): The neuropathology of chromosome 17-linked dementia. Ann Neurol 39:734–744.

Snowden JS, Neary D, Mann DMA (1996): Fronto-Temporal Lobar Degeneration: Fronto-Temporal Dementia, Progressive Aphasia, Semantic Dementia. New York: Churchill Livingstone.

Snowden JS, Neary D, Mann DMA, Goulding PJ, Testa HJ (1992): Progressive language disorder due to lobar atrophy. Ann Neurol 31:174–183.

Tonkonogy J, Barreira P (1989): Obsessive-compulsive disorder and caudate-frontal lesions. Neuropsychiatry Neuropsychol Behav Neurol 2:203–209.

Waldemar G, Bruhn P, Kristensen M, Johnsen A, Paulson OB, Lassen NA (1994): Heterogeneity of neocortical cerebral blood flow deficits in dementia of the Alzheimer type: A [^{99m}Tc]-d,1-HMPAO SPECT study. J Neurol Neurosurg Psychiatry 57:285–295.

Heutink P, Stevens M, Rizzu P, Bakker E, Kros JM, Tibben A, Niermeijer MF, van Duijn CM, Oostra BA, van Swieten JC (1997): Hereditary frontotemporal dementia is linked to chromosome 17q21-q22: a genetic and clinicopathological study of three Dutch families. Ann Neurol 41(2):150–159.

Verity A, Wechsler FV (1987): Progressive subcortical gliosis of Neumann: A clinicopathologic study of two cases with review. Arch Gerontol Geriatr 6:189–195.

Wilhelmsen K, Lynch T, Pavlou G, Higgins M, Nygaard T (1994): Localization of disinhibition-dementia-parkinsonism-amyotrophy complex to chromosome 17 q21–22. Am J Hum Genet 55:1159–1165.

Wilson DH, Chang AE (1974): Bilateral anterior cingulectomy for the relief of intractable pain (report of 28 patients). Confin Neurol 36:61–68.

CHAPTER 5

The Quantification of Behavior in Frontotemporal Dementia

ANDREW KERTESZ

Department of Clinical Neurological Sciences, St. Joseph's Health Centre, University of Western Ontario, London, Ontario N6A 4V2, Canada

INTRODUCTION

The function of the frontal lobe initially has been connected to language and intelligence for various reasons, not the least of which is the recognition of an evolutionary increase in size over other primates. Gall, Bouillaud and Broca all adopted the notion that increased frontal lobe size is associated with language as a uniquely human faculty. The extraordinary case of Phineas Gage, however, contributed to the change in thinking about frontal lobe function (Harlow, 1848, 1868). This case report described personality and behavioral changes in a previously conscientious workman who survived a penetrating injury when an explosion set a tamping iron through his maxilla and orbit, exiting in the mediodorsal frontal region. The description of his symptoms is worth reproducing here:

> "he is fitful, irreverent, indulging at times in the grossest profanity (which was not previously his custom), manifesting but little deference for his fellows, impatient of restraint or advice when it conflicts with his desires, at times pertinaciously obstinate, yet capricious and vacillating, devising many plans of future operation, which are no sooner arranged than they are abandoned in turn for others appearing more feasible. A child in his intellectual capacity and manifestations, he has the animal passions of a strong man. Previous to his injury, though untrained in the schools, he possessed a well-balanced mind, and was looked upon by those who knew him as a shrewd, smart business man, very energetic and persistent in executing all his plans of operation. In this regard, his mind was radically changed, so decidedly that his friends and acquaintances said he was 'no longer Gage'" (Harlow, p 339–340).

Subsequent cases contributed to the clinical pattern. Starr (1884) reported on 23 cases of frontal lobe lesions in which lack of self-control and inattention were the main deficits. A patient of Welt's (1888) with a penetrating injury to the orbitofrontal regions shown to be local-

Pick's Disease and Pick Complex, Edited by Andrew Kertesz and David G. Munoz
ISBN 0-471-17792-X ©1998 Wiley-Liss, Inc.

ized to the bilateral rectus gyrus and the right mesial inferior frontal gyrus became inappropriately jocular, aggressive, and malicious.

At the same time, animals with bilateral frontal lobe ablations were described as hyperactive, impulsive, and lacking affection and socialization (Ferrier, 1876; Goltz, 1892; Bianchi, 1895). Apathy and inattention were emphasized by Ferrier (1876). The function of the frontal lobes synthetizing emotive states with sensory motor input has been formulated by Bianchi: (1895):

> "The frontal lobes are the seat of coordination and fusion of the incoming and outgoing products of the several sensory and motor areas of the cortex . . . the frontal lobes would thus sum up into series the products of the sensorimotor regions, as well as the emotive states which accompany all the perceptions, the fusion of which constitutes what has been called the psychical tone of the individual. Removal of the frontal lobes does not so much interfere with the perceptions taken singly, as it does disaggregate the personality, and incapacitate for serializing and synthetizing groups of representations" (1895, p. 497–522).

This formulation of frontal lobe function has been replicated many times since, with several modern versions existing without reference to the original.

After World War I, investigators described frontal lobe injury particularly after gunshot wounds. The importance of character and personality changes produced by lesions of the frontal lobe was further elaborated by Feuchtwanger (1923). He distinguished the depressed type, in which the patient was apathetic and lacked concern. Others were psychopathic, antisocial, and hysteroid types. A third group was child-like and disinhibited. Kleist (1931, 1934) adopted a similar classification of frontal lobe injury. The apathetic type was slow, lethargic, and lacked initiative and spontaneity (abulia). This syndrome was associated with massive frontal lobe damage, although at times it was related to mesiofrontal involvement. The other type was characterized by restlessness, impulsivity, hyperkinesis, and explosiveness, and the lesion was usually orbitofrontal. Blumer and Benson's (1975) version of the same classification is "pseudodepressed" and "pseudopsychopathic."

Neurosurgical resections of frontal tumors and epileptogenic cortex provided further information concerning frontal lobe function. Many of the behavioral symptoms of frontal lobe disease come from this lesion material. Rylander (1939), describing frontal lobe resection in the patients of Olivecrona, the pioneering Swedish neurosurgeon, found lack of restraint, restlessness, and euphoria with orbitofrontal lesions. Ackerly and Benton (1948) described the primary sociopathy occurring in a young man who had congenital bilateral destruction of the frontal lobes and had grown up intellectually normal, but remained childish and lacking social appropriateness while retaining good verbal skills and an ingratiating, overly courteous manner toward adults. In this condition, tumors in the lateral and dorsolateral aspects of the frontal lobes are accompanied by focal epilepsy, head turning, grasping movements, and jackknifing of the body (Penfield and Jasper, 1954). At times, frontal lobe tumors present with pervasive disorganization of behavior, affective impairment, and cognitive changes resembling those of dementia (Strauss and Keschner, 1935; Hecaen, 1964). A patient with a frontal tumor became boastful, facetious, unexpectedly aggressive, nasty to his wife, impotent but constantly talking about sex, unable to plan daily activities, and unable to return to work. Despite this, he remained charming with strangers (Brickner, 1934).

Jacobsen (1936) described the chimpanzee "Becky," who often had "experimental neurosis," flying into a rage after failing to perform a task but becoming placid after a bilateral frontal lobotomy. Moniz (1936), inspired by these experiments, began to use lobotomy in humans to alleviate severe anxiety and psychosis, rendering them placid and sedate. After psychosurgery, however, inertia, lack of ambition, decreased consecutive thinking, indifference to others, and poor judgment were frequently seen (Freeman et al., 1942). Rylander (1948) eloquently described some of the patients who "lost their soul" after psychosurgery. "The deep feelings, the tenderness are gone. . . . She is shallow in some ways. . . . These patients can feel neither real happiness nor deep sorrow. . . . Something has died within them. . . ." Some patients lose ambition and efficiency after lobotomy. One dangerous and suicidal patient was hired as a cook by Dr. Rylander after a lobotomy. Originally she was clever, but she had difficulty using new recipes and began making ridiculous mistakes. She had difficulty in seeing the possibility of more than one solution to a problem. Going out to buy food, she might disappear for half a day, forgetting time and duties. Patients after lobotomy, leukotomy, and topectomy, as the various operations were called, had variable amounts of postoperative investigation. The results depended more on the premorbid disease and personality than on the extent and variety of the psychosurgery (Stuss and Benson, 1983a). The severe abulia and apathetic, uninterested behavior in some of these patients and the disinhibition in others deprived psychosurgery of its legitimacy.

The evolution of concepts regarding frontal lobe function in the 1960s and 1970s included the elaboration of frontal connections to the limbic lobe (Livingston, 1969; Nauta, 1971, 1973). Luria (1966, 1973) emphasized the importance of frontothalamic connections in selective arousal and gating of information. The frontal lobes were assigned the functions of planning, initiating, monitoring, and executing behavior. Nauta (1971) concluded that the prefrontal cortex is the ultimate target of sensory cascades and plays the role of synthesizing inner or visceral sensations, as well as external sensory domains. The bidirectional association of limbic and reticular activity with frontal structures provides a major role in arousal, motivation, and affect. Certain experimental paradigms such as response inhibition, delayed responses, delayed alternation, and short-term memory were associated with various prefrontal regions (Jacobsen, 1936; Mishkin, 1964). Frontal lobes were assigned functions such as short-term memory, polymodal integration, and temporal structuring of behavior (Goldman-Rakic, 1987; Fuster, 1989). The functional units of the dorsal convexity, orbitofrontal cortex, mesial prefrontal cortex, and their subcortical connections have been elaborated in animals using elegant tracer and metabolic studies (Friedman et al., 1990). Efforts have been made to find human equivalents of these functional systems through lesion studies, as well as through more recent functional activation (Cummings, 1993).

The attribution of personality and character changes to any anatomical location in the frontal lobe is complicated by variability in the size of the lesion, the type of pathology, and the extent of cortical versus subcortical involvement, in addition to the time course of the disease and the extent of damage to neighboring areas particularly to the anterior temporal lobe in head trauma and in frontotemporal degeneration. The definition of each frontal lobe syndrome varies greatly according to the complexity of the above-mentioned variables. As a result, there is no single frontal behavior disorder that recurs in all instances or could be considered the sine qua non of frontal lobe disease. Nevertheless, a great deal of interest in the quantification of impaired frontal function has resulted in many tests, especially in cognitive domains. In addition to briefly reviewing these test, this chapter emphasizes the quantification of personality alteration and behavior in frontal lobe dementia (FLD) or as it more recently renamed, frontotemporal dementia (FTD).

GENERAL INTELLIGENCE

An often noted paradox in testing frontal lobe-damaged patients is the relative preservation of intelligence, as measured by general intelligence tests (Feuchtwanger, 1923; Hebb, 1939). This was confirmed by testing several subsequent series of head-injured patients and in epilepsy surgery (Milner, 1964; Teuber, 1964; Black, 1976). The Columbia-Greystone studies (Mettler, 1949) also concluded that circumscribed surgical lesions do not decrease the intellectual function in lobectomy. One study suggested that after leukotomy, larger lesions were associated with higher IQ. The improved cognitive performance was attributed to recovery from psychotic symptoms in schizophrenics after psychosurgery (Stuss and Benson, 1983a). However, some studies showed a demonstrable loss with upper frontal lobe surgery involving sustained attention and problem-solving (Hamlin, 1970). Others also detected some deficits in intelligence with dorsolateral lesions, especially vocabulary, digit span, picture arrangements, and block design (Malmo, 1948; McFie and Thompson, 1972; Janowksy et al., 1989). These subtests may be influenced by difficulties in initiation and executive function.

MENTAL FLEXIBILITY, ABSTRACTION, AND CATEGORIZATION

In contrast to the relatively preserved visuospatial and verbal functions on intelligence tests, when abstraction, concept formation, and category shifting are tested, they are often found to be disturbed by frontal lesions. *The Wisconsin Card Sorting Test* (Grant and Berg, 1948) is one of the most commonly used tests to measure frontal lobe damage. This is a difficult test for many brain-damaged patients, and although high in sensitivity, it is low in specificity since it can be impaired from lesion locations other than the frontal lobes. Patients with dorsolateral frontal lobe resection displayed verbal sorting strategies but did not carry them out. Perseveration occurred equally with right- and left-sided lesions. Subsequently, this was also found to be the case in leukotomy patients and in those with lesions with medial frontal involvement (Stuss et al., 1981; Drewe, 1984). Perceptual shifting was shown to be impaired in other experiments, such as those involving Necker cube or Rubin's vase (Yacorzynski and Davis, 1945; Cohen, 1959; Miller, 1992). Similar results were found with the *Stroop Test,* which measures the ability to inhibit interference from a conflict of perceptual and verbal categories (Perret, 1974). Perseveration is the deficit side of mental flexibility or the ability to shift, and it is a common clinical and experimental symptom of frontal damage. It is defined as any situation in which elements of previous tasks or behaviors fuse or interfere with subsequent behavior, or when behavior cannot be terminated (Luria, 1966). Luria's go–no-go test is designed to test perseveration and response inhibition. Recurrent perseveration seems characteristic of patients with frontal lobe damage Vilkki (1989). Continuous perseveration, which is an inappropriate prolongation or repetition of behavior without interruption, is common in patients with basal ganglia damage (Sandson and Albert, 1984). Many patients with frontal lobe lesions have difficulty with abstract concepts and interpret everything literally. Objects, experiences, and whatever is said to them are taken at face value. This loss of abstract attitude is common with frontal lobe damage, although it appears with other lesions as well (Goldstein, 1944).

EXECUTIVE CONTROL, PLANNING, JUDGMENT, AND SELECTIVITY

Programming, regulation, and verification of activity were considered important frontal lobe functions (Luria, 1973). However, measuring these functions turned out to be difficult. Planning and organizing of activities can be tested with maze learning tests or shopping lists and itineraries to be carried out in an optimal sequence. Impulsivity, perseveration, and failure to respond to feedback are common findings in these tests in patients with frontal lobe excisions (Milner, 1964). A popularized problem-solving task is the Tower of Hanoi modified as the *Tow-*

er of London (Shallice, 1982). This high-level puzzle is suitable only for mildly affected patients. A model of executive function based on information processing principles was developed by Norman and Shallice (1986). This formulation suggested that the selection of actions triggered by the perceptual system is regulated by a set of inhibitory mechanisms, called *contention scheduling,* and by another set modulating the activation levels of the action schemata, called the *supervisory system.* Norman and Shallice postulated that the supervisory system involves planning, decision making, error correction, and shifting to novel sequences of actions. They explained difficulty with attention, inability to concentrate, and responding to irrelevant stimuli in the environment on the basis of damage to the supervisory system.

It is often said that patients with frontal lobe lesions lack judgment. This may be manifested in impulsive shopping, injudicious use of money, and errors in driving. Cognitive judgment was quantitated by Shallice and Evans (1978) and Smith and Milner (1984). Patients with frontal lesions had bizarre estimations of amounts, distances, and durations. Selectivity of action is another aspect of judgment, and it requires the appropriate inhibition of distracting stimuli. One clinical manifestation of this is inappropriate utilization behavior described by Lhermitte (1983). Patients with frontal lobe lesions utilized objects placed in their hands or in front of them despite instructions to the contrary. Imitation behavior occurs when the patient, without instructions, imitates the examiner's manners and gestures (echopraxia). Severe frontal lobe-damaged patients are often observed to explore compulsively and touch everything in their environment (hypermetamorphosis). In severe cases, there is an association with a grasp reflex. The combination of these behaviors is also called *environmental dependency,* usually reflecting extensive frontal damage. The utilization phenomenon has been explained as a failure of the supervisory system to provide inhibition and selectivity (Shallice et al., 1989). This phenomenon is akin to the alien hand syndrome, a disinhibited levitation or unilateral inability to use the arm appropriately in the absence of paralysis, at times seen in association with corticobasal degeneration. Impairment of initiating movement with the lower extremity results in gait apraxia or the so-called magnetic gait, in which the feet appear to be sticking to the ground (Denny-Brown, 1958).

ATTENTION AND DISTRACTIBILITY

Impaired attention and distractibility are prominent in frontal lobe symptomatology (Rylander, 1939; Goldstein, 1944; Hecaen, 1964). Luria and Homskaya (1964) found that frontal lobe-damaged patients could not maintain the orienting reflex. Motor impersistence was common in patients with right frontal lesions (Kertesz et al., 1985). Clinical tests of attention include the mental control test of the *Wechsler Adult Intelligence Scale* (*WAIS*), serial 7 subtraction, digit span forward and backward, the attention concentration index of the *Wechsler Memory Scale-Revised* (*WMS-R*), the *Trail-Making Test,* and the *Stroop Test.* A rather demanding sustained-attention task involving working memory and calculation is the *paced auditory serial addition task* (*PASAT*) (Gronwall, 1977). This is suitable only to detect subtle impairment in previously high-level individuals.

Electroencephalography and event-related potentials were also used to measure attention and distractibility. Sustained attention requires the suppression of irrelevant events in the environment. Focused sustained auditory attention generates negative evoked responses at 50 msec (*processing negativity*). Right frontal damage appears to interfere with this physiological activity. The P30 components of auditory evoked responses are disinhibited by prefrontal damage (Knight et al., 1989). P300 potentials, on the other hand, are generated by phasic attention capacity, which is also impaired by prefrontal lesions (Knight, 1990).

MEMORY: SHORT-TERM, WORKING, AND PROSPECTIVE

Memory functions in frontal lobe damage have been extensively studied. There is a consensus that recent and remote memory and learning are generally spared (Hecaen and Albert, 1978). On the other hand, short-term memory or working memory that integrates perceptual input and organizes motor and cognitive sequences is characteristically affected (Baddeley, 1986; Goldman-Rakic, 1987). Fuster (1985) postulated that the frontal lobe integrate information from recent past into behavior in the present and the near future. Short-term memory and preparatory motor circuits play essential roles in this integrated function and are considered to be represented in the dorsolateral prefrontal cortex, based on delayed response and delayed alternation tasks originating from animal experiments (Fulton and Jacobsen, 1935). Some of these experiments were carried out in patients with frontal lobe lesions, Huntington's chorea, and Korsakoff's disease (Freedman and Oscar-Berman, 1986). Visuospatial and attentional factors appear to be critical for delayed response, and short-term memory and response inhibition are essential for delayed alternation performance (Freedman and Oscar-Berman, 1986). In tasks with word list learning, patients with frontal lobe lesions have a disproportionately greater deficit in *recalling words* with relatively *preserved recognition memory*. This suggests that the frontal lobes are more important in retrieval than in encoding. Patients with frontal lobe deficits also had difficulty judging the recency of items presented (Milner, 1971). A similar deficit occurs in sequencing of words or objects (Shimamura et al., 1990). This has also been called *impairment of memory for temporal order.* Such an impairment was demonstrated even when the memory for the items remained intact. A similar deficit for the source of information and for the feeling of knowing something, or metamemory, was also found (Janowsky et al., 1989).

Prospective memory is also used to describe deficits in planning and organization, which may be considerable in frontal lobe patients without any impairment in declarative memory or learning. This is considered part of the *dysexecutive syndrome* (Braddeley and Wilson, 1988). Frontal lobe memory deficit has also been described as "forgetting to remember" due to the inability to follow external cues and rules, inattention, difficulty in sequencing, and susceptibility to distraction and interference (Hecaen and Albert, 1978).

INITIATION, DRIVE, AND EMOTIONS

Initiation of activity and drive are important frontal lobe functions. Apathy and lack of drive (abulia) are well-known features of frontal lobe disease. Some of these patients can talk about plans and projects, but they are unable to transform their words into action (Luria, 1973). They have to be reminded to carry out routine activities (aspontaneity). Motor impersistence can be observed during examination, as the patients will not sustain their gaze or hold the position of their limbs even for the brief periods required (Kertesz et al., 1985). In more severe cases, pathological inertia, unresponsiveness, or even mutism appears. The severe deficit may consist of difficulty initiating movements, completing motor sequences, or inhibiting inappropriate responses. The difficulty initiating action may also be called *akinesia* or *hypokinesia;* it may be present in the limbs and the eyes, and it may be unilateral (Bianchi, 1895; Heilman et al., 1985; Meador et al., 1986). More severe forms of frontal injury may result in akinetic mutism. In this condition there is very little spontaneous movement, and although patients seem alert and the eyes usually are open, they do not respond, speak, or display any emotion. They are usually incontinent and will eat and drink only if fed.

The supplementary motor area (SMA) in the parasagittal medial aspects of the frontal lobes has an important function in initiating movements of any kind. Cytoarchitectonically, this area represents a paralimbic extension from the adjacent limbic cortex such as the cingulate gyrus and has extensive reciprocal connections with it (Sanides, 1970; Damasio and Van Hoesen, 1983). It is also connected to the striatum via the subcallosal fasciculus (Yakovlev and Locke, 1961). Goldberg (1985) defined the role of the SMA in the selection and execution of specific movement sequences from the internal limbic drive. This is also defined as the external realization of intention brought about by projecting limbic outflow to motor executive regions via the SMA.

LANGUAGE

Lesions of the posterior portion of the third frontal convolution (F3) are well known to cause nonfluent aphasia, originally described by Broca. This area includes the foot of the premotor cortex, Brodmann areas 44 and 45. Persisting Broca's aphasia is usually seen with extension to the subcortical and parietal regions (Mohr et al., 1978; Kertesz, 1979). Patients with only Broca's area involved usually have a transient disturbance of articulation and speech output, with preserved comprehension. However, after recovery they may have a residual word fluency deficit and some persisting verbal apraxia. Subcortical connection and striatal damage can also produce a similar type of disturbance characterized by verbal apraxia and decreased fluency (Naeser, 1982; Damasio et al., 1982). Agrammatism is usually seen in larger, more persistent lesions, but syntactic processing is linked to short-term memory and posterior frontal lobe function (Nadeu, 1988). The articulatory network of language output usually includes a network of Broca's area, striatum, anterior insula region, and inferior central rolandic region (Kertesz, 1997).

When the dominant SMA is affected, language initiation is impaired. The importance of the SMA for speech on the left side was recognized by Penfield and Roberts (1959), who called in the *supplementary speech area.* Speech arrest can occur from stimulation in this region as frequently as from stimulation of the parasylvian language area. At times, even repetitive involuntary vocalization can be obtained from stimulation of this area (Brickner, 1940; Erickson and Woolsey, 1951). Epileptogenic tumors in the left SMA also produce vocalization and speech arrest during seizures (Sweet, 1951; Arseni and Botez, 1961). Reduction of spontaneous speech in patients with left frontal lobectomy for epilepsy has been reported (Milner, 1964). Tests of word fluency have been used to quantitate this phenomenon. The most consistent impairment is produced by left-sided frontal lesions, in particular from dorsolateral resection. Frontal lobe lesions impair letter fluency predominantly (the patient is asked to find words beginning with a certain letter), rather than in semantic categories (the patient is asked to generate the names of animals or tools) (Milner, 1964). Word fluency tasks may show impairment even when conversational speech is relatively fluent. The right hemisphere equivalent of the word fluency paradigms is design fluency, or the production of novel drawings (Jones-Gotman and Milner, 1977).

The syndrome of transcortical motor aphasia (TMA) is most often produced by lesions of the SMA on the left side (Goldstein, 1948; Arseni and Botez, 1961; Kornyey, 1975; Rubens, 1975). This syndrome is characterized by reduced fluency but relatively normal repetition and comprehension. A variable naming deficit is common, although naming appears relatively preserved and the written output is similar to the oral one. White matter lesions anterior and superior to Broca's area and dorsolateral convexity lesions have also produced various degrees of TMA (Freedman et al., 1984).

PERSONALITY, CHARACTER, AND SOCIAL CONTROL

Personality changes are most common with orbitofrontal damage. The example of Phineas Gage set the tone for many similar descriptions. Excessive and inappropriate facetiousness was described as *witzelsucht* by Oppenheim (1890). A similar term is *moria,* which is applied to the childish, jocular, euphoric behavior observed in frontal lobe patients. This hypomanic positive behavior, along with impulsiveness and fluctuating restlessness, appears resistant to correction by verbal means and may require sedation. Many patient who were more outspoken, less inhibited, and more irritable on some occasions had less initiative or interest and awareness at other times, alternating in a paradoxical fashion. Ruptured anterior communicating aneurysms, orbitofrontal tumors, and inferior frontal lobe infarction often produce this syndrome (Hunter et al., 1968; Logue et al., 1968; Bogousslavsky and Regli, 1990). Lishman (1968) summarized the behavioral symptoms after frontal damage including lack of judgment, reliability, and foresight, facetiousness, childish behavior, disinhibition, and euphoria.

Social competence is often somewhat impaired in frontal lobe disease, leading to a spectacular failure in all human relationships. A more recent case report of a frontal lobe meningioma describes the personality changes of unreliability, inability to complete work, tardiness, lack of productivity, and impairment of social behavior (Eslinger and Damasio, 1985). Damasio et al., (1990) found that subjects with bilateral ventromedial frontal lobe lesions had abnormal autonomic responses to socially meaningful stimuli, suggesting that such stimuli fail to activate somatic states previously associated with specific social situations marking the outcome of responses as appropriate or not. Ventromedial frontal lobe lesions caused inability to initiate, organize, and carry out normal activities (Anderson et al., 1992). These patients had poor decision making, financial mistakes, breakup of relationships, perseverative activities, and decreased spontaneity. They were also described as dependent and excessively talkative.

Emotional changes, particularly decreased emotional responsiveness or lability of emotions, in FLD are at times prominent. Motivation and emotions are highly correlated as orbitomedial and cingulate connections with the limbic lobe are affected. Frontal deficits are often characterized by severely impaired drive and apathy, as well as emotional indifference. As described above in the Introduction, emotional flatness is difficult to quantitate but it is often eloquently expressed in subjective narratives.

Quantitation of emotional changes and behavior after psychosurgery was attempted with the thematic appreciation test and matching facial expressions to emotional situations (Stuss and Benson, 1983b). The authors found a dissociation of perceptual and cognitive awareness in the emotional situations test. They also described disinhibition and dissociation between verbalization and the observed response. The behavior was influenced by premorbid illness and the localization, as well as by the extent of the frontal leukotomies on the computed tomography (CT) scan. The thematic appreciation test was insensitive to the effects of prefrontal leukotomy.

Some degree of lateralization of mood changes has been observed with localized brain damage. Right orbitofrontal lesions were more prone to result in anxiety and depression, while left dorsofrontal lesions were more prone to elicit abnormally increased anger and hostility. Orbitofrontal damage resulted in a chronic state of anxiety and a tendency toward obsessive/compulsive behavior. On the other hand, dorsofrontal patients appeared more introverted, apathetic, and depressed than controls. Starkstein and Robinson (1991) reported an increased incidence of depression with left frontal lesions, but more recently the lateralization of emotional deficits has been questioned.

FRONTAL LOBE DEMENTIA AND PICK'S DISEASE

Frontal lobe dementia (FLD), characterized by progressive personality change apathy, blunting of emotions, lack of insight, excessive eating, and disinhibition, has been described as a separate entity (Neary et al., 1986; Brun, 1987; Gustafson, 1987). Frontal lobe atrophy and progressive personality changes have been well-known features of Pick's disease (PiD) (Pick, 1904, 1906; Schneider, 1927; Löwenberg, 1935; Ferraro and Jervis, 1936; Constantinidis et al., 1974; Knopman et al., 1990). The definition of FLD consists of a mixture of clinical imaging and pathological criteria. The Lund and Manchester Groups (1994) achieved a consensus concerning the main features of what they began to call *frontotemporal dementia* (*FTD*). The core diagnostic features of FTD were loss of personal hygiene and social awareness, disinhibition, mental rigidity, hyperorality, perseveration, distractibility, utilization behavior, loss of insight, indifference, remoteness, inertia, and aspontaneity. Reduction of speech output, and finally mutism were considered common (see also Chapters by Miller, and Neary, Snowden and Mann in this volume).

COGNITIVE ASSESSMENT IN FLD

Neuropsychological test results in FLD patients were variable (Gustafson, 1987; Neary et al., 1986, 1988; Miller, et al., 1991), but frontal lobe functions generally showed poor performance, although there are important exceptions to this rule (Neary et al., 1986, 1988; Brun, 1987; Gustafson, 1987; Miller et al., 1991). We have studied 12 patients with FLD; their performance on neuropsychological tests was highly variable (Kertesz et al., unpublished). The most common frontal lobe deficits were perseveration on the Wisconsin Card Sorting Task, impaired word fluency, trail making, and picture arrangement from the WAIS-R. Some patients reached floor effect, while others were uncooperative and testing was incomplete. Three patients, however, had normal or near-normal scores on the frontal lobe function test despite a severe behavioral disturbance. These scores do not indicate some of the performance characteristics of the patients, which included perseveration, impersistence, and impulsive responses.

While memory loss and spatial deficit were characteristic of AD, they were relatively infrequent or mild in FLD. Many of these studies emphasized the manner of performance, in addition to the abnormal scores on the so-called frontal lobe tests. Frontal lobe patients are often impulsive, cursory, or amotivational, and answer only laconically and at times echolalically. Performance is often inconsistent and patchy. Recognition memory appears better than recall, and the patient tends to benefit from multiple-choice alternatives. Orientation and episodic memory are relatively well preserved. The relatives' complaint of forgetfulness is more like "forgetting to remember," which may not manifest itself during formal testing. There may be impaired tests scores on immediate and delayed recall of a story, yet the patient can recall personally relevant events, which is quite out of keeping with reduced test scores. This paradox contributes to the degree of variability in memory testing in FLD patients. Much of the variability depends on the stage of the illness; therefore, many of the patients, even in a single series, are not comparable.

Although drawings in FLD patients may be impoverished due to amotivational performance, visuospatial function is generally intact. The patients may be perseverative in drawing. At times copying can be compulsively faithful to detail. Visuospatial tasks requiring executive function, such as trail making, are impaired at an early stage, but block design and Raven's Coloured Progressive Matrices may be preserved. At times, echopraxia and utilization behavior are observed during neuropsychological testing.

Language was only mildly affected in early cases, although some logopenia and anomia were recorded in most of the patients. Performance on the Western Aphasia Battery (WAB) was sensitive to measure early anomic and fluency disturbances. Verbal fluency measures, especially word generation beginning with the same letter, were sensitive but intact in 20% of the cases. The Mini-Mental Status Examination, which is heavily weighted for language, was often normal in early cases. Altogether, the wide variability and relative insensitivity of neuropsychological testing leave a gap in the diagnostic definition of FLD. Behavioral quantitation may serve to fulfill this gap.

BEHAVIORAL QUANTITATION IN FRONTAL LOBE DEMENTIA

Quantitation of behavior has been attempted by Gustafson and Nielson (1982) in order to separate PiD from AD. The Manchester Group also assessed the symptoms of FLD in a retrospective study to correlate the clinical diagnosis with autopsy findings. Their results distinguished FLD and AD with a high degree of success (Barber et al., 1995). Lopez et al. (1996) found more symptoms of major depression, agitation, irritability, lability of mood, disinhibition, inertia, and social withdrawal in FTD patients, in contrast to AD patients, who displayed more signs of delusional psychosis. Gregory and Hodges (1996) reviewed the psychiatric symptomatology in FTD patients who had at least five of the core diagnostic features. Only 50% of the patients were diagnosed as having FTD at presentation, and a third received an initial psychiatric diagnosis such as schizophrenia, psychosis, depression with obsessive/compulsive features, alcohol dependency, and psychogenic memory impairment. A symptom inventory under the categories of self-monitoring, discontrol, self-neglect, self-centred behavior, and affective disorders was used by Lebert (1996) to differentiate frontotemporal dementia from Alzheimer's disease and vascular dementia. Miller et al. (1997) retrospectively evaluated the presence or absence of the Lund/Manchester items in 30 patients with FTD. The patients were selected on the basis of single photon emission computed tomography (SPECT) scans. Discriminant function showed a loss of hygiene, hyperorality, stereotypic and perseverative behavior, progressive reduction of speech and preserved spatial orientation differentiated FTD and AD subjects.

We constructed a 24-item frontal behavioral inventory (FBI), to target the most specific behaviors for optimum diagnostic accuracy for FLD to be used at the initial interview or for retrospective diagnosis (Kertesz et al., 1997). These items were selected from the core diagnostic features of the Lund/Manchester criteria and the most common symptoms in our FLD patients (Table 5.1). The inventory was designed as a series of structured questions scripted so that both the normal and abnormal negative aspects of the behaviors were included, giving the caregiver a choice (Table 5.2). If the caregiver seemed to hesitate or did not understand, the question was rephrased. Each item was scored on a scale of 4: 0 = none, 1 = mild or occasional, 2 = moderate, 3 = severe or most of the time.

The items were grouped as negative behaviors such as apathy, aspontaneity, indifference, inflexibility, concreteness, personal neglect, distractibility, inattention, loss of insight, logopenia, verbal apraxia, and alien hand. The last three items were included to capture specific motor and speech behaviors that may be associated with FLD. The second group of behaviors contained items of disinhibition such as perseveration, irritability, jocularity, irresponsibility, inappropriateness, impulsivity, euphoric restlessness, aggression, hyperorality, hypersexuality, utilization behavior, and incontinence. Since the time of the pilot study, modifications and additions have included replacing disinhibition because it referred to too many similar behaviors. The last five items represented behaviors usually seen at later stages of severe FLD. They are very disturbing to the families, and they are the most sensitive to discuss.

In a pilot study, the test was administered to 12 clinically diagnosed FLD patients, 16 patients with AD selected for early stages of illness at an outpatient clinic, and 11 patients with

TABLE 5.1   The Frequency of Symptoms in 12 Patients on History

Lack of insight	83%	Hyperorality	33%
Inappropiate remarks	75%	Irritability, impatience	33%
Perseveration	75%	Restlessness	33%
Logopenia, anomia	75%	Erratic or reckless driving[3]	33%
Personal neglect	66%	Argumentativeness	25%
Apathy	58%	Impulsiveness	25%
Forgetfulness[1]	58%	Incontinence	25%
Inattention, distractibility	58%	Aspontaneity	17%
Indifference (emotional flatness)	58%	Excessive touching	17%
Disorganization, inability to plan	50%	Hypersexuality	17%
Social withdrawal[2]	50%	Jocularity ("moria")	17%
Financial errors[3]	42%	Kleptomania	17%
Mental rigidity, concreteness	42%	Childishness	8%
Poor judgment	42%	Emotional lability	8%
Rambling[1]	42%	Paranoia	8%
Aggression	33%	Echolalia	8%

[1]Eliminated because of lack of specificity.
[2]Eliminated because of overlap with apathy.
[3]Overlap with poor judgment or impulsivity.

depressive dementia diagnosed by psychiatric assessment and depression inventories. AD patients met NINCDS-ADRD criteria. The severity of the dementia was defined by the scores on the Mattis Dementia Rating Scale (MDRS), and the groups were matched on this criterion. FLD patients were selected because of the striking behavior presentation, although at the later stages of the illness several of them developed a progressive logopenic disturbance, and one had typical motor neuron disease (MND) as well (see Chapter 19). Neuroimaging confirmed the presence of frontal lobe atrophy in 10/12 patients. Three patients had autopsy confirmation of Pick variant pathology, one with the corticobasal type and two with ubiquitin tau negative inclusions and clinical evidence of MND. A typical case description follows:

This 65-year-old man began to have stereotypic, compulsive movements of slapping his hands and repetitively banging walls. He cleared his throat and frequently paced back and forth. He began to make out-of-character remarks, wondering aloud how his daughter and son-in-law were having sex, remarking on a couple of birds chasing each other as having sex (he had formerly been shy and reserved). Sometimes he said things that were completely irrelevant to the questions asked. For example, someone would ask if he would like to go to the Dairy Queen and he would say, "No, I can't dance." He became easily distractible, and he would leave the stove burners on. He impulsively bought $2,000 worth of unneeded windows on phone solicitation. Inappropriately he would grab a stranger and start walking with them, or would make remarks about somebody having nice legs. He was uncharacteristically aggressive with his dog, throwing things at him, and he laughed without reason on several occasions. He retained good motor coordination, continuing to play tennis and to cross-county ski in the winter.

The initial diagnosis was an obsessive-compulsive disorder. Later he would not get out of bed, or properly eat or shave. He became less talkative than previously, and repeated questions in an echolalic fashion. He would eat a whole tub of ice cream for breakfast or a whole handful of candy at once. Sometimes he would put so much food in his mouth that he began to choke. He became incontinent or would come out of the bathroom with his pants still down. He required almost continuous supervision and care. Despite the symptoms, his memory remained reasonably good. He

TABLE 5.2   Frontal Behavioral Inventory (FBI)

Explain to the caregiver that you are looking for a change in behavior and personality. Ask the caregiver these questions in the absence of the patient. Elaborate if necessary. At the end of each question, ask about the extent of the behavioral change, and then score it according to the following: 0 = none, 1 = mild, occasional, 2 = moderate, 3 = severe, most of the time.

1. *Apathy*: Has s/he lost interest in friends or daily activities? _____
2. *Aspontaneity*: Does s/he start things on his/her own, or does s/he have to be asked? _____
3. *Indifference, Emotional Flatness*: Does s/he respond to occasions of joy or sadness as much as ever, of has s/he lost emotional responsiveness? _____
4. *Inflexibility*: Can s/he change his/her mind with reason or does s/he appear stubborn or rigid in thinking lately? _____
5. *Concreteness*: Does s/he interpret what is being said appropriately or does s/he choose only the concrete meanings of what is being said? _____
6. *Personal Neglect*: Does s/he take as much care of his/her personal hygiene and appearance as usual? _____
7. *Disorganization*: Can s/he plan and organize complex activiy or is s/he easily distractible, impersistent, or unable to complete a job? _____
8. *Inattention*: Does s/he pay attention to what is going on or does s/he seem to lose track or not follow at all? _____
9. *Loss of Insight*: Is s/he aware of any problems or changes, or does s/he seem unaware of them or deny them when discussed? _____
10. *Logopenia*: Is s/he as talkative as before or has the amount of speech significantly decreased? _____
11. *Verbal Apraxia*: Has s/he been talking clearly or has s/he been making errors in speech? Is there slurring or hesitation? _____
12. *Perseveration*: Does s/he repeat or perseverate actions or remarks? _____
13. *Irritability*: Has s/he been irritable or short-tempered, or is s/he reacting to stress or frustration as s/he always had? _____
14. *Excessive Jocularity*: Has s/he been making jokes excessively or offensively or at the wrong time? _____
15. *Poor Judgment*: Has s/he been using good judgment in decisions or in driving, or has s/he acted irresponsibily, neglectfully, or in poor judgment? _____
16. *Inappropriateness*: Has s/he kept social rules or has s/he said or done things outside of what is acceptable? Has s/he been rude or childish? _____
17. *Impulsivity*: Has s/he acted or spoken without thinking about the consequences, on the spur of the moment? _____
18. *Restlessness*: Has s/he been restless or hyperactive, or is the activity level normal? _____
19. *Aggression*: Has s/he shown aggression, or shouted at anyone or hurt them physically? _____
20. *Hyperorality*: Has s/he been drinking more than usual, eating excessively anything in sight, or even putting objects in his/her mouth? _____
21. *Hypersexuality*: Has his/her sexual behavior been unusual or excessive? _____
22. *Utilization Behavior*: Does s/he seem to need to touch, feel, examine, or pick up objects within reach and sight? _____
23. *Incontinence*: Has s/he wet or soiled him/herself (excluding physical illness, such as urinary infection or immobility)? _____
24. *Alien Hand*: Does s/he have any problem using a hand, and does it interfere with the other hand (excluding arthritis, trauma, paralysis, etc.)? _____

Total Score: _____

could recall what people were talking about, who was there, what people said, or what he heard in the news.

His wife committed suicide by taking an overdose of antidepressants, but when he learned of this he expressed no reaction. He was hospitalized a week later. Because of restlessness, pacing, and repetitive noisiness, he was given sedation, but this made him very sleepy. He was transferred to a psychiatric hospital, where a course of electroshock treatment initially seemed to reduce some of his behavioral disturbance. His urinary incontinence stopped and he appeared more aware of his surroundings, but again he declined despite another electroshock treatment. Because of recurrent agitation, Risperidone was started.

On examination two years after the onset, he appeared to be healthy but restless. He walked out of the office several times. He appeared laconic and echolalic, speaking in short sentences. He could recall information about past and even current events, but his comments were superficial, impulsive, and socially inappropriate. Formal neuropsychological testing was difficult because of his restlessness and inability to maintain attention. He gave impulsive answers to questions of orientation but selected the right date from a choice. He wrote full sentences, but they had no relationship to what was asked of him. He wandered off topic during conversations and had difficulty giving a full description of a picture. He did well on simpler comprehension tasks, although he experienced mild difficulty with multicomponent commands. His word fluency was low at 4 (normals = 20 or more) animals per minute. He was unable to imitate double alternating hand movements. He scored below the normal cutoff on tests of attention, initiation, perseveration, conceptualization, and memory of the Mattis Dementia Rating Scale (MDRS). His FBI score was 53. Magnetic resonance imaging (MRI) showed remarkable demarcated frontal lobe atrophy more on the right side.

The results of the pilot study indicated significantly higher FBI scores in the frontal group compared with the two control groups on the Analysis of Variance (ANOVA). No significant difference was found between patients with AD and depressive dementia (DD). The AD patients were older than the frontal and DD patients. Except for one, all FLD patients were in the presenile age group (under 65) at the onset of their illness. Analysis of the mean scores of each item indicated the frequency and severity of abnormal behaviors in all three groups (Figure 5.1). Loss of insight, personal neglect, and inflexibility were the most frequent negative behaviors. Perseveration and inappropriate remarks were the most common disinhibition phenomena.

FBI scores discriminated reliably between the FLD and control groups, with little overlap between them (Figure 5.2). This suggested cutoff points to operationalize the behavioral diagnosis of FLD. A sensitive, practical cutoff point is 27, including all FLD scores. There was only one false positive among the patients with DD. These patients could be identified by the vegetative symptoms of depression and positive depression inventories (Beck et al., 1961). All AD patients and most DD patients scored below 24. These cutoff points may serve as FBI criteria in grouping patients behaviorally for future studies.

There are numerous existing behavioral inventories that serve the more general purpose of exploring abnormal behavior in geriatric, psychiatric, or generally demented populations (Shader et al., 1974; Hersch et al., 1978; Schwartz, 1983; Reisberg et al., 1987; Niederehe, 1988; Mungas et al., 1989; Baumgarten et al., 1990; Drachman et al., 1992, Cummings et al., 1994). Geriatric scales often combine cognition behavior and activities of daily living, measuring the global extent of decline, but they do not discriminate specific behavior syndromes. The psychiatric behavioral scales also dilute the few frontal behaviors explored with symptoms of other psychiatric illness. Direct behavioral assessment of FLD patients uses items to detect motor or cognitive perseveration, verbal intrusions, disinhibition, loss of spontaneity, imita-

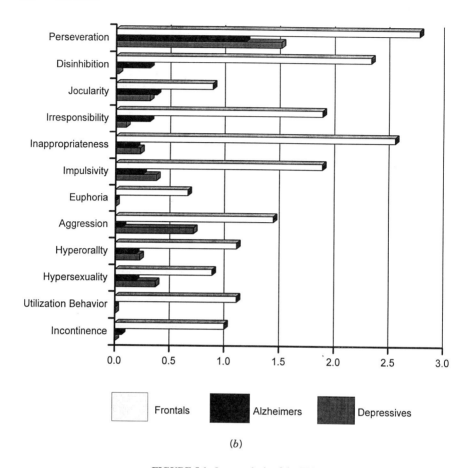

(b)

FIGURE 5.1. Item analysis of the FBI.

tion, and utilization behavior. Attempts have been made to formalize these frontal lobe signs in a "executive interview" (Royall et al., 1992). Such direct tests are often incorporated into a neurological examination and are complementary to the FBI.

Logopenia appears at later stages of FLD, at times associated with striking verbal and oro-facial apraxia. Hesitancy, dysprosody, substitutions and omissions of initial consonants, and at times stuttering behavior are seen. Since these occurred late in most of our FLD patients, the score on this item was the lowest on the FBI. When these symptoms appear as presenting features they are labeled *primary progressive aphasia (PPA)* (Mesulam, 1987) (see Chapter 6, this volume). A personality disorder often also appears in later stages of PPA (Kertesz et al., 1994). Therefore, the FBI may also be an important measurement tool in addition to a specific language task in PPA. Recently we surveyed a PPA group with the FBI, among others. The FBI scores were higher than those of the control groups but did not quite reach the level of FLD. Another group surveyed consisted of patients with vascular dementia (VAD), which often presents with features of FLD. These patients have achieved scores that are next to those of the

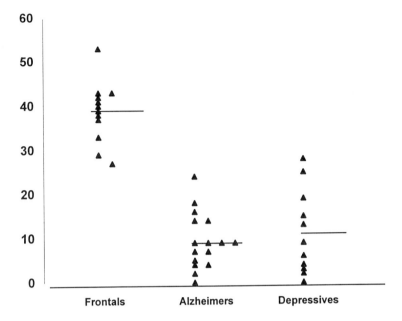

FIGURE 5.2. Scores for the FBI.

FLD groups (Table 5.3). This confirms the results of several studies suggesting a frontal type of neuropsychological deficit in VAD. This is not surprising, considering the extensive disconnection of frontal subcortical structures that is a feature of VAD. The prominence of disinhibition symptoms over apathy and withdrawal helps to distinguish FLD patients from those with VAD and DD.

In summary, in addition to neuroimaging and neuropathology, the quantitation of cognition and behavioral abnormalities is desirable in the diagnosis of FLD. Experienced clinicians recognize the complexity of frontal lobe deficit and interpret the neuropsychological findings with caution. A standardized behavioral inventory may prove most useful in the diagnosis of FLD and in the differential diagnosis of other syndromes resembling FLD, such as VAD or a depressive illness.

TABLE 5.3   FBI

	N	M/F	Age	FBI Score
AD	35	20/15	69.0 (8.8)	10.0 (6.9)
VAD	7	5/2	69.0 (8.9)	25.0 (10.7)
Frontals	13	11/2	58.8 (9.6)	37.5 (7.9)
DD	16	12/4	56.9 (11.2)	9.8 (8.5)
PPA	14	4/10	66.3 (6.2)	15.6 (11.4)
Total	85	52/33	64.7 (10.2)	16.7 (12.9)

REFERENCES

Ackerly SS, Benton AL (1948): Report of a case of bilateral frontal lobe defect. Res Publ Assoc Res Nerv Ment Dis 27:479–504.

Anderson SW, Damasio H, Tranel D, Damasio AR (1992): Cognitive sequelae of focal lesions in ventromedial frontal lobe. J Clin Exp Neuropsychol 14:83.

Arseni C, Botez MI (1961): Speech disturbances caused by tumors of the supplementary motor area. Acta Psychiatr Scand 36:379–299.

Baddeley AD (1986): Working Memory. Oxford: Oxford University Press.

Baddeley A, Wilson B (1988): Frontal amnesia and the dysexecutive syndrome. Brain Cogn 7:212–230.

Barber R, Snowden JS, Craufurd D (1995): Frontotemporal dementia and Alzheimer's disease: Retrospective differentiation using information from informants. J Neurol Neurosurg Psychiatry 59:61–70.

Baumgarten M, Becker R, Gauthier S (1990): Validity and reliability of the Dementia Behavior Disturbance Scale. J Am Geriatr Soc 38:221–226.

Beck AT, Ward CH, Mendelson M, Erbaugh JK (1961): An inventory for measuring depression. Arch Gene Psychiatry 4:561–571.

Bianchi L (1895): The functions of the frontal lobes. Brain 18:397–522.

Black FW (1976): Cognitive deficits in patients with unilateral war-related frontal lobe lesions. J. Clin Psychol 32:366–372.

Blumer D, Benson D (1975): Personality changes with frontal and temporal lobe lesions. In Benson DF, Blumer D (eds): Psychiatric Aspects of Neurologic Disease." New York: Grune & Stratton, pp 151–170.

Bogousslavsky J, Regli F (1990): Anterior cerebral artery territory infarction in the Lausanne Stroke Registry. Arch Neurol 47:144–150.

Brickner R (1934): An interpretation of frontal lobe function based upon the study of a case of partial bilateral frontal lobectomy. Res Publ Assoc Res Nerv Ment Dis 13:259–351.

Brickner R (1940): A human cortical area producing repetitive phenomena when stimulated. J Neurophysiol 3:128–130.

Brun A (1987): Frontal lobe degeneration of non-Alzheimer type. I. Neuropathology. Arch Gerontol Geriatr 6:193–208.

Cohen L (1959): Perception of reversible figures after brain injury. Arch Neurol Psychol 81:765–775.

Constantinidis J, Richard J, Tissot R (1974): Pick's disease: Histological and clinical correlations. Eur Neurol 11:208–217.

Cummings JL (1993): Frontal-subcortical circuits and human behavior. Arch Neurol 50:873–880.

Cummings JL, Mega M, Gray K, Rosenberg-Thompson S, Carusi DA, Gornbein J (1994): The neuropsychiatric inventory: Comprehensive assessment of psychopathology in dementia. Neurology 44:2308–2314.

Damasio AR, Damasio H, Rizzo M, Varney N, Gersh F (1982): Aphasia with nonhemorrhagic lesions in the basal ganglia and internal capsule. Arch Neurol 39:15–20.

Damasio AR, Tranel D, Damasio H (1990): Individuals with sociopathic behavior caused by frontal damage fail to respond autonomically to social stimuli. Behav Brain Res 41:81–94.

Damasio AR, Van Hoesen GW (1983): Emotional disorders associated with focal lesions of the limbic frontal lobe. In Heilman KM, Satz P (eds): Neuropsychology of Human Emotion. New York: Guilford Press, pp 85–110.

Denny-Brown D (1958): The nature of apraxia. J Nerv Ment Disord 126:9–33.

Drachman DA, Swearer JM, O'Donnell BF, Mitchell AL, Maloon A (1992): The Caretaker Obstreperous-Behavior Rating Assessment (COBRA) Scale. J Am Geriatr Soc 40:463–480.

Drewe EA (1975): An experimental investigation of Luria's theory on the effects of frontal lesions in man. Neuropsychologia 13:421–429.

Drewe EA (1984): The effect of type and area of brain lesion in Wisconsin Card Sorting test performance. Cortex 10:159–170.

Erickson TC, Woolsey CN (1951): Observations on the supplementary motor area of man. Trans Am Neurol Assoc 76:50–56.

Eslinger PJ, Damasio AR (1985): Severe disturbance of higher cognition after bilateral frontal lobe ablation: Patient EVR. Neurology 35:1731–1741.

Ferraro A, Jervis GA (1936): Pick's disease—Clinicopathologic study with report of two cases. Arch Neurol Psychiatry 36:739–767.

Ferrier D (1876): The Functions of the Brain. London: Smith and Elder.

Feuchtwanger E (1923): Die Funktionen des Stirnhirns, ihre Pathologie und Psychologie. Berlin: Springer.

Freedman M, Alexander MP, Naeser MA (1984): Anatomic basis of transcortical motor aphasia. Neurology 34:409–417.

Freedman M, Oscar-Berman M (1986): Comparative neuropsychology of cortical and subcortical dementia. Can J Neurol Sci 13:410–414.

Freeman W, Watts JW, Hunt T (1942): Psychosurgery. Baltimore: Thomas.

Friedman HR, Janas J, Goldman-Rakic PS (1990): Enhancement of metabolic activity in the diencephalon of monkeys performing working memory tasks: A 2-deoxyglucose study in behaving rhesus monkeys. J Cogn Neurosci 2:18–31.

Fulton JF, Jacobsen CF (1935): The functions of the frontal lobes: A comparative study in monkeys, chimpanzees and man. Adv Mod Biol 4:113–123.

Fuster JM (1985): The prefrontal cortex, mediator of cross-temporal contingencies. Hum Neurobiol 4:169–179.

Fuster JM (1989): The Prefrontal Cortex, 2nd ed. New York: Raven Press.

Goldberg F (1985): Supplementary motor area structure and function: Review and hypothesis. Behav Brain Sci 8:567–616.

Goldman-Rakic PS (1987): Circuitry of the prefrontal cortex and the regulation of behavior by representational memory. In Plum F (ed): Handbook of Physiology: The Nervous System, Vol 5. Bethesda, MD: American Psychological Society, pp 373–417.

Goldstein K (1944): The mental changes due to frontal lobe damage. J Psychol 17:187–208.

Goldstein K (1948): Language and Language Disturbances. New York: Grune & Stratton.

Goltz FL (1892): Der Hund ohne Grosshirn. Pflüger's Arch Gesamte Physiol 51:570–614.

Grant AD, Berg EA (1948): A behavioral analysis of reinforcement and ease of shifting to new responses in a Weigl-type card sorting problem. J Exp Psychol 38:404–411.

Gregory CA, Hodges JR (1996): Frontotemporal dementia: Use of consensus criteria and prevalence of psychiatric features. Neuropsychiatr Neuropsychol Behav Neurol 9:145–153.

Gronwall D (1977): Paced auditory serial addition task: A measure of recovery from concussion. Percept Mot Skills 44:367–373.

Gustafson L (1987): Frontal degeneration of non-Alzheimer type. II. Clinical picture and differential diagnosis. Arch Gerontol Geriatr 6:209–223.

Gustafson L, Nielson L (1982): Differential diagnosis of presenile dementia on clinical grounds. Acta Psychiatr Scand 65:194–207.

Hamlin RM (1970): Intellectual function 14 years after frontal lobe surgery. Cortex 6:299–307.

Harlow JM (1848): Passage of an iron bar through the head. Boston Med Surg J 39:389–393.

Harlow JM (1868): Recovery from the passage of an iron bar through the head. Publ Mass Med Soc 2:327–347.

Hebb DO (1939): Intelligence in man after large removals of cerebral tissue: Report of four left frontal lobe cases. J Gen Psychol 21:73–87.

Hecaen HJ (1964): Mental symptoms associated with tumors of the frontal lobe. In Warren JM, Akert K (ed): The Frontal Granular Cortex and Behaviour. New York: McGraw-Hill, pp 335–352.

Hecaen HJ, Albert ML (1978): Human Neuropsychology. New York: Wiley.

Heilman KM, Bowers D, Coslett B, Whelan H, Watson RT (1985): Directional hypokinesia: Prolonged reaction times for leftward movements in patients with right hemisphere lesions and neglect. Neurology 35:855–868.

Hersch EL, Kral VA, Palmer RB (1978): Clinical value of the London Psychogeriatric Rating Scale. J Am Geriatr Soc 26:348–354.

Hunter R, Blackwood W, Bull J (1968): Three cases of frontal meningiomas presenting psychiatrically. BMJ 3:9–16.

Jacobsen CC (1936): Studies of cerebral function in primates. Comp Psychol Monogr 13:1–68.

Janowsky JS, Shimamura AP, Kritchevsky M, Squire LR (1989): Cognitive impairment following frontal lobe damage and its relevance to human amnesia. Behav Neurosci 103:548–560.

Jones-Gotman M, Milner B (1977): Design fluency: The invention of nonsense drawings after focal cortical lesions. Neuropsychologia 15:643–652.

Karbe H, Kertesz A, Polk M (1993): Profiles of language impairment in primary progressive aphasia. Arch Neurol 50:193–201.

Kertesz A (1979): Aphasia and Associated Disorders. New York: Grune & Stratton.

Kertesz A (1982): Western Aphasia Battery. New York: Grune & Stratton

Kertesz A (1997): Recovery of aphasia. In Feinberg TE, Farah M (eds): Behavioral Neurology and Neuropsychology. New York: McGraw Hill, pp 167–182.

Kertesz A, Davidson W, Fox H (1997): Frontal behavioral inventory: Diagnostic criteria for frontal lobe dementia. Can J Neurol Sci 24:29–36.

Kertesz A, Hudson L, Mackenzie IRA, Munoz DG (1994): The pathology and nosology of primary progressive aphasia. Neurology 44:2065–2072.

Kertesz A, Nicholson I, Cancelliere A, Kassa K, Black SE (1985): Motor impersistence. Neurology 35:662–666.

Kleist K (1931): Gehirnpathologische und lokalisatorische Ergebnisse. 5. Das Stirnhirn im engeren Sinne und seine Störungen. Z Gesamte Neurol Psychiatry 131:442–452.

Kleist K (1934): Kriegsverletzungen des gehirns. Leipzig: Barth.

Knight RT (1990): ERPs in patients with focal brain lesions (abstract). Electroencephalogr Clin Neurophysiol 75:72.

Knight RT, Scabini D, Woods DL (1989): Prefrontal cortex gating of auditory transmission in humans. Br Res 504:338–342.

Knopman DS, Mastri AR, Frey WH, Sung JH, Rustan T (1990): Dementia lacking distinctive histologic features: A common non-Alzheimer degenerative dementia. Neurology 40:251–256.

Komyey E (1975): Aphasie transcorticale et echolalie: Le probleme de l'initiative de la parole. Rev Neurol 131A:347–363.

Lebert F (1996): Behavioral changes, non-cognitive assessment and management in frontotemporal dementia. In Pasquier F, Lebert F, Scheltens Ph. (eds): Frontotemporal Dementia. The Netherlands: ICG Publications, pp71–82.

Lhermitte F (1983): "Utilization behaviour" and its relation to lesions of the frontal lobes. Brain 106:237–255.

Lishman WA (1968): Brain damage in relation to psychiatric disability after head injury. Br J Psychiatry 114:373–410.

Livingston KE (1969): The frontal lobes revisited: The case for a second look. Arch Neurol 20:90–95.

Logue V, Durward M, Pratt TRC, Piercy M, Nixon WL (1968): The quality of survival after an anterior cerebral aneurysm. Br J Psychiatry 114:137–160.

Lopez OL, Gonzalez MP, Becker JT, Reynolds CF, Sudilovsky A, DeKosky ST (1996): Symptoms of depression and psychosis in Alzheimer's disease and frontotemporal dementia. Neuropsychiatry Neuropsychol Behav Neurol 9:154–161.

Löwenberg K (1935): Pick's disease—a clinicopathologic contribution. Arch Neurol Psychiatry 36:68–789.

Lund and Manchester Groups (1994): Clinical and neuropathological criteria for frontotemporal dementia. J Neurol Neurosurg Psychiatry 57:416–418.

Luria AR (1966): Higher Cortical Functions in Man. London: Tavistock.

Luria AR (1973): The frontal lobes and the regulation of behavior. In Pribram KH, Luria AR (eds): Psychophysiology of the Frontal Lobes. New York: Academic Press, pp 3–26.

Luria AR, Homskaya ED (1964): Disturbance in the regulative role of speech with frontal lobe lesions. In Warren JM, Akert K (eds): The Frontal Granular Cortex and Behaviour. New York: McGraw-Hill, pp 353–371.

Malmo RB (1948): Psychological aspects of frontal gyrectomy and frontal lobotomy in mental patients. Res Publ Assoc Res Nerv Ment Dis 27:537–564.

McFie J, Thompson JA (1972): Picture arrangement: A measure of frontal lobe function? Br J Psychiatry 121:547–552.

Meador K, Watson RT, Bowers D, Heilman KM (1986): Hypometria with hemispatial and limb motor neglect. Brain 109:293–305.

Mesulam MM (1987): Primary progressive aphasia—differentiation from Alzheimer's disease. Ann Neurol 22:533–534.

Mettler FA (1949): Selective Partial Ablation of the Frontal Cortex. New York: Paul B. Hoeber.

Miller BL, Cummings JL, Villanueva-Meyer J, Boone K, Mehringer CM, Lesser IM, Mena I (1991): Frontal lobe degeneration: Clinical, neuropsychological, and SPECT characteristics. Neurology 41:1374–1382.

Miller BL, Ikonte C, Ponton M, Levy M, Boone K, Darby A, Berman N, Mena I, Cummings JL (1997): A study of the Lund-Manchester research criteria for frontotemporal dementia: Clinical and single-photon emission CT correlations. Neurology 48:937–942.

Miller L (1992): Impulsivity, risk-taking, and the ability to synthesize fragmented information after frontal lobectomy. Neuropsychologia 30:69–79.

Milner B (1964): Some effects of frontal lobectomy in man. In Warren JM, Akert K (eds): The Frontal Granular Cortex and Behaviour. New York: McGraw-Hill, pp 313–334.

Milner B (1971): Interhemispheric differences in the localization of psychological processes in man. Br Med Bull 27:272–277.

Mishkin M (1964): Perseveration of central sets after frontal lesions in monkeys. In Warren JM, Akert K (eds): The Frontal Granular Cortex and Behaviour. New York: McGraw-Hill, pp 219–241.

Mohr JP, Pessin MS, Finkelstein S, Funkenstein HH, Duncan GW, Davis KR (1978): Broca: aphasia, pathologic and clinical. Neurology 28:311–324.

Moniz E (1936): Premiers essais de psycho-chirurgie. Technique et résultats. Lisboa Medi 12:152.

Mungas D, Weiler P, Franzi C, Henry R (1989): Assessment of disruptive behavior associated with dementia: The Disruptive Behavior Rating Scales. J Geriatr Psychiatry Neurol 2:196–202.

Nadeau SE (1988): Impaired grammar with normal fluency and phonology: Implications for Boca's aphasia. Brain 111:1111–1137.

Naeser MA (1982): Language behavior in stroke patients: Cortical vs. subcortical lesion sites on CT scans. TINS February 5: 53–59.

Nauta WJH (1971): The problem of the frontal cortex. Acta Neurobiol Exp 32:125–140.

Nauta WJH (1973): Connections of the frontal lobe with the limbic system. In Laitinen LV, Livingston RE (eds): Surgical Approaches in Psychiatry. Baltimore: University Park Press.

Neary D, Snowden JS, Bowen DM, Sims NR, Mann DMA, Benton JS, Northen YB, Yates DO, Davison AN (1986): Neuropsychological syndromes in presenile dementia due to cerebral atrophy. J Neurol Neurosurg Psychiatry 49:163–174.

Neary D, Snowden JS, Northen B, Goulding PJ (1988): Dementia of frontal lobe type. J Neurol Neurosurg Psychiatry 51:353–361.

Niederehe G (1988): Trims Behavioral Problem Checklist (BPC). Psychopharmacol Bull 24:771–773.

Norman D, Shallice T (1986): Attention to action: Willed and automatic control of behaviour. Center for human information processing (Technical Report No. 99). (Reprinted in revised form in Davidson RD, Schwartz GE, Shapiro D [eds]: Consciousness and Self-Regulation. New York: Plenum Press, pp 1–18.

Oppenheim H (1890): Zur pathologie der grosshirngeschwulste. Archiv für Psychiatrie 21:560–578.

Penfield W, Jasper HH (1954): Epilepsy and the Functional Anatomy of the Human Brain. Boston: Little, Brown.

Penfield W, Roberts L (1959): Speech and Brain Mechanisms. Princeton, NJ: Princeton University Press.

Perret E (1974): The left frontal lobe of man and the suppression of habitual responses in verbal categorical behaviour. Neuropsychologia 12:323–330.

Pick A (1904): Über primäre progressive Demenz bei Erwachsenen. Prag Med Wocheschr 29:417–420.

Pick A (1906): Über einen weiteren Symptomenkomplex im Rahmen der Dementia senilis, bedingt durch umschriebene stärkere Hirnatrophie (gemischte Apraxie). Vortag, gehalten im Wiener Vereine für Psychiatrie und Neurologie. Monatschr Psychiatry (Berl) 19:97–108.

Reisberg B, Borenstein J, Salob SP, Ferris SH, Franssen E, Georgotas A (1987): Behavioral symptoms in Alzheimer's disease: Phenomenology and treatment. J Clin Psychiatry 48(Suppl):9–15.

Royall DR, Mahurin RK, Cornell J (1992): Bedside assessment of executive cognitive impairment: The Executive Interview (EXIT). J Am Geriatr Soc 40:1221–1226.

Rubens AB (1975): Aphasia with infarction in the territory of the anterior cerebral artery. Cortex 11:239–250.

Rylander G (1939): Personality Changes After Operations on the Frontal Lobes: A Clinical Study of 32 Cases. Copenhagen: Munksgaard.

Rylander G (1948): Personality analysis before and after frontal lobotomy. Res Publ Assoc Res Nerv Ment Dis: 691–706.

Sandson J, Albert ML (1984): Varieties of perseveration. Neuropsychologia 22:715–732.

Sanides F (1970): Functional architecture of motor and sensory cortices in primates in the light of a new concept of neocortex evolution. In Noback CR, Montagna W (eds): The Primate Brain. New York: Appleton, pp 137–208.

Schneider C (1927): Uber Picksche Krankheit. Monatschr Psychiatr Neurol 65:230–275.

Schwartz GE (1983): Development and validation of the Geriatric Evaluation by Relatives Rating Instrument (GERRI). Psychol Rep 53:479–488.

Shader RI, Harmatz JS, Salzman C (1974): A new scale for clinical assessment in geriatric populations: Sandoz Clinical Assessment Geriatric (SCAG). J Am Geriatr S22:107–113.

Shallice T (1982): Specific impairments of planning. Philos Trans R Soc Lond B Biol Sci 298:199–209.

Shallice T, Burgess PW, Schon F, Baxter DM (1989): The origins of utilization behaviour. Brain 112:1587–1598.

Shallice T, Evans ME (1978): The involvement of the frontal lobes in cognitive estimation. Cortex 14:294–303.

Shimamura AP, Janowsky JS, Squire LR (1990): Memory for the temporal order of events in patients with frontal lobe lesions and amnesic patients. Neuropsychologia 28:803–814.

Smith ML, Milner B (1984): Differential effects of frontal-lobe lesions on cognitive estimation and spatial memory. Neuropsychologia 22:697–705.

Starkstein SE, Robinson RG (1991): The role of the frontal lobes in affective disorder following stroke. In Levin HS, Eisenberg HM, Benton AL (eds): Frontal Lobe Function and Dysfunction. New York: Oxford University Press, pp 228–303.

Starr MA (1884): Cortical lesions of the brain: A collection and analysis of the American cases of localized cerebral disease. Am J Med Sci New Series 87:366–391.

Strauss I, Keschner M (1935): Mental symptoms in cases of tumor of the frontal lobe. Arch Neurol Psychiatry 33:986–1007.

Stuss DT, Benson DF (1983a): Emotional concomitants of psychosurgery. In Heilman KM, Satz P (eds): Neuropsychology of Human Emotion. New York: Guilford Press, pp 111–140.

Stuss DT, Benson DF (1983b): Frontal lobe lesions and behavior. In Kertesz A (ed): Localization in Neuropsychology. New York: Academic Press, pp 429–454.

Stuss DT, Benson DF (1986): The Frontal Lobes. New York: Raven Press.

Stuss DT, Kaplan EF, Benson DF, Wier WS, Naeser MA, Levine HL (1981): Long-term effects of prefrontal leucotomy—An overview of neuropsychologic residuals. J Clin Neuropsychol 3:13–32.

Sweet W (1951): Discussion of Erickson and Woolsey. Trans Am Neurol Soc 76:55.

Teuber HL (1964): The riddle of frontal lobe function in man. In Warren JM, Akert K (eds): The Frontal Granular Cortex and Behavior. New York: McGraw-Hill, pp 410–444.

Vikki J (1989): Perseveration in memory for figures after frontal lobe lesions. Neuropsychologia 27:1101–1104.

Welt L (1888): Über Charakterveranderungen des Menschen infolge von Läsionen des Stirnhirns. Dtsch Arch Klin Med 42:339–390.

Yacorozynski GK, Davis L (1945): An experimental study of the functions of the frontal lobes in man. Psychosom Med 7:97–107.

Yakovlev PI, Locke S (1961): Limbic nuclei of thalamus and connections of limbic cortex. III. Corticocortical connections of the anterior cingulate gyrus, the cingulum, and subcallosal bundle in monkeys. Arch Neurol 5:364–400.

CHAPTER 6

Primary Progressive Aphasia

ANDREW KERTESZ

Department of Clinical Neurological Sciences, St. Joseph's Health Centre, University of Western Ontario, London, Ontario, N6A 4V2, Canada

INTRODUCTION

A series of patients with progressive language deficit, before other cognitive domains are involved, was described and subsequently named *primary progressive aphasia (PPA)* by Mesulam (1982, 1987). A cortical biopsy specimen from a patient from the original series showed only nonspecific pathology with lipofuscinosis, although Mesulam believed it could be related to diverse pathologies as long as the degeneration was focal, and he included Pick's disease (PiD) in the differential diagnosis. Since then, the term has been widely used, although similar patients were reported under variations of this term, such as *progressive aphasia without dementia* (Kirshner et al., 1987), *progressive nonfluent aphasia* (Turner et al., 1996), and *pure progressive aphemia* (Cohen et al., 1993).

Although both Pick (1892) and Alzheimer (1907) described their original patients as being significantly aphasic, the importance of language impairment in dementia has not been emphasized and documented systematically until recently (Appell et al., 1982; Bayles et al., 1982; Kertesz et al., 1986; Faber-Langendoen et al., 1988). Pick's (1892) conclusion was that "a more or less circumscribed type of aphasia could result from a single circumscribed atrophic process." Caron (1934), in his review of PiD, stated that the most common form is characterized by early development of aphasia, and others also emphasized early speech disturbance or aphasia in PiD (Malamud and Boyd, 1940; Lüers, 1947; Kosaka, 1976; Ohashi, 1983). The prominence of aphasic deficit in PiD was often overlooked, however, and textbooks emphasized the personality and behavioral changes in early PiD and even stated that aphasia is rarely a presenting feature (Tissot et al., 1985; APA, 1987). Mutism, on the other hand, is often mentioned, but rarely in sufficient detail to know how it begins or develops. Most patients go through a phase of word finding difficulty, and nonfluent aphasia of increasing severity before mutism.

Prominent language disturbance in dementia may be associated with a higher familial incidence (Folstein and Breitner, 1981; Seltzer and Sherwin, 1983) and presenile onset (Seltzer and

Pick's Disease and Pick Complex, Edited by Andrew Kertesz and David G. Munoz
ISBN 0-471-17792-X ©1998 Wiley-Liss, Inc.

Sherwin, 1983; Filley et al., 1986). A syntactic impairment was considered to be associated with earlier onset and more rapid progression of dementia (Becker et al., 1988). It is possible that a proportion of the early-onset patients with language impairment, in fact, have non-Alzheimer pathology and, in fact, PPA. In a dementia clinic, approximately 10% of patients present with progressive aphasia (Kertesz et al., 1986).

THE CLINICAL SYNDROME

The initial presentation of PPA often involves word-finding difficulty, or anomia. In this respect, PPA patients are not very different from Alzheimer disease (AD) patients, except that they have relatively preserved memory and nonverbal cognition. AD patients, by the time they present with word-finding difficulty, already have significant memory loss and disorientation, as well as constructional, visuospatial, and other cognitive impairments. As a rule, AD presentation involves a loss of episodic memory, with initial preservation of semantic memory and language. The relatively isolated language disturbance in the first 2 years of the illness, suggested by Mesulam as the operational definition of PPA, more or less distinguishes the two groups of patients. In many publications, however, this distinction is not adhered to and AD patients with prominent aphasia may be included in a PPA series. On the other hand, some of the pathologically proven cases of Pick complex have behavioral or extra-pyramidal features that appear before the 2-year deadline. Mesulam and Weintraub (1992) in their review, for instance, excluded the patients of Pick (1892) and Wechsler (1977) because they had early behavioral symptoms. Although the 2-year criterion may be arbitrary and may exclude patients who in fact have the disease, it seems useful for the clinical selection of PPA cases for prospective study in some instances.

The more typical clinical picture progresses from anomia to a nonfluent type of aphasia with increasing word-finding difficulty. Logopenia is defined as a phenomenon when the word-finding difficulty is prominent but the phrase length is longer than four words and syntax is preserved (Mesulam and Weintraub, 1992). Decreasing speech output involves spontaneous speech first, and repetition is affected to a less extent initially (Karbe et al., 1993). Sometimes the aphasic disturbance resembles Broca's aphasia with grammatical errors and phonemic paraphasias. The relative preservation of comprehension is typical, and nonverbal intelligence and memory are demonstrably maintained (Duffy and Petersen, 1992; Mesulam and Weintraub, 1992; Snowden et al., 1992; Karbe et al., 1993). Broca's aphasia with agrammatism is more characteristic of stroke patients, but it may also be seen in PPA as a transient stage, usually progressing with increasing word-finding difficulty to mutism. In a study of 10 patients with PPA, 9 were classified as anomic aphasic on the Western Aphasia Battery (WAB) (Karbe et al., 1993), with an average aphasia quotient (AQ) of 79.6 after an average duration of 2.3 years. Their language profiles were compared with those of stroke aphasics matched for severity and type of aphasia and with a control group of AD patients matched for the duration of illness. PPA patients had significantly lower AQ than comparably staged AD patients. PPA patients also tended to have lower fluency and lesser paraphasias than most stroke aphasics. In most of the subtests, however, no significant differences were found. Some of the nonverbal control tests, such as Raven's Coloured Progressive Matrices (RCPM) in patients with early PPA, were relatively preserved. Seven of these patients were followed at a yearly interval. At later stages, Broca's aphasia and then global aphasia was reached. Initially, fluency and naming deteriorated most rapidly, but eventually comprehension and repetition became impaired as well. At later stages, the patients failed nonverbal tests as well and were more likely to be called *demented*.

Naming errors in PPA were analyzed by Weintraub et al. (1990). They found more phonemic paraphasias, fewer circumlocutions, and more perceptual errors than in similar patients with AD. Snowden et al. (1992) combined all their patients with progressive language disorders with lobar atrophy. In addition to five nonfluent patients with preserved comprehension and five with fluent (semantic) aphasias (see below), they found a group of mixed patients in whom progressive loss of speech output was also associated with loss of comprehension. Writing was relatively preserved in some of the patients (Snowden et al., 1992; Karbe et al., 1993). Transcortical motor, anomic, Broca's, and global aphasic patterns were described in four patients with various degrees of left hemispheric dysfunction on single photon emission computed tomography (SPECT) and a variable rate of decline on the WAB (Cappa et al., 1996). In four presenile PPA patients, initial articulatory agility and grammatical form were mildly impaired, and productive language declined on subsequent testing. Detailed analysis of speech and language in these patients indicated variable profiles, with three of them resembling agrammatic Broca's aphasics and one having persistent word-finding difficulty with relatively little grammatical deficit (Thompson et al., 1997). The variations in the profiles of these patients may be related to the rate of decline or to the time of examination initially, as well as the length of the follow-up.

Other patients presented with stuttering or slow, dysprosodic speech and verbal apraxia, which included articulatory difficulty and phonological paraphasias. These patients were less likely to be mistaken for AD patients; however, the unexplained progressive articulatory disturbance in a younger person may be considered functional or hysterical (Kertesz et al., 1994). *Cortical dysarthria, anarthria, aphemia,* and *pure motor aphasia* are alternative terms used to describe this pattern. Writing and comprehension may be relatively preserved (Cohen et al., 1939). A number of cases of PPA with mainly dysarthria has been reported (Northen et al., 1990; Tyrell et al., 1991; McNeil et al., 1995). The articulatory impairment is characterized by particular difficulty with initial consonants, such as omission, repetition, and substitution. Although this condition is called *verbal apraxia,* it may occur with or without buccofacial or limb apraxia (Tyrell et al., 1991; Hart et al., 1997). A progressive limb apraxia can be a prominent feature (Fukui et al., 1996), indicating a clinical overlap between PPA and the apraxic-extrapyramidal syndrome of corticobasal degeneration (CBD). (For a further analysis of apraxia in Pick complex, see Chapter 10 in this volume.)

Mutism has been considered characteristic of PiD, and it tends to be the end stage of all forms of frontotemporal dementia (FTD), even those that start with behavioral abnormalities rather than language disturbance (Neary et al., 1988; Gustafson et al., 1990). Decreased speech output and mutism are core symptoms in the description of FTD, and there is a great deal of overlap between the descriptions of language deficit in FLD, PPA, and PiD. End-stage mutism also occurs in AD, but usually in a patient who already has a global dementia with loss of comprehension and of the basic functions of daily living (Appell et al., 1982). Mutism may not be considered an aphasic phenomenon in the end stages of the illness. The intermediate stages and its evolution are often not clear or defined. In PPD, FTD, and PPA, mutism occurs with relative preservation of comprehension, unlike the situation in global aphasia or severe AD.

A distinct, fluent form of PPA that is different from the more common non-fluent variety was described as *semantic dementia* by Snowden et al. (1989). These patients progressively lost the meaning of words but retained fluency and were able to carry on a conversation. Subsequent descriptions of this entity adopted this term (Hodges et al., 1992), although these patients are not demented in the usual sense. *Semantic aphasia* was a term used by Henry Head (1926) for a two-day disturbance of comprehension and naming. The picture is similar to that of transcortical sensory aphasia, in which articulation, phonology, and syntax remain intact but the patient does not comprehend well and has word-finding difficulty. *Transcortical sensory aphasia* was commonly used to describe patients with degenerative disease; this syndrome also appears in AD. However, patients with semantic dementia or primary progressive fluent aphasia differ significantly from the fluent aphasics of AD because they have relatively preserved episodic memory and autobiographical memory with loss of semantic memory in a rather selective fashion. Some very interesting studies showed that these patients retain information that has immediate relevance to their environment or to their person yet lose the meaning of other common things (Snowden et al., 1994). The behavior can be so dissociative that some of these patients are considered hysterical. They are able to carry on conversations concerning their relatives, their immediate environment, and recent events involving them, but when something less immediately relevant is discussed, they do not seem to be able to comprehend. The loss of meaning is similar in written language, but it has an additional consequence. The patients can read phonologically but not irregular words unless they know the meaning. Reading without meaning is also called *transcortical alexia,* and psycholinguistically it is categorized as surface alexia with regularization errors. The same regularization errors are seen in writing; therefore, the term *surface agraphia* is also applied to these patients. In other reports of fluent progressive aphasia, the semantic deficit is not emphasized (Poeck and Luzzatti, 1988; Parkin, 1993; Harasty et al. 1996). In Japan, similar patients are called *Gogi* ("word meaning") aphasia (Imura 1943; Tanabe et al., 1992). Face and object agnosia may be prominent and may precede the aphasic disturbance, although it may be conceptualized as optic aphasia rather than visual agnosia (Kertesz et al., 1992).

We have followed a patient with a progressive loss of meaning of objects with preserved phonology and syntax for 8 years (Kertesz et al. in press). The patient retained conversational speech, social skills, and orientation but showed severe anomia and comprehension deficit in all modalities. A frequency-dependent loss of meaning appeared consistent throughout all object categories. However, the relative preservation of visual categorization in all categories tested and the language-based categorization of animals suggested some fractionation of semantic memory. Relative preservation of autobiographical and personal memories versus semantic memory was a striking observation. Evidence of selective impairment of central semantic processing was obtained from experiments indicating item consistency of loss and the lack of semantic cueing. Neuroimaging evidence of left temporal lobe atrophy was similar to that in other cases labeled by the term *semantic dementia.* Neuropathological evidence suggests that these cases also belong to Pick complex (Hodges et al., 1992). (For further detail, see Chapter 7 in this volume.)

The age of onset of PPA is usually presenile (under 65), although there are numerous exceptions (Mesulam and Weintraub, 1992; Snowden et al., 1992; Karbe et al., 1993). A careful history is needed to determine the initial symptoms. When the patients are seen later in the illness, the duration is difficult to determine. The course is variable and usually quite prolonged, but sometimes patients who develop pathology in the basal ganglia or motor neurons progress quickly to mutism and develop difficulty with swallowing and choking; the course may be as little as 2 years from onset to death (Caselli et al., 1993; Kertesz et al., 1994). It is yet to be determined if rapid progression represents different patients with different pathology. However, most patients, whose symptomatic illness remains localized mainly in the cortical regions, progress very gradually over 6 or 7 years before they develop severe aphasia or mutism. Several patients, well after 10 years of illness, continue to function normally at home even though they are completely mute. In these cases, a considerable amount of comprehension, memory, visuospatial function, and motor function are retained. These patients can get around independently and carry out complex tasks, even though they are unable to talk. One of our younger patients, who managed to take care of her children and her household, was considered hysterical by the psychologist, speech pathologist, and neurologist before neuroimaging showed severe frontal atrophy, and the patient was diagnosed as having probable PiD (Kertesz et al., 1994). A frontal biopsy showing Pick bodies and swollen neurons confirmed the diagnosis, and autopsy 12 years after the onset of her illness confirmed these findings. Another patient, who managed to continue working well into the fifth year of his illness, was sent because of possible depression to a psychiatrist, who diagnosed his problem as PPA (Kertesz et al., 1994). The illness tends to be quite selective and of long duration, and global deterioration of the intellect does not occur as early or to the same extent as it does in AD.

Changes in behavior suggesting frontal lobe involvement often occur later on in the illness (Snowden et al., 1992; Kertesz et al., 1996; Frisoni et al., 1995). Apathy, irritability, and lack of insight occur commonly and may be misinterpreted as depression. One of our pathologically examined PPA patients received psychiatric treatment for depression and uncharacteristic aggression toward his wife (Kertesz et al., 1994). Six of 16 probable PPA patients followed in our clinic have developed hyperorality, utilization behavior, aggressiveness, emotional flatness, and bizarre obsessive behavior clearly indicating frontal lobe involvement that is outside the language network. The development of behavioral disturbance in PPA is probably more common than was hitherto recognized, and it is an important clinical feature supporting the close relationship of PPA to FLD and the Pick complex.

There are also patients with PPA who develop motor neuron disease (MND) with a rapid course and bulbar symptoms, such as increasing dysarthria and dysphagia, as indicated earlier, even though typical amyotrophy or spasticity may be absent (Neary et al., 1990; Caselli et al., 1993; Kertesz et al., 1994). Several cases of PPA and MND have been described pathologically with ubiquitinated silver and tau-negative inclusions in the dentate fascia and neocortical neurons, which several authors believe to be the hallmark of this variant (Cooper et al., 1995). However, there are patients with ubiquitin-positive pathology without MND (Tolnay and Probst, 1995).

Patients with PPA may develop extrapyramidal symptoms that are often unilateral and associated with severe apraxia and at times with the *alien hand,* a motor phenomenon of hesitation, neglect, disuse, and rigidity (and levitation). The motor component of the syndrome was described as corticonigral (Rebeiz et al., 1968) or *corticobasal degeneration* (*CBD*) (Gibb et al., 1989; Thompson and Marsden, 1992). The pathology appeared distinct, but, even the original description noted a significant overlap between the pathology of CBD and PiD (Rebeiz et al., 1968). Sporadic case reports of PPA with CBD have been published (Lang et al., 1992; Bergeron et al., 1996; Sakurai et al., 1996), and we have seen several patients with clinical PPA and FLD whose pathology was compatible with what is usually described as CBD (see chapter 19). In turn, many of the typical patients with CBD presenting with primarily extrapyramidal symptoms develop speech deficits, personality changes, and other features of PPA or FLD later on. Thus, CBD is one of the pathological substrates of PPA.

Standardized language testing is useful to diagnose and follow the course of the illness. It is particularly important to examine spontaneous speech for fluency and content and to document comprehension and naming, preferably with low- and high-frequency items and repetition. Reading and writing are also important, particularly a list of irregular words to detect surface or transcortical alexia. We used the WAB and have obtained considerable experience in documenting the type of language loss and the extent of deterioration across individuals in a large group of patients with PPA (Karbe et al., 1993). We also added a list of irregular words and nonwords to test for surface (transcortical) alexia and performed multimodality tests of naming, definitions, categorization, and comprehension of meaning to probe for semantic aphasia (Kertesz et al., in press). Additional psycholinguistic testing is of considerable interest in exploring the processing deficit, particularly in progressive fluent aphasia or semantic dementia (Hodges et al., 1992; Snowden et al., 1992, 1994; Parkin, 1993; Harasty et al., 1996).

A battery of nonverbal tests, block design, Raven's Coloured Progressive Matrices, a set of drawing tasks, copying from memory, and standard memory tests such as the Wechsler memory test or the California Verbal Learning Test (CVLT), depending on the stage of the patient, are useful to complete the neuropsychological profile. The Mini-Mental State Exam (MMSE) and the ADAS-Cog or Mattis Dementia Rating Scale (MDRS) are often used as global measures of staging of the dementia. However, variable results can be obtained, as the MMSE and ADAS-Cog are more heavily weighted for language and because lower total scores are seen in PPA patients than in those with AD in comparable stages, even though the patients are not generally demented (Weintraub et al., 1990; Karbe et al., 1993).

Neuroimaging abnormalities, such as left ventricular or sulcal atrophy, are relatively common in PPA, occurring in 65% of the published cases in the review of Mesulam and Weintraub (1992). Focal hypometabolism on positron emission tomography (PET) in the left temporal and parietal lobes (Chawluk et al., 1986; Croisile and Trillet, 1990; Tyrell et al., 1990; Yamamoto et al., 1990); and various other patterns, including asymmetrical temporal, frontal, and bifrontal hypometabolism on SPECT, were present (McDaniel et al., 1991; Snowden et al., 1992; Caselli et al., 1993; Cappa et al., 1996; Sakurai et al., 1996). Frontal opercular atrophy, anterior and superior temporal atrophy, and bifrontal and left temporoparietal atrophy were shown on the magnetic resonance imaging (MRI) scan in three patients with PPA by Caselli et al. (1992). These authors also commented that hypoperfusion with SPECT seemed to be even more extensive than atrophy on MRI.

The diagnostic role of neuroimaging in focal atrophies is clearly important. However, neuroimaging findings are neither specific nor 100% sensitive. Asymmetry of the ventricular and sulcal atrophy is often considered a normal variant. There are several issues, however, that require clarification, such as the structures commonly affected, the extent of atrophy, the best modality to document it, and its correlation with the clinical manifestations. We have made the presumptive diagnosis of PPA in 34 patients on the basis of prominent speech and language symptoms. We have further divided this group into 19 probable PPA patients, who fulfill the stricter criteria of PPA, on the basis of relatively preserved memory and visuospatial function historically, and in some documented neuropsychologically on the initial examination and on follow-up. The other group of 15 patients had a history in which it was either doubtful that the initial symptom was memory loss or forgetting proper names and dates as the feature of early anomia, or fluent aphasia was the major clinical feature for years. This group was designated as having possible PPA. Computed tomography (CT), MRI, and SPECT scans in this population were scored separately by two independent observers. In case of discrepancies, a consensus was reached. Significant left more than right atrophy was noted in both groups. A pairwise comparisons for each of the anatomical structures between the probable and possible PPA groups showed no significant differences, except that the left frontal horn and occipital horn were significantly more atrophied in the probable PPA group. There was a trend toward more atrophy of all the structures in the probable PPA group. These results suggested that the possible PPA group also has focal, asymmetrical atrophy. Focal atrophy on MRI or CT, affecting the left temporal and parietal lobes, is a hallmark of PPA, and it was seen in all of the probable PPA cases (Kertesz, in press) (Figure 6.1).

Our understanding of the pathological substrate of PPA has improved considerably as an increasing number of cases have accumulated. However, it is only with the relatively recent application of the concept of *Pick complex* that the diverse descriptions can be seen to conform to a consonant pattern. The initial reports emphasized nonspecific findings such as lipofuscinosis (Mesulam, 1982) and spongiform change in layers II and III of the cortex, as the characteristic alteration of PPA (Kirshner et al., 1987), as it is seen in virtually all cases. Confusion between this superficial linear spongiosis, restricted to the upper cortical layers, and the spon-

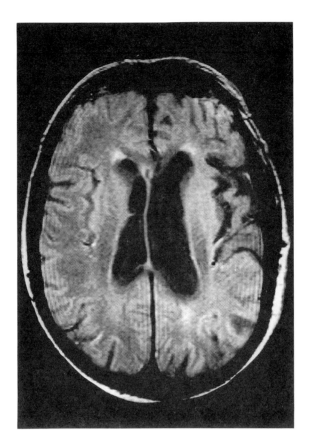

FIGURE 6.1. Severe left hemispheric atrophy involving frontal, central, and temporal areas in a patient with progressive logopenia and nonfluent aphasia. Case report in Karbe et al. (1993). Reprinted from Archives Neurology 1993;50:196. Copyright American Medical Association.

giosis throughout the cortex characteristic of the transmissible encephalopathies is the most likely explanation of the reports of PPA due to Creutzfeldt-Jakob disease. The spongiosis of the latter disease involves the basal ganglia, whereas the spongiosis in PPA is restricted to the cortex. Prion proteins, as determined by immunohistochemistry and Western blotting, have not been reported.

Others, including our group, described AD pathology in PPA (Pogacar and Williams, 1984; Benson and Zaias, 1991; Karbe et al., 1993). Some of these cases, however, appear to represent the coexistence of Pick complex abnormalities with moderate-minor AD-type pathology similar to that seen in many nondemented elderly individuals. Characteristically, the AD-type pathology, consisting of abundant senile plaques, predominantly diffuse, and rare neurofibrillary tangles, is spread throughout the cortex, contrasting with the focal distribution of Pick complex-type abnormalities such as the spongiform change. In other patients, the language disturbance appears later and is a manifestation of AD. The prominent aphasia is not primary, and it is accompanied by other deficits. In these cases, the initial history of memory loss may have been overlooked or underreported. Pathological descriptions of focal AD have appeared sporadically, but its clinical correlation with PPA is not convincing (Tariska, 1970). Posterior cortical atrophies are more likely to be associated with AD. Some of these reports of PPA note the presence of senile plaques, but the superficial cortical vacuolation, gliosis, neuronal loss, and even ballooned neurons are overlooked or considered nonspecific pathology.

Many cases of PPA turned out to be PiD with classical silver-staining globose Pick bodies and ballooned, achromatic neurons called *Pick cells* (Malamud and Boyd, 1940; Wechsler et al., 1982; Holland et al., 1985; Graff-Radford et al., 1990, Kertesz et al., 1994). In addition to the cases published as PPA (Kertesz et al., 1994), this category includes patients in whom such a diagnosis can be made retrospectively. For example, one of the two patients with partial atrophy of the brain presented by Rosenfeld (1909) had characteristic PPA, with relatively well-preserved mentation in other domains, and PiD established on autopsy. Wechsler (1977) published the first modern case of presenile dementia presenting with aphasia; subsequently, the autopsy also showed PiD (Wechsler et al., 1982). PPA, therefore, can be seen with the following histopathological variants: First is PiD, as defined by the presence of argyrophilic, tau-immunoreactive round inclusions in the neurons of the dentate gyrus of the hippocampus, as well as in other hippocampal, neocortical, and subcortical sites. In addition, Pick cells are always present. There is gliosis and spongiform change in layers II and III of the cortex. Second, the CBD type of pathology is characterized by the combination of cortical ballooned neurons (Pick cells) and argyrophilic and tau-immunoreactive clusters of astrocytic processes (*glial plaques*), a dense network of argyrophilic threads in the white matter, cortex, and basal ganglia, and globose or ring-like neurofibrillary tangles in the substantia nigra (*corticobasal inclusion bodies*) and other sites. *Dementia of motor neuron type* is characterized by the presence of ubiquitin-positive but tau-negative and nonargyrophilic cytoplasmic inclusions in the granular cell layer of the dentate gyrus, as well as other cortical and subcortical sites. Not all these patients develop clinical or pathological evidence of amyotrophic lateral sclerosis (ALS). Finally, the descriptive term *dementia lacking distinctive histology,* so called due to the absence of inclusions, nevertheless consistently shows superficial linear spongiosis in the cortex, gliosis, and neuronal loss, sometimes accompanied by the presence of scattered, ballooned neurons in the deep layers.

Attempts to treat PPA aimed to control symptoms or, in a few instances, to influence the disease process itself pharmacologically. Most of the drugs used were already approved medications, usually for Parkinson's disease or depression. These attempts to use Levodopa, Selegiline, or Prozac have not altered the course of the disease. Other drugs, such as nootropics, have also been tried. In our pilot study, the results of Cerebrolysin, a nootropic nerve growth-promoting factor given by intravenous injection for 4 weeks, has been inconclusive, with no dramatic clinical effect seen. So far, it appears to be easily administered and has no obvious side effects. More extensive clinical trials are required with this drug and with similar medications, either to prevent the progression of degeneration (such as Selegiline in Parkinson's disease) or to enhance remaining function, such as Cerebrolysin. Until proper randomized clinical trials are carried out, these drugs cannot be considered efficacious, considering the variability and the relatively long clinical course of PPA.

Speech pathologists have an important role in diagnosing and counseling patients, but extensive speech therapy is not justified according to our current knowledge. Patients can be taught compensatory strategies, such as the use of writing pads if writing is preserved, and the patient and family can be helped to adjust to the condition. Education of the family concerning the nature of the illness, the relatively slow deterioration, and the relatively preserved writing and nonverbal cognition is very helpful. Families appreciate counseling beyond the diagnosis itself. It should be emphasized that the patient can often lead a very useful and productive life despite the progressive speech output deficit. We are presently carrying out a study of pragmatics or family communication in progressive aphasia and hope to utilize the results of this study in creating programs for families to compensate for the slowly progressive output disorder.

In the final stages of the disease, dysarthria and dysphagia often become prominent, and counseling by clinicians experienced in dysphagia management becomes important. These patients may have a combination of bulbar, pseudobulbar, and extrapyramidal disorders at the end stages of their illness resembling partly motor neuron disease and partly Parkinson's disease. These complex motor disorders can be quite challenging to diagnose and manage.

FAMILIAL OCCURRENCE

Familial occurrence of PPA suggests an important genetic component for this degenerative disease similar to other varieties of PiD. A large family with a prominent language disturbance was described by Malamud and Waggoner (1943). Another large PiD family with 25 affected members had a mostly frontal presentation, but some of them had progressive aphasia and mutism (Schenk, 1958–1959). The study of this family has been republished recently, with linkage to chromosome 17 (Heutink et al., 1997) (see also Chapter 18 in this volume). In a family of Italian heritage, 4 of 10 members in a single generation developed dementia, bulimia, aphasia, and occasionally parkinsonian signs (Kim et al., 1981). Pathology with loss of cortical cell status, spongiosis, and astrocytosis were seen, which were considered nonspecific. *Hereditary, dysphasic dementia* was described by Morris et al. (1984), showing pathological features of PiD, as well as neuritic plaques and subcortical pathology of Lewy body formation in the substantia nigra, in addition to a striking spongiform degeneration of the superficial cortical layers. The authors considered this a distinct entity and discussed its relationship to PiD and AD. Three subsequent generations of the family were affected; of the 10 members affected, 4 had autopsy. The patients had a combination of progressive language disorder that resulted in a mute state within 5 years and additional features suggesting frontal lobe deficits or extrapyramidal symptoms. In a few of the members, corticospinal, motor neuron tract abnormalities were also found. Neary et al. (1993) described two brothers with familial progressive aphasia. They both became ill in their early 60s. In one of them, the illness remained purely an aphasic disturbance for 7 years, when he developed behavioral disorders. In the second sibling, a behavioral disorder occurred within months of the onset of the language difficulty. In the first case, the SPECT scan showed hypometabolism in the left hemisphere; in the second, bilateral anterior reduction in uptake was observed. Frontotemporal atrophy was found subsequently on postmortem examination. Histologic examination showed neuronal loss, gliosis, and superficial cortical spongiform change. Brown et al. (1996) described two families in which 14 individuals developed a dementia, aphasia, and neuropathological examination of one member from each family revealed swollen, achromatic neurons and corticobasal inclusion bodies.

REFERENCES

Alzheimer A (1907): Über eine eigenartige Erkrankung der Hirnrinde. Allg Z Psychiatry 64:146–148.

American Psychiatric Association (APA) (1987): Diagnostic and Statistical Manual of Mental Disorders (DSM-III-R). Washington, DC: American Psychiatric Association.

Appell J, Kertesz A, Fisman A (1982): A study of language functioning in Alzheimer patients. Brain Lang 17:73–91.

Bayles KA (1982): Language function in dementia. Brain Lang 16:265–280.

Becker JT, Huff FJ, Nebes RD, Holland A, Boller F (1988): Neuropsychological function in Alzheimer's disease: Pattern of impairment and rates of progression. Arch Neurol 45:263–268.

Benson DF, Zaias BW (1991): Progressive aphasia: A case with postmortem correlation. Neuropsychiatry Neuropsychol Behav Neurol 4:215–223.

Bergeron C, Pollanen MS, Weyer L, Black SE, Lang AE (1996): Unusual clinical presentations of cortical-basal ganglionic degeneration. Ann Neurol 40:893–900.

Brown J, Lantos P, Roques P, Fidani L, Rossor MN (1996): Familial dementia with swollen achromatic neurons and corticobasal inclusion bodies: A clinical and pathological study. J Neurol Sci 135:21–30.

Brun A (1987): Frontal lobe degeneration of the non-Alzheimer type: I. Neuropathology. Arch Gerontol Geriatr 6:193–208.

Cappa SF, Perani D, Messa C, Miozzo A, Fazio F (1996): Varieties of progressive non-fluent aphasia. Ann NY Acad Sci 777:243–248.

Caron M (1934): Etude clinique de la maladie Pick. Paris: Vigot.

Caselli RJ, Jack CR, Petersen RC, Wahner HW, Yanagihara T (1992): Asymmetric cortical degenerative syndromes: Clinical and radiologic correlations. Neurology 42:1462–1468.

Caselli RJ, Windebank AJ, Petersen RC (1993): Rapidly progressive aphasic dementia and motor neuron disease. Ann Neurol 33:200–207.

Chawluk JB, Mesulam M, Hurtig H, Kushner M, Weintraub S, Saykin A, Rubin N, Alavi A, Reivich M (1986): Slowly progressive aphasia without generalized dementia: Studies with positron emission tomography. Ann Neurol 19:68–74.

Cohen L, Benoit N, Van Eeckhout P, Ducarne B, Brunet P (1993): Pure progressive aphemia. J Neurol Neurosurg Psychiatry 56:923–924.

Cooper PN, Jackson M, Lennox G, Lowe J, Mann DMA (1995): τ-Ubiquitin and αB-crystallin—immunohistochemistry define the principal causes of degenerative frontotemporal dementia. Arch Neurol 52:1011–1015.

Croisile B, Trillet M (1990): Cerebral blood flow and transient global amnesia. J Neurol Neurosurg Psychiatry 53:361.

Duffy JR, Petersen RC (1992): Primary progressive aphasia. Aphasiology 6:1–15.

Faber-Langendoen K, Morris JC, Knesevich JW, LaBarge E, Miller P, Berg L (1988): Aphasia in senile dementia of the Alzheimer type. Ann Neurol 223:365–370.

Filley CM, Kelly J, Heaton RK (1986): Neuropsychologic features of early and late-onset Alzheimer's disease. Arch Neurol 43:574–576.

Folstein MF, Breitner JCS (1981): Language disorder predicts familial Alzheimer's disease. Johns Hopkins Med J 149:145–147.

Frisoni GB, Pizzolato G, Zanetti O, Bianchetti A, Chierichetti F, Trabucchi M (1995): Corticobasal degeneration: Neuropsychological assessment and dopamine D2 receptor SPECT analysis. Eur Neurol 35:50–54.

Fukui T, Sugita K, Kawamura M, Shiota J, Nakano I (1996): Primary progressive apraxia in Pick's disease: A clinicopathologic study. Neurology 47:467–473.

Gibb WRG, Luthert PJ, Marsden CD (1989): Corticobasal degeneration. Brain 112:1171–1192.

Graff-Radford NR, Damasio AR, Hyman BT, Hart MN, Tranel D, Damasio H, Van Hoesen GW, Rezai K (1990): Progressive aphasia in a patient with Pick's disease: A neuropsychological, radiologic, and anatomic study. Neurology 40:620–626.

Gustafson L (1987): Frontal lobe degeneration of non-Alzheimer type: II. Clinical picture and differential diagnosis. Arch Gerontol Geriatr 6:209–223.

Gustafson L, Brun A, Holmkvist AF, Risberg J (1985): Regional cerebral blood flow in degenerative frontal lobe dementia of non-Alzheimer type. J Cereb Blood Flow Metab 5:(Suppl 1):141–142.

Gustafson L, Brun A, Risberg J (1990): Frontal lobe dementia of non-alzheimer type. In Wurtman RJ, Corkin S, Growdon J, Ritter-Walker E (eds): Alzheimer's Disease. New York: Raven Press, pp 65–71.

Harasty JA, Halliday GM, Code C, Brooks WS (1996): Quantification of cortical atrophy in a case of progressive fluent aphasia. Brain 119:181–190.

Hart RP, Beach WA, Taylor JR (1997): A case of progressive apraxia of speech and non-fluent aphasia. Aphasiology 11:73–82.

Head H (1926): Aphasia and Kindred Disorders of Speech. Cambridge: Cambridge University Press.

Heutink P, Stevens M, Rizzu P, Bakker E, Kros JM, Tibben A, Niermeijer MF, van Duijn CM, Oostra BA, Van Swieten JC (1997): Hereditary frontotemporal dementia is linked to chromosome 17q21–q22: A genetic and clinicopathological study of three Dutch families. Ann Neurol 41:150–159.

Hodges JR, Patterson K, Oxbury S, Funnell E (1992): Semantic dementia: Progressive fluent aphasia with temporal lobe atrophy. Brain 115:1783–1806.

Holland AL, McBurney DH, Moossy J, Reinmuth OM (1985): The dissolution of language in Pick's disease with neurofibrillary tangles: A case study. Brain Lang 24:36–58.

Imura T (1943): Aphasia: Characteristic symptoms in Japanese. Psychiatr Neurol Jap 47:196–218.

Karbe H, Kertesz A, Polk M (1993): Profiles of language impairment in primary progressive aphasia. Arch Neurol 50:193–201.

Kertesz A, Appell J, Fisman M (1986): The dissolution of language in Alzheimer's disease. Can J Neurol Sci 13:415–418.

Kertesz A, Davidson W, McCabe P: Primary progressive semantic aphasia. J Int Neuropsychol Soc (in press).

Kertesz A, Hudson L, Mackenzie IRA, Munoz DG (1994): The pathology and nosology of primary progressive aphasia. Neurology 44:2065–2072.

Kertesz A, Polk M, Kirk A (1992): Visuoverbal dissociation and semantic deficit in dementia. J Clin Exp Neuropsychol 4:374.

Kim RC, Collins SH, Parisi JE, Wright AW, Chu YB (1981): Familial dementia of adult onset with pathologic findings of a "non-specific" nature. Brain 104:61–78.

Kirshner HS, Tanridag O, Thurman L, Whetsell WO (1987): Progressive aphasia without dementia: Two cases with focal spongiform degeneration. Ann Neurol 22:527–532.

Knopman DS, Mastri AR, Frey WH II, Sung JH, Rustan T (1990): Dementia lacking distinctive histologic features: A common non-Alzheimer degenerative dementia. Neurology 40:251–256.

Kosaka K (1976): On aphasia of Pick's disease—A review of our own 3 cases and 49 autopsy cases in Japan (in Japanese). Seishin Igaku 18:1181–1189, as quoted by Ohashi (1983).

Lang AE, Bergeron C, Pollanen MS, Ashby P (1992): Parietal Pick's disease mimicking cortical-basal ganglionic degeneration. Neurology 44:1436–1440.

Lüers T (1947): Ueber den Verfall der Sprache bei der Pickschen Krankheiten. (umschriebene Atrophie der Grosshirnrinde). Z Gesamte Neurol Psychiatry 179:94–131.

Lund and Manchester Groups (1994): Clinical and neuropathological criteria for frontotemporal dementia. J Neurol Neurosurg Psychiatry 57:416–418.

Malamud N, Boyd DA (1940): Pick's disease with atrophy of the temporal lobes: A clinico-pathological study. Arch Neurol Psychiatry 43:210–222.

Malamud N, Waggoner RW (1943): Genealogic and clinicopathologic study of Pick's disease. Arch Neurol Psychiatry 40:288–303.

McDaniel KD, Wagner MT, Greenspan BS (1991): The role of brain single photon emission computed tomography in the diagnosis of primary progressive aphasia. Arch Neurol 48:1257–1260.

McNeil MR, Small SL, Masterson RJ, Tepanta RD (1995): Behavioral and pharmacological treatment of lexical-semantic deficits in a single patient with primary progressive aphasia. Am J Speech Lang Pathol 4:76–93.

Mesulam MM (1982): Slowly progressive aphasia without dementia. Ann Neurol 11:592–598.

Mesulam MM (1987): Primary progressive aphasia—differentiation from Alzheimer's disease. Ann Neurol 22:533–534.

Mesulam MM, Weintraub S (1992): Primary progressive aphasia: Sharpening the focus on a clinical syndrome. In Boller F, Forette F, Khachturian Z, Poncet M, Christen Y (eds): Heterogeneity of Alzheimer's Disease. Berlin, Heidelberg: Springer-Verlag, pp 43–66.

Morris JC, Cole M, Banker BQ, Wright D (1984): Hereditary dysphasic dementia and the Pick-Alzheimer spectrum. Ann Neurol 16:455–466.

Neary D, Snowden JS, Bowen DM, Sims NR, Mann DMA, Benton JS, Northen B, Yates DO, Davison AN (1986): Cerebral biopsy in the investigation of presenile dementia due to cerebral atrophy. J Neurol Neurosurg Psychiatry 49:157–162.

Neary D, Snowden JS, Mann DMA (1993): Familial progressive aphasia: Its relationship to other forms of lobar atrophy. J Neurol Neurosurg Psychiatry 56:1122–1125.

Neary D, Snowden JS, Mann DMA, Northen B, Goulding PJ, Macdermott N (1990): Frontal lobe dementia and motor neurone disease. J Neurol Neurosurg Psychiatry 53:23–32.

Neary D, Snowden JS, Northen B, Goulding P (1988): Dementia of frontal lobe type. J Neurol Neurosurg Psychiatry 51:353–361.

Northen B, Hopcutt B, Griffiths H (1990): Progressive aphasia without generalized dementia: A case study. Aphasiology 4:55–65.

Ohashi H (1983): An aphasiologic approach to Pick's disease. In Hirano A, Miyoshi K. (eds): Neuropsychiatric Disorders in the Elderly. Tokyo: Igaku-Shoin, pp 132–135.

Parkin AJ (1993): Progressive aphasia without dementia—A clinical and cognitive neuropsychological analysis. Brain Lang 44:201–220.

Pick A (1892): Über die Beziehungen der senilen Hirnatrophie zur Aphasie. Prag Med Wochenschr 17:165–167.

Poeck K, Luzzatti D (1988): Slowly progressive aphasia in three patients. Brain 111:151–168.

Pogacar S, Williams RG (1984): Alzheimer's disease presenting as slowly progressive aphasia. RI Med J 67:181–185.

Rebeiz JJ, Kolodny EH, Richardson EP (1968): Corticodentatonigral degeneration with neuronal achromasia. Arch Neurol 18:20–33.

Rosenfeld M (1909): Die partielle Grosshirnatrophie. J Psychol Neurol 14:115–130.

Sakurai Y, Hashida H, Uesugi H, Arima K, Murayama S, Bando M, Iwata M, Momose T, Sakuta M (1996): A clinical profile of corticobasal degeneration presenting as primary progressive aphasia. Eur Neurol 36:134–137.

Schenk VWD (1958–1959): Re-examination of a family with Pick's disease. Ann Hum Genet 23:325–333.

Seltzer B, Sherwin I (1983): A comparison of clinical features in early and late-onset primary degenerative dementia. Arch Neurol 40:143–146.

Snowden JS, Goulding PJ, Neary D (1989): Semantic dementia: A form of circumscribed cerebral atrophy. Behav Neurol 2:167–182.

Snowden JS, Griffiths H, Neary D (1994): Semantic dementia: Autobiographical contribution to preservation of meaning. Cogn Neuropsychol 11:265–288.

Snowden JS, Neary D, Mann MA, Goulding PJ, Testa HJ (1992): Progressive language disorder due to lobar atrophy. Ann Neurol 31:174–183.

Tanabe H, Ikeda M, Nakagawa Y, et al. (1992): Gogi (word meaning) aphasia and semantic memory for words. High Brain Funct Res 12:153–167.

Tariska I (1970): Circumscribed cerebral atrophy in Alzheimer's disease: A pathological study. In Wolstenhome GEW, O'Connor M (eds): Alzheimer Disease and Related Conditions. London: J & A Churchill, pp 51–69.

Thompson CK, Ballard KJ, Tait ME, Weintraub S, Mesulam M (1997): Patterns of language decline in non-fluent primary progressive aphasia. Aphasiology 11:297–321.

Thompson PD, Marsden CD (1992): Corticobasal degeneration. In Baillière T (ed): Ballière's Clinical Neurology. pp 677–686. London: Baillière Tindall.

Tissot R, Constantinidis J, Richard J (1985): Pick's disease. In Frederiks JAM (ed): Handbook of Clinical Neurology, Vol 46. Amsterdam: Elsevier Science, pp 233–246.

Tolnay M, Probst A (1995): Frontal lobe degeneration: Novel ubiquitin-immunoreactive neurites within frontotemporal cortex. Neuropathol Appl Neurobiol 21:492–497.

Turner RS, Kenyon LC, Trojanowski JQ, Gonatas N, Grossman M (1996): Clinical, neuroimaging, and pathologic features of progressive nonfluent aphasia. Ann Neurol 39:166–173.

Tyrell PJ, Kartsounis LD, Frackowiak RSJ, Findley LJ, Rossor MN (1991): Progressive loss of speech output and orofacial dyspraxia associated with frontal lobe hypometabolism. J Neurol Neurosurg Psychiatry 54:351–357.

Tyrell PJ, Warrington EK, Frackowiak RSJ, Rossor MN (1990): Heterogeneity in progressive aphasia due to focal cortical atrophy. Brain 113:1321–1336.

Wechsler AF (1977): Presenile dementia presenting as aphasia. J Neurol Neurosurg Psychiatry 40:303–305.

Wechsler AF, Verity A, Rosenschein S, Fried I, Scheibel AB (1982): Pick's disease. A clinical, computed tomographic, and histologic study with Golgi impregnation observations. Arch Neurol 39:287–290.

Weintraub S, Rubin NP, Mesulam M (1990): Primary progressive aphasia: Longitudinal course, neuropsychological profile, and language features. Arch Neurol 47:1329–1335.

Yamamoto H, Tanabe H, Kashiwagi A, Ikejiri Y, Fukyuama H, Okuda J, Shiraishi J, Nishimura T (1990): A case of slowly progressive aphasia without generalized dementia in a Japanese patient. Acta Neurol Scand 82:102–105.

CHAPTER 7

Semantic Dementia

JOHN R. HODGES, PETER GARRARD, and KARALYN PATTERSON

University of Cambridge Neurology Unit, Addenbrooke's Hospital (J.R.H., P.G.) Cambridge CB2 2QQ, United Kingdom, and MRC Applied Psychology Unit, 15 Chaucer Road, Cambridge (J.R.H., K.P.) CB2 2EF, United Kingdom

INTRODUCTION

In tracing the origins of the term *semantic dementia,* it is necessary to draw on three initially separate bodies of neurological and neuropsychological literature: those relating to Pick's disease (PiD), progressive aphasia, and semantic memory impairment.

Although the name of Arnold Pick is most often associated with progressive frontal lobe degeneration, one of his earliest published case reports drew attention to the association between progressive aphasia and temporal lobe atrophy (Pick, 1892). This celebrated paper describes a 71-year-old man with a 2-year history of gradual behavioral deterioration and a later disturbance of speech and language in whom a post-mortem examination showed diffuse atrophy of the left hemisphere, particularly marked in the temporal region. It was only in subsequent papers (Pick, 1906) that Pick turned his attention to the clinical syndromes associated with frontal atrophy. In 1911 Alois Alzheimer, shortly after describing the intraneuronal plaques and extracellular tangles associated with his name, reported neuronal swelling and argyrophilic inclusions in a patient with focal lobar atrophy (Alzheimer, 1911). These distinctive histological features later become known as *Pick cells* and *Pick bodies.*

The first half of this century saw a profusion of reports in PiD, most of which concentrated on the pathological features (Lowenberg et al., 1939; Akelaitis, 1944; Neumann, 1949; Malamud and Boyd, 1997). Over the same period, clinical interest began to shift from the temporal to the frontal lobes, but among the early case reports are a number of descriptions of the phenomena associated with temporal lobe atrophy. Following the terminology of the day, such patients were described as exhibiting *psychic blindness, transcortical sensory aphasia,* or *amnesia verborum* (Pick, 1904; Mingazzini, 1914). It is unclear what degree of descriptive precision is invested in these terms but, as we shall see, they seem peculiarly appropriate to clinical features that can now be united under the heading of *semantic dementia.*

Pick's Disease and Pick Complex, Edited by Andrew Kertesz and David G. Munoz
ISBN 0-471-17792-X ©1998 Wiley-Liss, Inc.

The period after 1950 is characterized by a general lack of interest, at least among neurologists, in dementia syndromes. To take up the story of semantic dementia, it is therefore necessary to turn to the neuropsychological literature. Warrington was among the first to appreciate the scientific potential of studying the pattern of cognitive deficits shown by patients with neurodegenerative diseases. She described three patients with progressive anomia accompanied by a loss of word and picture comprehension in the absence of deficits in the phonological or syntactic aspects of language, perceptual or visuospatial abilities, or day-to-day (episodic) memory. Drawing on Tulving's newly proposed psychological distinction (Tulving, 1972) between memory for experienced events and knowledge about the world (*episodic* and *semantic memory* in his terminology), she argued that these patients exhibited selective breakdown of semantic memory (Warrington, 1975). This novel formulation represented a departure from the earlier practice of classifying such patients as having either visual associative agnosia (De Renzi et al., 1969) or transcortical sensory aphasia and took into consideration the fact that their difficulties spanned both verbal and visual domains.

Schwartz et al. (1979) described a very similar patient, W.L.P., a few years later and again documented a profound loss of semantic knowledge in the presence of a relatively well-preserved appreciation of the syntactic aspects of language. While these studies had a profound impact on cognitive and experimental neuropsychology, their relevance to studies of dementia in general, and to PiD in particular, went largely unnoticed. Warrington's patients were simply said to have "cerebral atrophy" and W.L.P. "a form of dementia." Essentially all authorities would now agree on a diagnosis of semantic dementia in each of these patients. Moreover, two of Warrington's patients were subsequently shown at postmortem to have classic Pick's pathology (Hodges et al., 1992).

We turn, then, to the third piece of this jigsaw puzzle: primary progressive aphasia. In 1982, neurological interest in the progressive aphasic syndromes was rekindled by Mesulam's publication of six cases of progressive deterioration of language in the absence of generalized dementia (Mesulam, 1982). With one exception,[1] these patients had in common a predominant disturbance of language output characterized by anomia, with preservation of language comprehension in at least one modality (spoken or written). In spontaneous discourse, word production was noted to be sparse in four, and in all cases computed tomography (CT) scanning demonstrated focal atrophy of the left perisylvian region.

Interest in these syndromes grew rapidly, and within a decade over 100 cases had been added to the literature. One insight to emerge from this wealth of clinical material was that progressive aphasia is a far from homogeneous entity (Tyrrell et al., 1990). Quite apart from the variety of sites of cortical damage and histological patterns, there were also obvious clinical differences. Although anomia was an almost universal finding, the degree of disturbance of the semantic, syntactic, and phonological aspects of spoken and written language abilities varied considerably from individual to individual. One of the clearest ways of subdividing patients is according to whether their spontaneous speech is fluent or nonfluent. Patients with nonfluent progressive aphasia have deficits in the phonological and syntactic aspects of language, and in some respects resemble classic Broca's aphasics. By contrast, it became apparent that patients with progressive fluent aphasia do not conform to the complementary syndrome of Wernicke's aphasia but rather show a progressive loss of knowledge of word meaning of the type classically found in amnestic aphasia (Poeck and Luzzatti, 1988). A key paper in the further characterization of the cognitive deficit underlying the progressive anomia and word comprehension seen in such patients was that of Snowden et al. (1989). This report describes three patients

[1]A 17-year-old female who presented with pure word deafness and showed only limited progression over the next 10 years.

TABLE 7.1 **Core Features of Semantic Dementia**

1. Selective impairment of semantic memory causing severe anomia, impaired spoken and written single-word comprehension, reduced generation of exemplars on category fluency tests, and an impoverished fund of general knowledge about objects, people, and the meanings of words.
2. Relative sparing of other components of language output and comprehension, notably syntax and phonology.
3. Normal perceptual skills and nonverbal problem-solving ability.
4. Relatively preserved autobiographical and day-to-day (episodic) memory.

with a progressive breakdown in the semantic components of language, evidenced by a loss of appreciation of the meanings of both words and objects. In all patients, spontaneous speech was anomic but fluent (i.e., normal with respect to articulation, phonation, prosody, syntax, and rate of production). Following Warrington (1975) and Schwartz et al. (1979), they interpreted this pattern of findings as indicating a loss of language at the level of representational knowledge and proposed the term *semantic dementia* to encapsulate the key features of the syndrome.

In 1992 five very similar cases were reported by Hodges et al. (1992), who proposed criteria for the diagnosis of semantic dementia (see Table 7.1), drew attention to the consistent association with left temporal lobe atrophy, and suggested that this form of progressive aphasia represented a form of PiD. More recently, we have contrasted the neuropsychological profile of semantic dementia with that found in patients with progressive nonfluent aphasia (Hodges and Patterson, 1996), and have also explored aspects of the organization of semantic memory and related cognitive domains in these patients (Graham et al., 1995; Graham and Hodges, 1977).

The remainder of this chapter will deal with the major clinical features of the syndrome of semantic dementia before going on to discuss some of the theoretical neuropsychological issues it also serves to highlight.

CLINICAL FEATURES

Progressive problems with language occur in the context of dementia of Alzheimer type (DAT) (Appell et al., 1982; Bayles and Tomoeda, 1983; Nebes, 1989; Chertkow and Bub, 1990; Hodges et al., 1990, 1991); progressive nonfluent aphasia, and semantic dementia. Table 7.2 summarizes the principal clinical differences between these three groups of patients. It is easily appreciated that there is potential for considerable overlap between these groups (Pogacar and Williams, 1984), though many of the borderline cases can be assigned to another clinical category on the basis of longitudinal clinical and neuropsychological evaluation.

The majority of individuals in all three groups present with symptoms of memory difficulty, and an important first task for the clinician is to establish whether this refers to problems with recalling words and/or names (semantic memory) or events (episodic memory). Most patients with semantic dementia, or their relatives, will recognize the phrase *word-finding difficulties* as being an appropriate description of their problems, and a few also report the progressive decline in word comprehension that is apparent on formal testing. Anomia is also a well-recognized feature of DAT, but it is rarely a prominent feature early on and is virtually always overshadowed by impairment of new learning. The opposite pattern (loss of semantic knowledge with relatively preserved episodic memory) strongly favors a diagnosis of semantic dementia. Patients with semantic dementia are well oriented and demonstrate good recall

TABLE 7.2 Comparison of the Clinical Features of Semantic Dementia, Progressive Nonfluent Aphasia, and DAT

	Semantic Dementia	Progressive Nonfluent Aphasia	Alzheimer-Type Dementia
Age at onset	Commonly <65	Commonly <65	Usually >65
Disease progression	Generally rapid	Slow	Variable
Spontaneous speech	Fluent and grammatically correct, but empty of content words	Labored and telegraphic, with long word-finding pauses and frequent phonological and grammatical errors	Initially normal in most instances
Paraphasias	Semantic	Phonological	Semantic (early) Phonological (late)
Comprehension			
Single words	Impaired	Intact	Initially intact
Syntax	Intact	Impaired	Initially intact
Repetition	Normal for single words	Phonemic errors	Generally intact
Episodic memory	Preserved for recent events	Intact	Severely impaired early in course
Frontal "executive" functions	Intact in early stages	Intact	May be impaired
Visuospatial and perceptual skills	Intact	Intact	Often impaired from early in course, sometimes severely
Behavior	Appropriate initially, but frontal features invariably appear later	Appropriate until very late	Normal in early stages but commonly disturbed in later stages
General neurological findings	Usually none	Buccofacial apraxia and unilateral limb signs commonly seen	Usually normal until the late stage
MRI findings	Focal temporal lobe atrophy, often worse on the left	Left perisylvian atrophy	Hippocampal atrophy

of recent life events, even though their language difficulties result in poor performance on bedside and formal tests of verbal memory. We have recently shown that the apparent preservation of episodic memory is in fact temporally modulated: while memory for recent autobiographical events is indeed spared, patients show marked impairment in recalling early life memories. This pattern is the opposite of that found in DAT patients, who perform particularly poorly on tests of recent autobiographical memory (Graham and Hodges, 1997).

Disturbance of personality, behavior, and social conduct often occurs in the later stages of the disease, either because of the development of advanced bilateral temporal lobe atrophy resulting in emergence of the Klüver-Bucy syndrome (sexual disinhibition and hyperorality) (Cummings and Duchen, 1981; Mendez et al., 1993) or because of spread of the pathology to involve the frontal lobes. There is certainly some clinical overlap between progressive frontal lobe atrophy and semantic dementia—we have encountered patients with features of both syndromes at presentation—and the Lund and Manchester groups have proposed that cases of focal frontal and/or temporal lobar atrophy should be regarded as forming part of a unifying clinical spectrum, which they have termed *fronto-temporal lobar degeneration* (Brun et al., 1994). In the future, this may turn out to be an anatomically correct description of the natural history of certain types of degenerative brain disease but, as illustrated in Figure 7.1, it obscures differences that remain important to unresolved issues of clinical taxonomy.

With regard to features of the language disturbance in semantic dementia, patients' speech is superficially normal, with preservation of syntactic constructions. Word-finding pauses and semantic errors may be prominent, but phonological errors never occur. At the most advanced stages, when the vocabulary has been reduced to a few words and phrases, grammatical structure may still be remarkably good, though highly stereotyped. In sharp contrast, progressive nonfluent aphasics have halting and distorted, or "telegraphic," speech and a tendency to make syntactic and prominent phonological errors (Mesulam, 1982; Mesulam and Weintraub, 1992; Grossman et al., 1996; Hodges and Patterson, 1996). Their ability to understand spoken or written language is, by comparison, relatively preserved. The following transcripts of spontaneous speech from (1) a nonfluent aphasic and (2) a patient with semantic dementia serve to illustrate these differences. (The phonological errors of the nonfluent patient are underlined, with our interpretation of the likely target word shown in parentheses.)

> 1. **Examiner**: *Could you tell me something about your holiday in Norway?*
> **Patient**: *Er* [holding up nine fingers] *nides* (= nine days) *and an aeropload* (= aeroplane) *have flow and a mawnd bandelez and er the* (unintelligible) *When we came out a coach and took ud* (= us) *all round hoadle* (= hotel) *three days and er we a coach er two days and a splip ote and er ote five days it was all right.* (giving "thumbs up" sign).

> 2. **Patient** (on being a shown a picture of a soldier): *Oh gosh, this seems to be, oh come on, try to remember the name; I know what they are 'cause there's, oh gosh, I'm saying there's three of these, so it's not the two and three, it's the one which, er . . . Some of them will be in Britain because, er, you know with our stuff in Britain, some of them are also outside Britain, some of them are also in Britain as well. What d'you call them again because N.'s son, no not son, his brother, he's one of these as well. So tell me what these are . . . .*

Single-word repetition is typically well preserved in semantic dementia, while ability to repeat sentences (McCarthy and Warrington, 1987) or short strings of unrelated words (Patterson et al., 1994) may depend on the patient's level of comprehension: with strings of words for which the patient's knowledge of meaning is degraded, migration of phonological segments may occur (e.g., *mint, rug → rint, mug*). Patients with semantic dementia are good at reading "regular" words, whose pronunciations can be determined by knowledge of typical spelling-to-sound correspondences. By contrast, many patients with semantic dementia tend to "regularize" pronunciation when reading exception words (e.g., reading *pint* to rhyme with *mint, flint*, etc.)—a pattern of reading impairment termed *surface dyslexia* (Hodges et al., 1992). The reading errors in surface dyslexia depend strongly on both word frequency (Patterson and Hodges, 1992) and degree of irregularity (Patterson et al., 1997). For instance, the word *have* (a high-frequency exception word) is rarely regularized (to rhyme with *cave, save*, etc.), while a lower-frequency exception word such as *pint* often yields regularization errors. We have argued that both the phonological errors in multiword repetition and the regularization errors in reading may be due to reduced interactive activation between semantic and phonological representations (Patterson et al., 1997). In addition to the reading disorder, patients typically demonstrate an analogous disorder of writing—surface dysgraphia (i.e., a disproportionate difficulty in written and oral spelling of words with an atypical sound-to-spelling correspondence), for example, spelling *honest* as *onnist*.

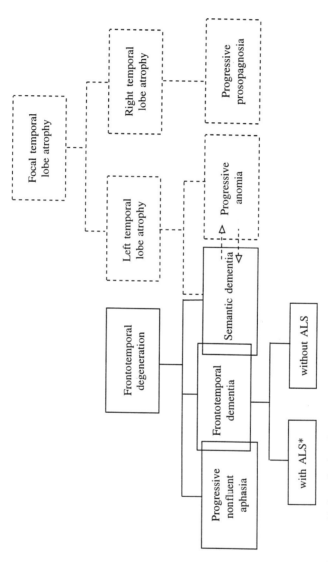

* Amyotrophic lateral sclerosis

FIGURE 7.1. *Solid lines*: classification of lobar atrophy syndromes under the rubric of frontotemporal lobar degeneration following the Lund and Manchester groups (1994). Dotted lines: other clinically important related headings.

One practical implication of surface dyslexia concerns the patients' poor performance on the low-frequency irregular words of the National Adult Reading Test (NART) (Nelson, 1982). Estimates of premorbid IQ are often based on the NART, but in semantic dementia this would obviously lead to an underestimation of intellectual ability.

Inventories such as the Mini Mental State Examination (MMSE) (Folstein et al., 1975) have traditionally been used to screen for cognitive deficits in the setting of the neurology clinic or bedside examination. However, although they are valuable in documenting the severity and progression of dementia, they are insensitive tools and poorly discriminant of the various clinically important domains of cognitive functioning. Many patients with semantic dementia, and indeed in the early stages of DAT, score above 24/30 on the MMSE, the traditional cutoff score for normality.

In the assessment of patients with progressive aphasia or suspected DAT, it is much better to use specifically targeted clinical tests. Perhaps the simplest of these are letter and category fluency tests. In the former, a subject is asked to think of as many different words as possible within a minute, excluding proper names, beginning with a given letter (*F, A,* and *S* are usually used). In semantic category-based fluency tests, subjects generate as many examples as possible from given categories (e.g., animals, household items, fruit). Normal subjects generate 20 or more examples from each category and slightly fewer words on the letter fluency task. In semantic dementia (and to a lesser extent in DAT) there is disproportionate impairment of category fluency. In nonfluent progressive aphasia and subcortical dementias (e.g., progressive supranuclear palsy, Huntington's disease) the opposite pattern is seen, reflecting greater phonological and executive demands of the letter-based test (Rosser and Hodges, 1994).

Confrontation naming is always impaired in semantic dementia; patients show substantial deficits on standard tests of naming such as the Boston Naming Test (Kaplan et al., 1983) and often fail to score at all on more stringent tests (such as the Graded Naming Test). In contrast to patients with nonfluent aphasia, their errors are typically of the semantic variety—either superordinate (calling all four-legged creatures "animal") or category coordinate (calling a giraffe a "horse" or a window a "door"). They also show a tendency to use high-frequency prototypical labels (e.g., "dog" or "cat" for most animals). Visuoperceptual errors (calling a glove a "hand"), however, are typically absent. Since the naming deficit reflects a central disorder of semantic knowledge, patients are equally or even more impaired on tests of naming to definition (e.g., "what do we call the small green animal that hops about in ponds?").

Understanding of conversational language may appear normal but, when formally tested, patients are typically impaired on tests of single-word comprehension such as word–picture matching, with a tendency to choose semantically related foils. For instance, when faced with an array consisting of six pictures of animals and asked to "point to the tiger" they may choose a lion or even a cat.

Other tests of semantic knowledge on which these patients are impaired include generating definitions in response to a spoken word and verifying semantic attributes (Warrington, 1975; Hodges et al., 1992). It should be noted that the deficit is *not* confined to verbally based tests of semantics; patients also show marked impairment on purely pictorial tasks such as the Pyramids and Palm Trees Test (Howard and Patterson, 1992), as well as tests of picture sorting (Hodges et al., 1992), color knowledge (Hodges et al., 1992), and knowledge about people using pictures of famous faces. These findings provide compelling evidence that the disorder is one of central semantic knowledge.

Scores on tests of semantic knowledge are sometimes disproportionately higher for one category of items than another; the most extensively documented dissociations are between living things and manufactured items (Warrington, 1975; McCarthy and Warrington, 1988; Barbarotto et al., 1995) and between concrete and abstract nouns (Breedin et al., 1994). As noted above, performance on semantic tasks appears to be sensitive to the frequency and familiarity of the test items (*dog, cat,* and *horse* are always more likely to be named, understood, and defined than *goat, crocodile,* and *hippopotamus*), and an explanation of class-specific impairment based on word and concept familiarity has been advanced (Funnell and Sheridan, 1992). One problem with this position, however, is that the direction of the advantage does not always conform to its predictions. For instance, abstract nouns are in general much less frequently encountered in spoken language than concrete nouns, and some classes of manufactured items (such as vehicles) are far more frequently encountered than almost any living creature, yet examples of both of these dissociations favoring the *less* familiar category have been documented (Sacchett and Humphreys, 1992; Gainotti et al., 1995). Possible explanations for category-specific advantages in terms of the cognitive organization of knowledge will be discussed in more detail in the next section.

In contrast to the breakdown in word meaning, there is usually preservation on tests that assess the comprehension of syntax, such as the Test for the Reception of Grammar (TROG) (Bishop, 1989), which uses a simple vocabulary (*boy, dog, red, big, chase,* etc.) to form increasingly complex sentences (i.e., from simple, two-element sentences such as *the dog is sitting* to embedded sentences such as *the boy the dog chases is big*).

Normal or near-normal performance is also seen on tests of auditory-verbal short-term memory (digit span), nonverbal problem solving (Raven's Progressive Matrices [Raven, 1962]), visuospatial abilities (Rey-Osterreith complex figure [Lezak, 1983], judgment of line orientation [Benton et al., 1983]), and nonverbal memory (e.g., memory for designs or the faces component of the Recognition Memory Test [Warrington, 1984]). A summary of the core neuropsychological features of semantic dementia is presented in Table 7.2.

Although the clinical and neuropsychological picture of patients with focal temporal lobe atrophy most commonly conforms to the profile of semantic dementia outlined above, variant forms have also been described. Some patients with left-sided atrophy may show a purely anomic syndrome with very poor naming in the absence of any major semantic or phonological deficits. One such patient (F.M.) has been the subject of intense investigation and has been characterized as showing insufficient activation of phonology by meaning (Graham et al., 1995). A second patient (V.H.) presented with a progressive prosopagnosia that evolved into a loss of person-specific semantic knowledge (Evans et al., 1995). The initial locus of damage in the latter case was the right temporal lobe. This raises questions about the role of the right hemisphere in semantic processing, which will be considered in more detail later.

PROGNOSIS

The prognosis for patients with semantic dementia is variable. In our experience, based on approximately 20 patients seen over the last 6 years, the outlook is generally poor, with rather rapid progression: of the five patients we reported in 1992 (Hodges et al., 1992), two have since died and two others have progressed to a state of fairly advanced global dementia. Over time, the disease spreads to involve nonsemantically based aspects of cognition (e.g., spatial abilities, short-term memory). Changes in behavior, personality, and social conduct are also prominent, and many of the features that characterize dementia of the frontal lobe type appear with time. A recurring theme, observed in several of our patients who have reached this stage, is a striking fixation on food and time, resulting in absolute rigidity in matters connected with meals and mealtimes. J.L., for instance, began to insist on eating king prawns at the same Chinese restaurant every Saturday and sometimes, in his impatience to get to the restaurant, would advance all the clocks in the house to the usual departure time (Hodges et al., 1995). Similar observations are mentioned in one other series of patients with severe bilateral temporal lobe atrophy, all with PiD confirmed at post mortem (Cummings and Duchen, 1981).

RADIOLOGICAL FINDINGS

The role of structural and functional brain imaging in the differential diagnosis of neurodegenerative diseases remains to be fully established. CT is generally helpful in excluding other forms of pathology but is insensitive to the presence of focal lobar atrophy. In semantic dementia, magnetic resonance imaging (MRI) has shown that the focus of atrophy is the pole and the inferolateral regions of one or both temporal lobes. The left temporal lobe is invariably involved, but the disease is frequently bilateral (see Figure 7.2). In contrast to the often striking atrophy of the temporal neocortex, the hippocampus and parahippocampal gyrus are usually spared, at least in the early stages of the disease—a finding that is relevant to the preservation of recent episodic memory, discussed earlier.

Cases in which serial imaging has been performed suggest that, with progression of the disease, the tendency is toward additional involvement of the contralateral hemisphere (Graff-Radford et al., 1990). In our series, the majority of cases with bilateral disease show more left-

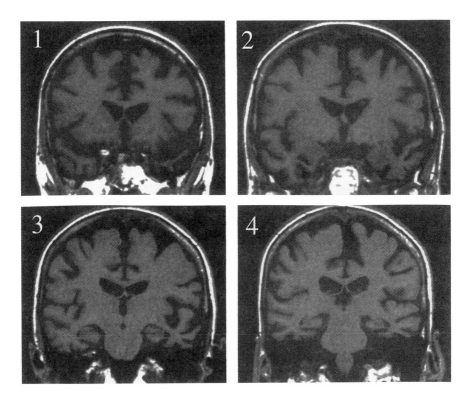

FIGURE 7.2. Coronal T_1-weighted MR images through the temporal lobes showing atrophy of the left pole and anterior temporal region (1, 2). In the more posterior cuts (3, 4) the atrophy involves the inferolateral region. Note the sparing of the hippocampus.

sided atrophy; this preponderance of left-sided cases, which has been commented on before (Mansvelt, 1954), remains unexplained. It has been argued that symptoms referable to the right temporal lobe are of less functional significance; but if the higher frequency of left-sided cases only reflects this difference, then there should be no disparity, as left temporal lobe atrophy should just as frequently follow right temporal lobe atrophy as precede it. Differential vulnerability of the two hemispheres to the disease process therefore cannot be ruled out at this stage.

In addition to indicating the site of the atrophy, MRI scanning is helpful in documenting its progression over time, as well as the concomitant involvement of other brain regions, particularly with the development of features that cannot be ascribed to temporal lobe dysfunction. Precision in judging the degree of atrophy is, however, difficult, and proper quantification of both the degree of atrophy and the site of maximal involvement must therefore await formal validation of a volumetric technique akin to that used in structural assessments of the hippocampi (Fox et al., 1996).

Functional imaging techniques such as single photon emission computed tomography (SPECT) and positron emission tomography (PET), which detect changes in regional brain metabolism, are potentially much more sensitive methods. Early reports documented a marked heterogeneity in the pattern of results obtained (Kempler et al., 1990; Tyrrell et al., 1990); but such studies were hampered by the fact that the clinical heterogeneity of the progressive aphasic syndromes was not appreciated until later. In particular, the study of Tyrrell et al. contained six patients with progressive aphasic syndromes, at least two of whom had semantic dementia, while another two clearly showed signs of the nonfluent variety. In our series, all patients have shown focal left hypoperfusion on SPECT, often before changes are apparent on MRI (Sinnatamby et al., 1996). In one of our patients with advanced semantic dementia (P.P.), PET changes were confined to the left temporal and inferior parietal regions (Patterson et al., 1994).

PATHOLOGY

A fully developed account of the relationship between aphasic syndromes, other focal lobar atrophies, and the diseases that give rise to them is made difficult not only by the problems of clinical classification, but also by the variety of pathological processes that might underlie a single clinical and radiological picture. The three main histological patterns commonly described in pathological discussions of focal lobar atrophy are (1) nonspecific spongiform degeneration or microvacuolation and neuronal loss; (2) the same changes with additional histological markers of PiD (i.e., intraneuronal argyrophilic inclusion bodies and/or ballooned neurons); and (3) the amyloid plaques and neurofibrillary tangles characteristic of Alzheimer's disease(AD).

In semantic dementia, the focus of pathology is invariably found to be the left temporal lobe, particularly the polar region and the inferolateral aspects, though reports vary over exactly which structures are involved and which spared. Most cases demonstrate abnormalities in both the white and gray matter of the temporal lobes, with some showing additional changes in the orbitomedial frontal and/or parietal regions. (Cummings and Duchen, 1981). The question of whether the hippocampal formation is consistently involved remains open; some cases are reported as showing prominent and severe atrophy and inclusion bodies in this region (Graff-Radford et al., 1990) and others complete normality (Scheltens et al., 1990; Scholten et al., 1994; Harasty et al., 1996). Similar considerations apply to the basal ganglia. Table 7.3 summarizes the pathological findings in all known published cases meeting the clinical criteria for semantic dementia in which histological data are available. It can be seen that the majority of cases reported to date have shown non-Alzheimer pathology, and in a proportion Pick bodies have been present.

TABLE 7.3 Summary of All Published Cases of Semantic Dementia[1] with Pathological Diagnoses

Patient ID Sex Age at Onset Duration of Illness	Clinical Syndrome [Authors' Diagnosis]	Imaging Data	Path
Warrington (1975) E.M. Female 58 ? years	Deteriorating memory for 3 yr; fluent speech with impoverished vocabulary; severe anomia; circumlocutions; impaired single-word comprehension. [Selective loss of semantic memory]	Air encephalogram: mild cortical atrophy	probable PiD (Warrington, personal communication)
Do. C.R. Male 59 8 years	Loss of professional knowledge (industrial chemistry) resulting in retirement 1 yr earlier; fluent speech with occasional word-finding difficulty; mildly disordered syntax; severe anomia; impaired single-word comprehension; later, Kluver-Bucy syndrome [Selective loss of semantic memory]	CT: diffuse ventricular enlargement and sulcal widening (Cummings and Duchen, 1981)	PiD (Cummings and Duchen, 1981)
Cummings & Duchen (1981) Case 2 Female 61 10 years	Difficulty remembering names of people, places, and things for 18 mo; personality change; word-finding difficulty in spontaneous speech; hyperoral; later, akinetic-rigid syndrome [Kluver-Bucy syndrome and prominent language impairment]	CT: dilatation of lateral ventricles and widening of cerebral sulci, most markedly in left anterior temporal region	PiD
Do. Case 5 Male 47 11 years	Gradual personality change; word-finding difficulties and problems understanding spoken language; anomic [Kluver-Bucy syndrome and prominent language impairment]	Air encephalogram: dilated ventricles, cortical atrophy, worse on left.	PiD
Poeck & Luzzatti (1988) Case 2 (H.S.) Male 56	Forgetfulness and word-finding problems; fluent, stereotypic, clichéd speech; impaired single-word comprehension; surface dysgraphia, surface dyslexia; progressed to highly automatized speech, akinetic rigid	CT: marked bilateral temporal lobe atrophy, more marked on the left. MRI: D0.	DLDH (Schwartz et al., 1997)

(continued)

Table 7.3 (continued)

Patient ID / Sex / Age at Onset / Duration of Illness	Clinical Syndrome [Authors' Diagnosis]	Imaging Data	Path
14 years	state, and Kluver-Bucy syndrome (De Bleser et al., 1996) [Primary progressive aphasia]		Awaited
McCarthy & Warrington (1988) T.O.B. Male 61 10 years	Deteriorating expressive language and comprehension for 4 yr; fluent speech with impoverished vocabulary; severe anomia; circumlocutions; impaired single-word comprehension [Semantic dementia]	CT: normal MRI: left perisylvian atrophy PET: hypometabolism in left posterior frontal, superior middle, and inferior temporal regions (Tyrrell et al., 1990)	
Graff-Radford et al (1990) Male 59 6 years	Difficulty recalling names of people and objects; fluent, grammatical speech; severe anomia; intact single-word comprehension [Progressive fluent aphasia]	MRI: atrophy of anterior one-third of both temporal lobes; severe on left, moderate on right SPECT: reduced rCBF in left temporal lobe only	PiD
Hodges et al. (1992) P.P. Female 66 5 years	Difficulty remembering names of people, places, and things for 2 yr; fluent, grammatical speech with severe word-finding difficulty and frequent semantic paraphasias; severe anomia; impaired single-word comprehension; letter-by-letter alexia [Semantic dementia]	MRI: atrophy, more marked in left hemisphere, particularly around sylvian fissure PET: left inferior frontal and temporoparietal hypometabolism	PiD (Hodges, unpublished data)

Reference / Patient	Clinical features	Imaging	Histology
Do. J.L. Male 60 5 years	Difficulty remembering names of people, places, and things for 2 yr; fluent grammatical speech with occasional word-finding difficulty and semantic paraphasias; severe anomia; impaired single-word comprehension; surface dyslexia and dysgraphia; later, some features of Kluver-Bucy syndrome. [Semantic dementia]	MRI: striking atrophy of both temporal lobes, more marked on the right SPECT: bilateral temporal lobe hypoperfusion	PiD (Hodges et al., 1995)
Snowden et al. (1992) Case 7 (E.B.) Female 58 5 years	Difficulties with word finding and recognizing previously familiar people for 2 yr; fluent, grammatical speech; anomia; impaired single-word comprehension; surface dyslexia and dysgraphia. [Progressive fluent aphasia]	CT: widening of both sylvian fissures; ventricular enlargement SPECT: bifrontal hypoperfusion	DLDH
Scheltens et al. (1994) Male 59 13 years	Difficulties comprehending spoken language, and spontaneous paraphasias for 5 yr; fluent but meaningless speech; anomia; impaired single-word comprehension; later, behavioral disturbance [Progressive fluent aphasia]	CT: progressive widening of both sylvian fissures MRI: severe bilateral temporal lobe atrophy	DLDH
Scholten et al. (1994) Female 60 10 years	Word-finding difficulty for 4 yr; fluent, grammatical circumlocutory speech; anomic; impaired single-word comprehension. [Progressive fluent aphasia]	MRI: bilateral temporal lobe atrophy, more pronounced on the left	DLDH
Harasty et al. (1994) E.M. Female 65 4 years	Difficulty remembering names and aspects of daily activities; semantic difficulties in conversation; intact syntax, grammar, and phonology; later, signs of disinhibition requiring institutional care. [Progressive fluent aphasia]	None reported	DLDH

Abbreviations: PiD = Pick's disease; DLDH = dementia lacking distinctive histology.

[1] We include under this heading cases that appear retrospectively to meet diagnostic criteria for semantic dementia.

EXPERIMENTAL ASPECTS

A disease process that selectively and progressively disrupts semantic knowledge while leaving other areas of cognition largely intact represents a valuable experimental model for the neuropsychological study of language and memory. Over the past 5 years, the study of patients with semantic dementia has been of enormous value in approaching some of the fundamental issues surrounding the organization of knowledge in the brain. We will deal here with two such issues.

The Cognitive Organization of Knowledge

It was observed earlier that patients with semantic impairment show a distinctive pattern of errors on naming tests, characterized by the occurrence of semantically related labels. Moreover, longitudinal evaluation has revealed that the type of semantic error may change in an orderly fashion with progression of the disease (Hodges et al., 1995). For example, at presentation a patient may respond to a picture of an elephant with an appropriate circumlocution (such as "a large African animal") or a semantically close associate (such as "giraffe"); months later, the response may change to the name of a highly familiar exemplar from the appropriate category (such as "horse"); and at very late stages, only the category name (i.e., "animal") may be produced. A parallel finding is that on tests of attributional knowledge, such as picture or word sorting, failure to judge finer-grained distinctions (e.g., sorting animals into fierce and nonfierce varieties) often precedes failure on category-level decisions (e.g., sorting animals into land animals, birds, and water creatures), and performance on superordinate-level distinctions (e.g., sorting items into living things and artifacts) is preserved until relatively late (Hodges et al., 1995). These phenomena have been interpreted by some as representing evidence of a hierarchical structure in the organization of semantic knowledge (Warrington, 1975).

A hierarchically structured system can be visualized as a branching tree, at the origin of which is the most inclusive, and at the periphery the most selective, designation of knowledge about a concept. This idea, first proposed by Collins and Quillian (1969), was originally based on the reaction times of normal subjects when performing categorization tasks. The tendency for patients with semantic dementia to apply a few superordinate labels to a wide range of distinct exemplars is cited as evidence that the process of categorization stops at the limits of a disintegrating hierarchy, in which the most peripheral elements are most vulnerable to damage.

One problem with the hierarchical model is that it necessitates duplication of knowledge in cases where not all attributes of an exemplar are also attributes of its immediate superordinate. For instance, a tiger is both carnivorous and fierce, but since neither of these attributes necessarily implies the other, they would have to contribute to the individual cognitive representations of every exemplar to which they applied. The fact that most attributional knowledge is of this sort implies an extreme degree of redundancy. An alternative model, that of the distributed feature network, allows semantic attributes to be represented uniquely by proposing that higher-order concepts reside in the largely shared structure for category coordinates in their patterns of activation across collections of attribute units (Smith et al., 1974). This model has additional advantages: in addition to reflecting the physical properties of the apparently unstructured cortical neuronal network, it can be modeled in working computer simulations, allowing for the generation of predictions that can be further tested in living systems (McClelland et al., 1995). Preservation of the superordinate at the expense of finer-grained knowledge, as seen in semantic dementia, is predicted by the distributed network model because even in a network that had lost many individual attribute "nodes," category coordinates would still contain units in common, and these would allow judgments about category membership to be supported long after more fine-grained knowledge had dissappeared.

Any adequate model of semantic organization must also account for the phenomenon of category-specific semantic impairment, alluded to earlier. The occurrence of semantic memory impairment selectively affecting some categories of knowledge while leaving others relatively intact has been most extensively documented in patients who have suffered focal damage to either the temporal lobes (as a consequence of herpes simplex virus encephalitis [Warrington and Shallice, 1984; Pietrini et al., 1988; Sartori and Job, 1988] or semantic dementia [McCarthy and Warrington, 1988]) or the frontoparietal regions (usually after a large middle cerebral artery territory infarct) (Warrington and McCarthy, 1983; Hillis and Caramazza, 1991; Sacchett and Humphreys, 1992). The former group of patients often demonstrate selective loss of knowledge about biological kinds (animals, fruit, vegetables, etc.), while the latter may show a disproportionate impairment (though usually less striking) in the domain of manufactured objects (tools, vehicles, utensils, etc.). At the simplest level, this could be interpreted as suggesting that the neural representations of different categories are located in separate cortical regions. An alternative hypothesis, however, is that the weighting of attributes critical to the identification of items in these two broad domains differs. According to this view, some categories, dominated by natural kinds, are distinguished primarily in terms of their perceptual attributes, and others, dominated by artifacts, are distinguished in terms of their functional features (Saffran and Schwartz, 1994; Garrard et al., 1977; Lambon Ralph et al., 1997). Comparing the process of deciding whether an animal is a tiger or a leopard with that of determining whether a vessel is a vase or a bottle is a striking illustration of this idea. Thus, a loss of perceptual attributes would lead to a disproportionate impairment on tests of semantic knowledge pertaining to living things.

Support for the perceptual–functional dichotomy as a basis for category specificity came initially from a group study of patients with category-specific semantic impairment, in whom the impaired categories did not always respect the living–manufactured distinction (Warrington and McCarthy, 1987). In particular, body parts were found to segregate with artifacts, while fabrics, precious stones, and musical instruments behaved more like biological kinds. A distinction cast in terms of the relative importance of perceptual and functional attributes in the representation of these categories may account for these unusual patterns of dissociation.

The observation that selective loss of knowledge about natural kinds often results from damage to inferior temporal lobe structures, and loss of artifact knowledge from frontoparietal lesions, suggests that the former pattern should occur in the context of semantic dementia, in which the pathology involves predominantly the inferolateral temporal lobe (see above). Occasional single case reports have upheld this prediction (McCarthy and Warrington, 1988; Barbarotto et al., 1995), but there are no published group data on the subject. A possible confounding factor, to which Funnell and Sheridan have drawn attention, is the contribution of the nonsemantic variables of concept familiarity and age of acquisition to the vulnerability of different concepts. Unpublished data from our series of semantic dementia patients (all of whom have predominantly inferolateral temporal lobe atrophy) suggests a mild group advantage for artifacts. Figures 7.3a and 7.3b show the average naming and spoken word comprehension performances of nine patients on two different sets of 32 items from the Snodgrass and Vanderwaert corpus of line drawings (Snodgrass and Vanderwart, 1980). In each set, 16 items are drawn from biological categories and 16 from categories of manufactured objects. These biological and manufactured subgroups are matched in one set for familiarity and in the other for age of acquisition. On confrontation naming, there was a significant group difference ($p < 0.05$) between the biological and manufactured items only on the age of acquisition matched set (Figure 7.3b), suggesting that concept familiarity may be an important predictor of name retrieval. By contrast, on the word–picture matching test there was a significant difference for both sets of items.

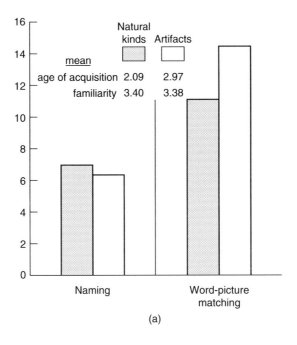

(a)

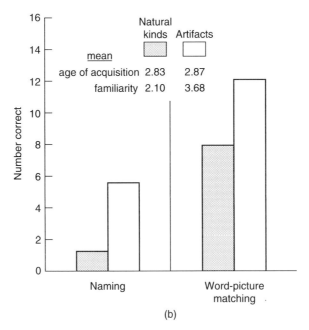

(b)

FIGURE 7.3. (a) Comparison of correct responses to 16 living and 16 manufactured items from a famil-
iarity-matched stimulus set. (b) Comparison of correct responses to 16 living and 16 manufactured items
from an age-of-acquisition-matched stimulus set.

This pattern of findings implies that the linguistic variables important to processes of picture naming and word–picture matching are partially distinct. Moreover, although the size of the advantage is unspectacular when compared to some documented cases (perhaps because of the substantial degree of overall semantic impairment in the patient population), the similarity between the patterns of category selectivity in semantic dementia and the reported HSVE cases, both of which have damage concentrated in the temporal lobes, supports the idea that this region has a special role in the identification of natural kinds, perhaps along the lines of the functional–perceptual distinction proposed by a number of theorists.

Differing Roles for Right and Left Temporal Lobes?

Evans et al. (1995) reported the case of a patient (V.H.) with a 12- year history of progressive difficulty in recognizing familiar faces, together with MRI evidence of focal atrophy of the right temporal lobe. The problem had become apparent to friends and relatives only over the 2 years prior to referral. Formal testing demonstrated consistent, progressive loss of knowledge about famous people, with complete preservation of general semantic memory. This finding was in keeping with two previous reports of selective person-specific knowledge in association with right temporal lobe damage secondary to HSVE in one case (Ellis et al., 1989) and lobectomy in the other (Hanley et al., 1989).

A selective deficit such as this can be explained in a number of ways: (1) a high-level visuoperceptual disorder selectively interfering with face recognition; (2) a disorder of processing affecting categories that consist of an infinite number of unique instances; or (3) disturbance of a specialized system for processing person-specific knowledge, analogous to the general semantic memory breakdown seen in left temporal lobe atrophy. By documenting the integrity of high-level perceptual analysis (including judgments of facial expressions and eye/gaze) and normal performance on a test of knowledge of famous buildings, Evans et al. argued that V.H. had a specific deficit of person-specific semantic information, and that this was the result of damage to a specialized cognitive system dependent on the right temporal lobe. Over time, V.H. has shown impairment on more general tests of semantic memory, particularly when she is required to access knowledge or names from the visual modality.

The study of V.H. raises issues about the contribution of the right hemisphere to the processing and representation of both person-specific and more general semantic knowledge. In the first place, it is not completely clear whether general semantic knowledge can be independently disrupted by an abnormality affecting the right temporal lobe alone. With the exception of V.H., all of our patients with predominantly right-sided disease also had changes on the left at the time of presentation, so comparisons with those patients showing left-sided changes must be interpreted with caution. Second, if the right temporal lobe *does* contribute to the processing of semantic information, how might its functions be separable from those of the left lobe? The variations that are evident among individuals from our series suggest a number of different patterns.

First, there is considerable variability in the degree of anomia (both in spontaneous speech and in tests of confrontation naming) in proportion to semantic impairment, as measured by performance on nonnaming based tests of semantic knowledge (word–picture matching, picture sorting, Pyramids and Palmtrees, etc.). In F.M. (Graham et al., 1995), a patient with left temporal lobe atrophy whose deficit (profound progressive anomia in the face of *very* mild and—for many years—nonprogressive semantic impairment) has been interpreted as resulting from insufficient activation of phonology by meaning, this pattern perhaps represents one extreme. The majority of the left temporal lobe patients in our series have had very obvious semantic impairment, which is nonetheless often accompanied by disproportionately severe

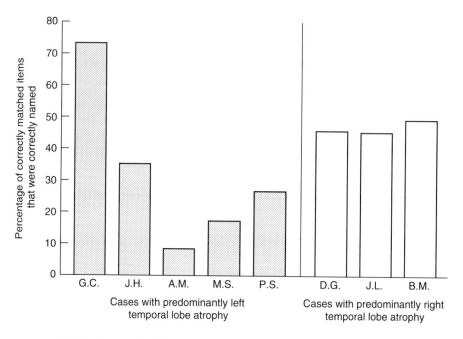

FIGURE 7.4. Severity of naming deficit relative to semantic deficit (number of items correctly named as a percentage of the number correct on word–picture matching).

anomia. By contrast, in those with predominantly right-sided atrophy, the naming deficit, though definitely present, is less severe (see Figure 7.4). This suggests that although the system specialized for activating names of objects may be localized to the left temporal neocortex, semantic knowledge itself may be more bilaterally represented.

Second, the process and/or efficiency of assessing semantic knowledge from visual and verbal stimuli may be very different. One way of examining this is to compare the performance of individual patients on the visual (picture-based) and verbal (word-based) versions of the Pyramids and Palm Trees Test (Howard and Patterson, 1992). This test requires subjects to match a stimulus item with a semantically related target in preference to a semantically unrelated foil; for example, when presented with *pyramid* as the stimulus item, the subject has to choose between *palm tree* and *fir tree* as a response. Performance on the test therefore depends on preserved access to associative semantic knowledge. The response is made by pointing and requires no verbal output. Normal controls show a maximum error rate of 2–3% in both picture and word conditions. Within our patient group there are some individuals who perform better on the picture-based version and others on the word-based version of this task. With few exceptions, the former have predominantly left-sided temporal lobe atrophy and the latter predominantly right. The fact that there can be an advantage for either modality, plus the apparent association between direction of advantage and side of predominant atrophy, suggests at least partially separate and specialized processes for comprehending pictures and words (Shallice, 1988), though the precise roles of these systems remain unspecified. The most transparent interpretation is perhaps that the right temporal lobe is important in accessing semantics from visual information and the left from verbal information. An alternative interpretation, however, is that these results simply reflect a subtle disturbance of high-level visual processing dependent on the right hemisphere and a similar disturbance in the analysis of word forms dependent on the left. The application of appropriately designed neuropsychological tasks to a carefully chosen population of patients should eventually allow these issues to be resolved.

REFERENCES

Akelaitis AJ (1944): Atrophy of basal ganglia in Pick's disease. Arch Neurol Psychiatry 51:27–34.

Alzheimer A (1911): Uber eigenartige Krankheitsfalle des spateren Alters. Z Gesamte Neurol Psychiatrie 4:356–385.

Appell J, Kertesz A, Fisman M (1982): A study of language functioning in Alzheimer patients. Brain Lang 17:73–91.

Barbarotto R, Capitani E, Spinnler H, Trivelli C (1995): Slowly progressive semantic impairment with category specificity. Neurocase 1:107–119.

Bayles KA, Tomoeda CA (1983): Confrontational naming impairment in dementia. Brain Lang 19:98–114.

Benton AL, DesHamsher K, Varney NR, Spreen O (1983): Contributions to Neuropsychological Assessment. New York: Oxford University Press.

Bishop DVM (1989): Test for the Reception of Grammar, 2nd ed. Manchester: University of Manchester.

Breedin SD, Saffran EM, Coslett HB (1994): Reversal of the concreteness effect in a patient with semantic dementia. Cogn Neuropsychol 11:617–660.

Brun A, Englund B, Gustafson L, Passant U, Mann DMA, Neary D, Snowden JS (1994): Clinical and neuropathological criteria for frontotemporal dementia. J Neurol Neurosurg Psychiatry 57:416–418.

Chertkow H, Bub D (1990): Semantic memory loss in dementia of Alzheimer's type. Brain 113:397–417.

Collins AM, Quillian MR (1969): Retrieval time from semantic memory. J Verbal Learning Verbal Behav 8:240–247.

Cummings JL, Duchen LW (1981): Kluver-Bucy syndrome in Pick's disease: Clinical and pathologic correlations. Neurology 31:1415–1422.

De Bleser R, Weis, J, Schwartz M (1996): Primary progressive aphasia: A 14 year follow-up study. Brain Lang 55:76–78.

De Renzi E, Scotti G, Spinnler H (1969): Perceptual and associative disorders of visual recognition: Relationship to the site of the cerebral lesion. Neurology 19:634–642.

Ellis AW, Young AW, Critchley EMR (1989): Loss of memory for people following temporal lobe damage. Brain 112:1469–1483.

Evans JJ, Heggs AJ, Antoun N, Hodges JR (1995): Progressive prosopagnosia associated with selective right temporal lobe atrophy. A new syndrome? Brain 118:1–13.

Folstein MF, Folstein SE, McHugh PR (1975): Mini-mental state: A practical guide for grading the mental state of patients for the clinician. J Psychiatr Res 12:189–198.

Fox NC, Warrington EK, Freeborough PA, Hartikainen P, Kennedy AM, Stevens JM, Rossor MN (1996): Presymptomatic hippocampal atrophy in Alzheimer's disease: A longitudinal MRI study. Brain 119:2001–2007.

Funnell E, Sheridan J (1992): Categories of knowledge? Unfamiliar aspects of living and nonliving things. Cogn Neuropsychol 9:135–153.

Gainotti S, Silveri MC, Daniele A, Giustolisi L (1995): Neuroanatomical correlates of category-specific semantic disorders: A critical survey. Memory 3:247–264.

Garrard P, Perry RJ, Hodges JR (1997): Disorders of semantic memory. J Neurol Neurosurg Psychiatry 62:431–435.

Graff-Radford NR, Damasio AR, Hyman BT, Hart MN, Tranel D, Damasio H, Van Hoesen GW, Rezai K (1990): Progressive aphasia in a patient with Pick's disease: A neuropsychological, radiologic and anatomic study. Neurology 40:620–626.

Graham KS, Hodges JR (1997): Differentiating the roles of the hippocampal complex and the neocortex in long-term memory storage: Evidence from the study of semantic dementia and Alzheimer's disease. Neuropsychology 11:77–89.

Graham KS, Patterson K, Hodges JR (1995): Progressive pure anomia: Insufficient activation of phonology by meaning. Neurocase 1:25–38.

Grossman M, Mickanin J, Onishi K, Hughes E, D'Esposito M, Ding X-S, Alavi A, Reivich M (1996): Progressive nonfluent aphasia: Language, cognitive, and PET measures contrasted with probable Alzheimer's disease. J Cogn Neurosci 8:135–154.

Hanley JR, Young AW, Pearson NA (1989): Defective recognition of familiar people. Cogn Neuropsychol 6:179–210.

Harasty JA, Halliday GM, Code C, Brooks WS (1996): Quantification of cortical atrophy in a case of progressive fluent aphasia. Brain 119:181–190.

Hillis A, Caramazza A (1991): Category specific naming impairment and comprehension: A double dissociation. Brain 114:2081–2094.

Hodges JR, Graham N, Patterson K (1995): Charting the progression in semantic dementia: Implications for the organisation of semantic memory. Memory 3:463–495.

Hodges JR, Patterson K (1996): Nonfluent progressive aphasia and semantic dementia: A comparative neuropsychological study. J Int Neuropsychol Soc 2:511–524.

Hodges JR, Patterson K, Oxbury S, Funnell E (1992): Semantic dementia: Progressive fluent aphasia with temporal lobe atrophy. Brain 115:1783–1806.

Hodges JR, Salamon DP, Butters N (1990): Differential impairment of semantic and episodic memory in Alzheimer's and Huntington's diseases: A controlled prospective study. J Neurol Neurosurg Psychiatry 53:1089–1095.

Hodges JR, Salmon DP, Butters N (1991): The nature of the naming deficit in Alzheimer's and Huntington's disease. Brain 114:1547–1558.

Hodges JR, Salmon DP, Butters N (1992): Semantic memory impairment in Alzheimer's disease: Failure of access or degraded knowledge? Neuropsychologia 30:301–314.

Howard D, Patterson K (1992): Pyramids and Palm Trees: A Test of Semantic Access from Pictures and Words. Bury St. Edmunds, UK: Thames Valley Publishing.

Kaplan E, Goodglass H, Weintraub S (1983): The Boston Naming Test. Philadelphia: Lea and Febiger.

Kempler D, Metter EJ, Rieger WH, Jackson CA, Benson DF, Hanson WR (1990): Slowly progressive aphasia: Three cases with language, memory, CT and PET data. J Neurol Neurosurg Psychiatry 53:987–993.

Lambon Ralph MA, Patterson K, Hodges JR (1997): The relationship between naming and semantic knowledge for different categories in dementia of Alzheimer's type. Neuropsychologia 35:1251–1260.

Lezak MD (1983): Neuropsychological Assessment. New York: Oxford University Press.

Lowenberg K, Boyd DA, Salon DD (1939): Occurrence of Pick's disease in early adult years. Arch Neurol Psychiatry 41:1004–1020.

Malamud N, Boyd DA (1997): Pick's disease with atrophy of the temporal lobes: A clinicopathologic study. Arch Neurol Psychiatry 43:210–222.

Mansvelt J (1954): Pick's Disease. A Syndrome of Lobar Cerebral Atrophy, Its Clinico-anatomical and Histopathological Types. Utrecht: These.

McCarthy R, Warrington EK (1987): The double dissociation of short term memory for lists and sentences. Brain 110:1545–1563.

McCarthy R, Warrington EK (1988): Evidence for modality specific meaning systems in the brain. Nature 334:428–430.

McClelland JL, McNaughton BL, O'Reilly RC (1995): Why are there complementary learning systems in the hippocampus and neocortex: Insights from the successes and failures of connectionist models of learning and memory. Psychol Rev 102:419–457.

Mendez MF, Selwood A, Mastri AR, Frey WH (1993): Pick's disease versus Alzheimer's disease: A comparison of clinical characteristics. Neurology 43:289–292.

Mesulam MM (1982): Slowly progressive aphasia without generalized dementia. Ann Neurol 11:592–598.

Mesulam MM, Weintraub S (1992): Primary progressive aphasia: Sharpening the focus on a clinical syndrome. In Boller F (ed): Heterogeneity of Alzheimer's Disease. Berlin and Heidelberg: Springer-Verlag, pp 43–66.

Mingazzini G (1914): On aphasia due to atrophy of the cerebral convolutions. Brain 36:493–524.

Nebes RB (1989): Semantic memory in Alzheimer's disease. Psychol Bull 106:377–394.

Nelson HE (1982): National Adult Reading Test (NART): For the Assessment of Premorbid Intelligence in Patients with Dementia. Windsor, UK: NFER-Nelson.

Neumann MA (1949): Pick's disease. J Neuropathol Exp Neurol 8:255–282.

Patterson K, Graham N, Hodges JR (1994): The impact of semantic memory loss on phonological representation. J Cogn Neurosci 6:57–69.

Patterson K, Hodges JR (1992): Deterioration of word meaning: Implications for reading. Neuropsychologia 30:1025–1040.

Patterson K, Plaut DC, McClelland JL, Seidenberg MS, Behrman M, Hodges JR (1997): Connections and disconnections: A connectionist account of surface dyslexia. In Reggia J, Berndt R, Ruppin E. (eds): Neural Modelling of Cognitive and Brain Disorders. New York: World Scientific, pp 177–201.

Pick A (1892): Uber die Beziehungen der senilen Hirnatrophie zur Aphasie. Prager Med Wochenschr 17:15–17.

Pick A (1904): Zur symptomatologie der linksseitigen Schlaffenappenatrophie. Monatsschr Psychiatrie Neurol 16:378.

Pick A (1906): Uber einen witeren Symptomenkomplex im Rahmen der Dementia senilis, bedingt durch umschriebene starkere Hirnatrophie (gemischte Apraxia). Monatsschr Psychiatrie Neurol 19:97–108.

Pietrini V, Nertempi P, Vaglia A, Revello M, Pinna V, Ferro-Milone F (1988): Recovery from herpes simplex encephalitis: Selective impairment of specific semantic categories with neuroradiological correlation. J Neurol Neurosurg Psychiatry 51:1284–1293.

Poeck K, Luzzatti C (1988): Slowly progressive aphasia in three patients: The problem of accompanying neuropsychological deficit. Brain 111:151–168.

Pogacar S, Williams RS (1984): Alzheimer's disease presenting as slowly progressive aphasia. RI Med J 67:181–185.

Raven JC (1962): Coloured Progressive Matrices Sets A, AB, B. London: HK Lewis.

Rosser A, Hodges JR (1994): Initial letter and semantic category fluency in Alzheimer's disease, Huntington's disease, and progressive supranuclear palsy. J Neurol Neurosurg Psychiatry 57:1389–1394.

Sacchett C, Humphreys GW (1992): Calling a squirrel a squirrel but a canoe a wigwam: A category specific deficit for artifactual objects and body parts. Cogn Neuropsychol 9:73–86.

Saffran EM, Schwartz MF (1994): Origins of paraphasias in deep dysphasia: Testing the consequences of a decay impairment to an interactive spreading activation model of lexical retrieval. Brain Lang 47:609–660.

Sartori G, Job R (1988): The oyster with four legs: A neuropsychological study on the interaction between vision and semantic information. Cogn Neuropsychol 5:105–132.

Scheltens P, Hazenberg GJ, Lindeboom J, Valk J, Wolters EC (1990): A case of progressive aphasia without dementia: A case of "temporal" Pick's disease? J Neurol Neurosurg Psychiatry 53:79–80.

Scheltens P, Rivka R, Kamphorst W (1994): Pathologic findings in a case of primary progressive aphasia. Neurology 44:279–282.

Scholten IM, Kneebone AC, Denson LA, Field CD, Blumberg P (1995): Primary progressive aphasia: Serial linguistic, neuropsychological and radiological findings with neuropathological results. Aphasiology 9:495–516.

Schwartz M, De Bleser R, Poeck K, Weis J (1997): Primary progressive aphasia: A 14 year follow up study with neuropathological findings. Brain (in press).

Schwartz MF, Marin OSM, Saffran EM (1979): Dissociations of language function in dementia: A case study. Brain Lang 7:277–306.

Shallice T (1988): From Neuropsychology to Mental Structure. Cambridge: Cambridge University Press.

Sinnatamby R, Antoun NA, Freer CEL, Miles KA, Hodges JR (1996): Neuroradiological findings in primary progressive aphasia: CT, MRI and cerebral perfusion SPECT. Neuroradiology 38:232–238.

Smith EE, Shoben EJ, Rips L (1974): Structure and process in semantic memory: A featural model for semantic decisions. Psychol Rev 81:214–241.

Snodgrass JG, Vanderwart MA (1980): A standardised set of 260 pictures: Norms for name agreement, familiarity and visual complexity. J Exp Psychol [Gen] 6:174–215.

Snowden JS, Goulding PJ, Neary D (1989): Semantic dementia: A form of circumscribed cerebral atrophy. Behav Neurol 2:167–182.

Snowden JS, Neary D, Mann DMA, Goulding PJ, Testa HJ (1992): Progressive language disorder due to lobar atrophy. Ann Neurol 31:174–183.

Tulving E (1972): Episodic and semantic memory. In Tulving E, Donaldson W (eds): Organisation of Memory. New York: Academic Press, pp 382–403.

Tyrrell PH, Warrington EK, Frackowiak RSJ, Rossor MN (1990): Heterogeneity in progressive aphasia due to cortical atrophy: A clinical and PET study. Brain 113:1321–1336.

Warrington EK (1975): Selective impairment of semantic memory. Q J Exp Psychol 27:635–657.

Warrington EK (1984): Recognition Memory Test. Windsor, UK: NFER-Nelson.

Warrington EK, McCarthy R (1983): Category specific access dysphasia. Brain 106:859–878.

Warrington EK, McCarthy R (1987): Categories of knowledge: Further fractionations and an attempted integration. Brain 110:1273–1296.

Warrington EK, Shallice T (1984): Category specific semantic impairments. Brain 107:829–853.

CHAPTER 8

The Movement Disorders of Corticobasal Degeneration

PETER A. LeWITT

Departments of Neurology, and Psychiatry and Behavioral Neuroscience, Wayne State University School of Medicine, and The Clinical Neuroscience Program, West Bloomfield, MI 48322

INTRODUCTION

Since 1960, several new movement disorders with unique patterns of neuronal degeneration have entered into the literature of neurology. Like progressive supranuclear palsy and the disorder now termed *multiple system atrophy,* corticobasal degeneration (CBD) has become the subject of increasing awareness and study. CBD is a rare disorder of neuronal degeneration that occurs in later life and is probably greatly underdiagnosed (Riley et al., 1990; Litvan et al., 1997). Prior to its first published description in 1967, clinicians had been aware of patients whose motor impairment seemed parkinsonian but lacked full congruence with the usual clinical syndrome of idiopathic Parkinson's disease. Such patients were usually designated as having *parkinsonian-plus* syndromes, but this appellation was often unsatisfactory because the resemblance to the features of idiopathic Parkinson's disease was only superficial. In the 1960s, most survivors of encephalitis lethargica pandemic were reaching the end of their life spans, and so there were fewer patients whose tremors, bradykinesia, and other movement disorders could be attributed to von Enconomo's disease. Pathologists at that time were also busy codifying criteria for more definitive diagnoses of Parkinson's disease and other neurodegenerative conditions, and began to recognize multiple patterns of neurodegenerative change even within similar clinical syndromes.

Thirty years ago, a short report from a clinical meeting appeared entitled "Corticodentatonigral Degeneration with Neuronal Achromasia: A Progressive Disorder of Late Adult Life." The author was a neurology trainee at the Massachusetts General Hospital, Jean Rebeiz, who worked with Edward Kolodny and E.P. Richardson, Jr., to describe the clinical and pathological features of three cases. A more complete report was published 1 year later. Rebeiz and colleagues (1968) described a unique pattern of motor impairment that, to their knowledge, had

Pick's Disease and Pick Complex, Edited by Andrew Kertesz and David G. Munoz
ISBN 0-471-17792-X ©1998 Wiley-Liss, Inc.

not previously appeared in the medical literature. The three patients in this report each had a progressive disorder with limb rigidity, slowness, tremor, and apraxia that began unilaterally. Other features mentioned included vertical or horizontal gaze disturbances, cerebellar deficits, and long-tract pyramidal signs. Each patient had histological changes of swollen and poorly staining (achromatic) neurons. The distribution and severity of the neuronal pathology were compatible with the range of impairments observed in each case. Although these findings were similar to changes found in pellagra and in Pick's disease, the authors realized that the severe extrapyramidal and cortical disorder was not typical of either condition.

Despite the unique clinical features of their cases, the authors commented on the pathological similarity to Pick's disease. In addition to the usual pattern of selective lobar atrophy, rare cases of Pick's disease had been known to have extensive degenerative involvement of the basal ganglia (von Braunmühl, 1930). These cases and another with striatal involvement (Winkelman and Book, 1948) each lacked, on clinical examination, any motor features of extrapyramidal impairment. Rebeiz and colleagues were apparently unaware of other cases in the medical literature with similarities to theirs. For example, one case described to have the pathology of Pick's disease had movement disorders suggestive of extrapyramidal involvement (prominent, involuntary facial grimacing and irregular tongue protrusions) (van Bogaert, 1934). A clumsy gait (Löwenberg, 1936) and a generalized rigid, contractured state (van Husen, 1934) have also been described in patients seemingly with Pick's disease pathology. Another report by Akelaitis (1944) was even more suggestive of CBD in that the patient developed slow, dysarthric speech, a rigid facial expression, decreased blink rate, cogwheel rigidity in the arms, tremor of the hands and tongue, and a tendency toward shuffling and propulsive gait. The patient in this case, who also developed a progressive dementia, had asymmetrical atrophy of the basal ganglia and prominent histological features of Pick's disease. Since the pathology of CBD seems to overlap (or else may be difficult to distinguish from) that of Pick's disease and possibly other neurodegenerative disorders, these examples in the literature may be earlier instances of the syndrome definitively established by Rebeiz and colleagues many years later.

Three decades after their report, the disorder now commonly termed corticobasal degeneration has remained an elusive condition that may be unrecognized in life. Even the pathological features of this disorder are subtle enough to be overlooked by a pathologist not familiar with CBD. Descriptions of CBD histopathology did not appear in textbooks of neuropathology for some time after the 1968 publication by Rebeiz and colleagues. The clinical syndrome also escaped much attention in the clinical literature of neurology over the two decades after its initial description. Even movement disorder specialists have not become attuned to CBD until recently. For example, a typical case presented in narrative and videotaped form was unrecognized at a large meeting on "Unusual Movement Disorders" at the 1985 American Academy of Neurology meeting. During that same year, this author met with E.P. Richardson, Jr., who commented that the absence of further publications on this topic led him to question whether "corticodentatonigral degeneration" was actually a novel disorder. Dr. Richardson's concerns were relieved by the publication later that year of highly similar cases (Scully et al., 1985; Watts et al., 1985).

Subsequent reports (Gibb et al., 1989; Watts et al., 1989; Greene et al., 1990; Lippa et al., 1990; Riley et al., 1990; Eidelberg et al., 1991; Mitani et al., 1993; Rinne et al., 1994; Oda et al., 1995; Rey et al., 1995; Boeve et al., 1996a; Massman et al., 1996; Mizuno et al., 1996; and Tokumaru et al., 1996, among others) have added many more clinically similar cases with pathological verification to the medical literature. Several reviews have appeared (Thompson and Marsden, 1992; Lang et al., 1993; Watts et al., 1994), and an international meeting on the topic was held recently (Movement Disorder Society Symposium on Cortical-Basal Ganglionic Degeneration and Its Relationship to Other Asymmetrical Cortical Degeneration Syndromes,

1996). The syndrome of CBD has become increasingly recognized over the past 10 years, as indicated by clinical reports accumulating from around the world (e.g., LeWitt et al., 1989; Maraganore et al., 1992; Feifel et al., 1994; Marti and Carrera, 1994; Muhiddin et al., 1994; Brunt et al., 1995; Markus et al., 1995; Ford and Fahn, 1996; Saint-Hilaire et al., 1996). Initially, the occurrence of CBD's core features (unilateral rigidity, bradykinesia, cortical sensory deficit, and apraxia) was thought to be pathognomonic for the pathology of neuronal loss with pale, swollen neurons. Subsequently, the spectrum of clinical variants and alternative pathologies was recognized, as discussed below.

The search for the identity of CBD is evident in the evolution of its nomenclature. Rebeiz and colleagues originally used the term *corticodentatonigral degeneration with neuronal achromasia* to emphasize the distribution of parietal, frontal, and subcortical neuronal dropout, gliosis, and pale, swollen neurons not taking up histological stains. Two of their cases had pathological changes seen in dentate nuclei in addition to the cortical and subcortical pathology. This author reviewed these cases (Rebeiz et al., 1968) with the study's original neuropathologist, Dr. Richardson, who commented that the neuronal changes in the dentate nucleus were not as robust as neuronal degeneration seen elsewhere. Dentate nucleus pathology has not been observed in subsequent neuropathological studies of cases otherwise closely resembling those in the original report. For this reason, a clinicopathological conference report (Scully et al., 1985) revised this disorder's nomenclature to *corticonigral degeneration with neuronal achromasia.* Subsequently, Watts and colleagues (1985) introduced the term *corticobasal ganglionic degeneration* (which has been shortened to *corticobasal degeneration*). Both terms have been used widely, as has *cortical-basal ganglionic degeneration* (Riley et al., 1990). Other descriptions of this disorder, such as *progressive dystonia with apraxia* (LeWitt et al., 1989), *progressive asymmetric rigidity with apraxia* (Maraganore et al., 1992), and *Rebeiz's syndrome* (Parashos et al., 1996), have not been adopted. It remains to be learned if this disorder might acquire the eponym of the early-twentieth-century composer Maurice Ravel, whose progressive neurological disorder was linked recently to CBD (Baeck, 1996).

THE TYPICAL CLINICAL SYNDROME OF CBD

CBD is generally slowly progressive, with asymmetric apraxia, bradykinesia, rigidity, and usually one or more additional features such as a supranuclear pattern of eye movement disorder, tremor or myoclonic jerks, and the alien limb phenomenon. Eventually, most cases of CBD will evolve fully into this distinctive clinical syndrome. However, its earliest stages can easily be confused with Parkinson's disease or other parkinsonian disorders, especially if clinicians are not familiar with the unique combinations of deficits that characterize this rare syndrome. In recent years, it has become clear that cases highly typical of idiopathic Parkinson's disease can nonetheless present a diagnostic challenge. In a series of 100 patients initially thought to have Parkinson's disease, almost one-fifth were found to have a different pathology at autopsy (Hughes et al., 1992). The difficulties of diagnostic certainty about CBD are discussed below.

The syndrome described by Rebeiz and colleagues (1967, 1968) in three cases is characteristic of most CBD, and the report's clear and detailed descriptions would be difficult to improve on. CBD is generally characterized by unilateral or highly asymmetrical motor impairment developing insidiously over the course of weeks to months. The prominent occurrence of a useless, rigid, and dystonic arm flexed at the elbow and wrist, with fingers extended, is quite typical of CBD. Tremulousness or jerking can also be an early sign. Almost one-third of the patients in one series presented with a disturbance of gait (Rinne et al., 1994). The earliest symptoms in most cases are subtle, and the patient may have great difficulty explaining how a limb has become stiff, clumsy, or otherwise awkward. It is rare for bilateral involvement or for an ipsilateral arm and leg to be affected simultaneously. Often the initial signs and symptoms affect just the hand or a portion of it. A progressive loss of function in gripping tasks or in finger dexterity may be experienced long before objective testing might reveal rigid and dystonic features. While reaching for an object, an affected arm may be intermittently or constantly tremulous, sometimes with irregular jerking. With further progression, an abnormal posture or sustained flexion of the forearm becomes evident. Other features may be present, such as athetosis, involuntary lifting upward of the arms held outstretched, or the alien limb phenomenon (see below).

Characteristic of CBD are volleys of myoclonus elicited by touch or other stimulation of the limb. Myoclonus may also arise from tapping the face or during a voluntary motion. Apraxia may be evident in carrying out or demonstrating tasks (see below). Deficits of cortical sensory function or dysesthesias (especially a sense of numbness on the affected side) may be early complaints. Other signs of parietal impairment may include motor neglect or hemispatial neglect and constructional disturbance. Occasionally, these can be presenting features, mimicking sensory deficits on a peripheral basis (Rinne et al., 1994). Sometimes, spontaneous pains or dysesthesias can occur. When the disorder affects right limbs in right-handed individuals, there may be changes evident in the voice such as a soft, droning quality or dysfluency. In two reported cases, apraxia of speech was the presenting feature of clinically diagnosed CBD (Rosenfield et al., 1991); other oral-motor functions were intact.

Deficits from CBD tend to evolve slowly over months to years. It may be difficult to gauge much change over the course of several months. In one study, involvement of the other ipsilateral limb or contralateral spread occurred after a median of 3.5 years (Rinne et al., 1994). Most patients worsen with greater rigidity, further loss of functional capabilities such as one or more patterns of gait disturbance (Abe et al., 1995), development of myoclonus, and increasingly bilateral involvement. At this point, the fully developed disorder usually can be differentiated from other established categories of movement disorder. At this stage, the rigid limbs or face can take on a dystonic quality. The slowness and stiffness may be major factors in the progressive loss of function, although apraxia, dysarthria, or dysphagia can be the predominant source of disability. Falls, inability to provide self-care, and progression in dementia are typical outcomes.

Patients with CBD display deficits highly consistent with the focal, unilateral involvement of frontal and parietal cortical regions (together with damage to nigrostriatal projections). A progressive dementia can be the earliest aspect of this disorder (Bergeron et al., 1996; Brown et al., 1996). Even with severely advanced motor impairment, the sensorium can be normal, with the patient imprisoned in a body unable to move or to be positioned comfortably. Communication abilities can deteriorate to a greater extent than in more common forms of parkinsonism. Changes in behavior may develop that are consistent with frontal lobe damage, such as pseudobulbar crying or laughter, excessive emotionalism, or loss of socially appropriate responses. In the face of deterioration in motor and communicative abilities, it can be difficult for the examiner to recognize the decline in cognition that often occurs several years into the illness. Frontal lobe-type dementia and progressive aphasia, which can develop in the first 3 years of the disorder, will be discussed in the following chapter.

With progression of motor deficits, patients can adopt a forward-flexed or tilted posture. The gait can be slow and hesitant, especially on the affected side. Falling can occur in any direction, and some patients have toppling with backward pull, as can be observed in Parkinson's disease. Other neurological findings in CBD include abnormality of eye movements, as described below. Some patient have hyperactive muscle stretch reflexes or Babinski signs (unilateral or bilateral), but these reflexes can be normal. Grasp, snout, and other regressive oral-facial reflexes can also be released in this disorder.

CBD generally begins in the sixth or seventh decade (although this author follows one patient whose disorder began at age 42). Apart from advancing age, there are no obvious health risk factors for CBD. The majority of cases have no familial or environmental clustering. One case report described progressive apraxia and other features of CBD in a patient whose identical twin was clinically unaffected with this disorder after 7 years (Caselli et al., 1996). Though discordant on clinical grounds, neuropsychological testing and positron emission tomography (PET) provided evidence of cortical hemispheric asymmetry that might be consistent with a subclinical CBD disease state. Stronger evidence for the possible hereditary occurrence of CBD comes from two families in which several cases each of progressive dementia and both the clinical and pathological features of CBD developed (Brown et al., 1996). Both sexes can develop CBD in roughly equal proportions; several series report slightly more affected women than men. The heterogeneity in clinical expression among cases of CBD is common to several other neurodegenerative disorders. The progression of disabilities can vary. When CBD is the proximate cause of death, patients were generally bed-bound and suffering from the impact of paralysis, rigidity, dementia, and dysphagia. The time from onset to the latter condition has often been from 5 to 10 years.

TESTING TO SUPPORT THE DIAGNOSIS OF CBD

Apart from the clinical syndrome, evidence of CBD may be lacking on various types of testing. Neuroimaging with computed tomography (CT) or magnetic resonance imaging (MRI) can be normal, though some cases show asymmetrical or focal atrophy in the frontal and parietal regions. In other instances there may be a more generalized, though asymmetrical, picture of cortical atrophy. Such changes can be especially prominent in the peri-Rolandic gyri, and atrophy of basal ganglia structures can also be recognized (Tokumaru et al., 1996). Cortical atrophic changes on CT or MRI scans can be absent in cases with long-standing and otherwise prominent clinical syndromes. In some instances, cases of CBD lacking cortical atrophy may nonetheless show a major loss of cortical metabolic activity, as measured with 2-deoxyglucose PET or single photon emission computed tomography (SPECT) scans (Okuda et al., 1992). Neuroimaging by means of PET (Watts et al., 1989; Riley et al., 1990; Eidelberg et al., 1991; Sawle et al., 1991; Gimenez-Roldan et al., 1994; Brunt et al., 1995; Nasagawa et al., 1996) and SPECT (Okuda et al., 1992; Frisoni et al., 1995; Markus et al., 1995) has also helped to characterize the metabolic "landscape" of CBD. In most instances, imaging the uptake pattern of 2-deoxyglucose reveals a marked decrease in parietal and frontal cortex activity contralateral to the side on which the limbs are affected. With 18-fluorodopa, decreased uptake contralateral to the side of maximal bradykinetic and rigid features can be found in putamen and caudate structures. Studies of regional cerebral blood flow have compared cases of CBD to Parkinson's disease and found asymmetrical reductions in the caudate, putamen, and thalamus, as well as in the parietal and frontal regions. Even in cases with clinically unilateral involvement with this disorder, the abnormalities in blood flow were bilateral (Markus et al., 1995).

The electroencephalogram reveals no pathognomonic patterns in CBD, and most cases show no more than mild slowing or asymmetry. In one study, a correlation to atrophic changes on neuroimaging studies occurred in only one-third of cases (Westmoreland et al., 1996). The latencies and interpeak amplitudes of somatosensory-evoked potentials are not distinctively abnormal in CBD, although an index of asymmetry can reveal changes not found in progressive supranuclear palsy (Miwa et al., 1996).

Other motor aspects of CBD, including apraxia and myoclonus, have also been analyzed extensively, as described below. The study of cases with CBD's typical features of unilateral, progressive dystonic rigidity and apraxia has shown that other pathology (such as Alzheimer's disease, Pick's disease, or progressive supranuclear palsy) occasionally may be found. In addition, the distinctive neuronal changes described by Rebeiz and colleagues can be associated with progressive dementia without an extrapyramidal or apraxic disorder (Clark et al., 1986).

Like most other neurodegenerative disorders, CBD has no obvious etiological factors. Abnormal tau proteins and the characteristic argyrophilic intraneuronal inclusions, while highly specific for CBD (Feany et al., 1996), do not arise from known mechanisms of neuronal loss. Studies of the brain have revealed that the pale, ballooned neurons typical of CBD are immunoreactive for antibodies against heme oxygenase-1, a possible marker of oxidative stress (Castellani et al., 1995). Unlike idiopathic Parkinson's disease, olfactory function is not impaired in CBD (Wenning et al., 1995).

SPECIFIC MOTOR IMPAIRMENTS IN CBD

Rigidity

The rigidity in CBD can develop to the intensity suggestive of contracture. Usually the rigidity is similar in both agonist and antagonist muscles, and neither clasp-knife nor cogwheeling features are found. The muscle stiffness does not vary or trigger muscle spasms, although myoclonic jerking or tremor can be superimposed. Fisted rigidity of hand clenching can be intense enough to drive the fingernails deep into the skin of the palm.

Eye Movements

Although they may be normal early in the disorder, most patients eventually develop some abnormality of eye movements. The clinical exam can demonstrate difficulties in generating voluntary pursuit and in saccades, which can be slow and jerky. Rottach and colleagues (1996) found saccade latency to be increased in CBD patients in contrast to findings in patients with idiopathic Parkinson's disease, progressive supranuclear palsy, or multiple system atrophy. In the CBD patients (who had been affected with the disorder for 3–6 years), gain in initial upward saccades was reduced. Slow vertical saccades (the hallmark of progressive supranuclear palsy) were also present in one of the three CBD patients. Another study found increased latency of eye movements to visible targets in CBD (Vidailhet et al., 1994). The major abnormality of eye movements in CBD was a marked increase in reflexive horizontal saccade latency, with normal accuracy. These authors found that saccade latency was proportional to the severity of apraxia. Vidailhet and colleagues (1994) concluded that analysis of saccades permitted clear differentiation of CBD from striatonigral degeneration, progressive supranuclear palsy, and Parkinson's disease. However prominent the eye movement findings may be, CBD patients are rarely bothered by them except when apraxia of eyelid opening or upper facial myoclonus is present, as is rarely the case (Stell and Bronstein, 1994).

Speech and Bulbar Impairment

Many patients with the syndrome of CBD experience a progressive loss of communication abilities. A recent study categorizing these problems found that of 16 patients with CBD features, 7 had mild and 3 had moderately impaired language (Seal et al., 1996). Half of the patients in this series had evidence of bulbar dysfunction (six with dysarthria and four with significant degrees of aspiration, as well as slowing of speech production and swallowing). The extent of language changes is reviewed in Chapter 9.

Apraxia and Its Relationship to Other Motor Impairments

Apraxia is found in most cases of CBD (Lindholm et al., 1996) and can occur in several different patterns (Okuda et al., 1992). The damage to the parietal cortex in this disorder likely accounts for disturbances in spatial problem-solving tasks that can be prominent features of CBD (Stark et al., 1996). Three studies have provided a thorough evaluation of the neuropsychological profile of CBD, with special attention to the occurrence of apraxia. Massman and colleagues (1996) analyzed the characteristics of apraxia in 21 CBD patients with the clinical syndrome of CBD (including 1 whose diagnosis was confirmed by autopsy). Only mild features of dementia were present in the patients in this series, and both immediate and delayed recall tended to be preserved. Tests of sustained attention and verbal fluency brought out the most prominent deficits in the CBD group. Compared to Alzheimer's disease patients (either with or without features of parkinsonism), the CBD patients had a distinct pattern of deficits on neuropsychological testing. Only a few errors were made on testing of motor and cognitive flexibility. However, the CBD patients showed impairments on several tests of motor functioning, including uni- and bimanual motor programming, tapping tasks, and tests of praxis. These functional deficits were consistent with the predominant sites of neuronal pathology in CBD (particularly in the left parietal region and the frontal lobes). The pattern of impairments is compatible with a relative sparing of discrete frontal lobe regions mediating set-shifting functions. Despite the usually asymmetrical impairment of motor involvement in CBD, most patients did not exhibit a corresponding asymmetry in the type or severity of cognitive impairments or in manual praxis. However, patients with left-sided onset of this disorder tended to be more impaired on this side than in their right hand.

Another study focused on the nature of apraxia in CBD (Leiguarda et al., 1994). This investigation tested the least affected limb in 10 patients. Seven were impaired on testing for ideomotor praxis and for movement imitation. Together with ideomotor apraxia, four subjects were impaired on tests of sequential arm movements. Features of ideational apraxia were prominent in three of the subjects also affected with ideomotor apraxia and with other types of cognitive deficit. Among the five patients presenting with CBD involving right-sided limbs, all had ideomotor apraxia of their left hand. In contrast, only two of the five patients with left-sided onset of symptoms demonstrated apraxic features of right-sided limbs. These results were consistent with pathological change in the left cerebral cortical hemisphere as the basis for the disorders of praxis in CBD. In this study, the alien limb phenomenon was observed only in those patients also affected with ideomotor apraxia. Ideomotor apraxia correlated well with deficits on both the Mini-Mental State Examination and the picture arrangement test (a task sensitive to frontal lobe dysfunction). Two of the three patients with ideomotor apraxia and ideational apraxia showed relatively severe cognitive impairments.

Results of the latter study were similar to observations in 15 patients also with the clinical diagnosis of CBD (Pillon et al., 1995). As in the report of Massman and colleagues (1996), this study contrasted the findings with the results of similar neuropsychological testing in Alzheimer's disease patients, as well as in those with progressive supranuclear palsy. The CBD patients were moderately demented. The nature of cognitive impairments in CBD differed from those observed in Alzheimer-type dementia. A "dysexecutive" pattern of impairment in the CBD patients was as severe as that observed in progressive supranuclear palsy, indicative of the subcortical-frontal dysfunction in both disorders. In contrast to the patients with progressive supranuclear palsy, however, CBD patients had fewer demonstrations of utilization behavior (responses linked to a release of parietal lobe function). The encoding of information seemed more impaired in CBD than did retrieval tasks. Other findings included altered performance by the CBD patients in the control and activation of simple movements, in the temporal organization of movements, and in tasks requiring posture reproduction, gesture evocation and imitation, and object-use gestures. Some of the CBD patients had evidence of bucco-facial apraxia, but this tended to be milder than the degree of limb apraxia observed.

With the development of rigidity and bradykinesia, the functional impairments of cortical function can be difficult to recognize. In this instance, the mobile limbs on the other side, though seemingly uninvolved, may nonetheless reveal subtle features of apraxia or other types of neuropsychological deficit. It is not clear to what extent the decreased activation of cerebral cortex by damaged basal ganglia (Frisoni et al., 1995) might add to the functional deficits caused by degeneration in cortical neurons. One study provided evidence that the apraxic disorder can be understood as more than just the impairment of the motor program for limb movement (Caselli et al., 1996).

Alien Limb Syndrome

Some cases of CBD display a behavioral disturbance resulting from cortical damage and termed *alien hand syndrome*. This disorder is characterized by the patient's failure to recognize a limb (often a hand or an arm), especially when visual contact is eliminated. As the syndrome progresses, patients may fully reject perceiving the limb or other body parts as entities belonging to them (Doody and Jankovic, 1992). The alien limb may wander involuntarily or may grasp items. These movements may seen to be an "overflow" activation of the affected limb when the other limb is engaged in specific tasks. There also may be a slow, spontaneous levitation of the affected limb (Brunt et al., 1995). In other circumstances, the limb actually carries out movements spontaneously, with a deviant character inappropriate to the situation. The alien limb may compete with or interfere with the unaffected limb's tasks or may act autonomously (seemingly without the patient's willed behavior). In association with this syndrome, CBD patients may display obligate grasp reflexes and cortical reflex myoclonus. A recent series of 36 patients found almost half of them developing alien limb 1 to 2 years after the onset of the disorder (Rinne et al., 1994). Alien limb can be a presenting feature of CBD (Halliday et al., 1995).

Myoclonus

Repetitive jerking in limb or facial muscles in CBD is compatible in most instances with myoclonus. These involuntary movements can be brought out both during action and by sensory stimulation. Myoclonus is often focal, usually involving an arm, initially the hand, and occurring in almost half of the cases of CBD (Thompson, 1995–1996). In a series of 36 CBD cases (14 with myoclonus), myoclonic jerks corresponded to highly synchronous bursts (12–16 Hz) lasting for 25–50 msec and created by simultaneous activation of agonist and antagonist muscles (Thompson et al., 1994). This study used a variety of electrophysiological techniques to characterize the myoclonus of CBD. Back-averaging studies provided no evidence of a preceding cortical discharge before myoclonic jerks. In contrast to the usual patterns of cortical reflex myoclonus, the secondary component of the cortical somatosensory evoked potential was not enlarged and the latency was appropriately 10 msec shorter (Thompson, 1995–1996). Magnetic brain stimulation revealed normal onset latencies to muscle responses (Thompson et al., 1994). However, cortical sensory evoked responses were abnormal for most patients studied, especially in morphologic studies of the parietal conduction component (both on the myoclonic and nonmyoclonic sides). These findings are in keeping with the sites of predilection for pathology in CBD. When an entire limb was involved in each burst of repetitive myoclonus, recordings showed an orderly proximal-to-distal recruitment of limb muscles (suggesting activation through the fast-conducting corticospinal tract). The latency of reflex myoclonus was only 1–2 msec longer than the sum of afferent and efferent conduction to the cortex. Thompson and colleagues (1994) concluded that myoclonus results from a pathological enhancement of a direct sensory input to cortical motor regions, in contrast to other forms of cortical reflex myoclonus (such as those associated with cerebellar degeneration or focal cortical lesions). In their studies, cutaneous or mixed nerve stimulation, muscle stretch, and taps to affected limbs each elicited reflex myoclonus. The intensity of cutaneous stimulation could be below the threshold necessary for perception of the stimulus. Although each repetition of myoclonus could possibly be the consequence of feedback from the previous muscle contraction, studies with magnetic stimulation of the motor cortex indicated that the repetitive volleys were mediated by cortical excitability independent of afferent feedback.

Kato and colleagues (1994) also investigated transcranial magnetic stimulation in four cases with the clinical diagnosis of CBD. In contrast to 5 cases with Parkinson's disease and 10 normal controls, the excitability of the motor cortex in the CBD cases was increased due to damaged cortical inhibitory mechanisms. The inhibitory potential occurred at 4.5 ± 12.5 msec, much less than the 129 ± 30 msec in controls or the 171 ± 57 msec in the Parkinson's disease subjects.

Another study by Brunt and colleagues (1995) characterized features of myoclonus, which had developed early in the course of the illness. After going through a phase of action tremor and progressive rigidity in the arm, the two patients in this study then began to exhibit slow, rhythmic myoclonus during attempts at arm movements and after various types of sensory stimulation at several sites in the myoclonic segment. The electrophysiological characterization of myoclonus showed trains of repetitive, highly synchronized discharges of short duration. One of the patients had spontaneous myoclonic discharges that could be reset by peripheral and central stimulation, and a jerk-locked cortical potential could be elicited. Somatosensory evoked cortical potentials showed abnormal parietal curves with reduced N20 amplitudes and lacking giant sensory-evoked response characteristics. Later-evoked response components also tended to be abnormal. The latencies of the cortical responses, as well as the duration and distribution pattern of the jerks, corresponded to cortical reflex myoclonus due to contralateral parietal cortex damage.

ALTERNATIVE NEUROPATHOLOGICAL ENTITIES WITH THE CLINICAL SYNDROME OF CBD

Among patients with unilaterally developing rigidity, bradykinesia, apraxia, myoclonus, and cortical-type sensory deficits, other pathological entities have been described. In a study of 80 cases of progressive asymmetrical rigidity (with or without apraxia), Boeve and colleagues (1996a) had the opportunity to study 8 cases pathologically and added another to their series of alternative pathologies. Of five cases thought to be "probably" or "definitely" CBD on clinical grounds only one actually had the pathology of this disorder. Another highly typical case was found to have only the pathology of Alzheimer's disease. This situation has been reported on several other occasions (LeWitt et al., 1989; Ceccaldi et al., 1995; Eberhard et al., 1996; Factor et al., 1996), including an instance of the alien hand syndrome and other features suggestive of CBD (Ball et al., 1993). The series of Boeve and colleagues (1996c) included a further case strongly suggestive of NBD but showing at autopsy only markedly asymmetrical degenerative changes in the frontal and parietal regions with status spongiosis. Two other cases in this series also had status spongiosis. In another report, the pathology of patients with CBD-like features consisted of mild neuronal loss in pigmented brainstem neurons, asymmetrical dropout of neurons, gliosis, and status spongiosis affecting parietal, frontal, and cingulate cortices (Boeve et al., 1996a). In another case, the only pathology was nonspecific, patchy degenerative changes in neocortical, subcortical, and pigmented brainstem structures. Argyrophilic substantia nigra inclusions and various abnormalities of tau-immunoreactive (and ubiquitin-nonreactive) lesions are characteristic of CBD pathology (Feany et al., 1996) but can be lacking in otherwise typical clinical cases (Kawasaki et al., 1996).

An additional disease entity that can underlie the clinical syndrome of typical CBD is that of Pick's disease, as discussed above. Cases have been described with the full histopathological spectrum of this disorder, such as Pick bodies. In one case (Lang et al., 1994), a patient developed unilateral rigidity and bradykinesia, resting and action tremor, apraxia, impersistence of eyelid closure, unilateral alien hand phenomenon, and a cortical-type sensory deficit. Fukui and colleagues (1996) described a case with gradual onset of impairment in speech, dexterity, and other motor functions. The patient displayed action and postural myoclonus in cranial and arm musculature, asymmetrical limb rigidity, and a progressive loss of verbal output and comprehension. Apraxic features (buccofacial, limb clumsiness, and ideomotor apraxia of the limbs and trunk) became prominent together with increasing rigidity. The pathology of focal atrophy and neuronal dropout included no gliosis or neuronal achromasia and only rare Pick bodies. Other cases have been described in which asymmetrical parietal lobe atrophy and Pick's disease pathology have been found, strongly resembling CBD but lacking pale, swollen neuronal changes typical of CBD (Cambier et al., 1981; Rajput, 1996). In other instances, the overlap of pathological changes made difficult the clear differentiation of these two disorders (Jendroska et al., 1995; Feany et al., 1996).

The pathology of progressive supranuclear palsy has also been reported in cases mimicking CBD. Although the two disorders can be usually distinguished on clinical grounds (Gimenez-Roldan et al., 1994), several cases have been reported with apparent overlap between the two disorders (Boeve et al., 1996c; Li et al., 1996; Takahashi et al., 1996). In another case with a progressive dystonic apraxia and cortical sensory deficit, the only changes in extraocular motor disturbances were "delayed and slow" eye movements (Saint-Hilaire et al., 1996). The implication of these observations is that degenerative pathology that affects parietal and frontal cortices asymmetrically may result in a syndrome clinically indistinguishable from that of CBD with neuronal achromasia. Furthermore, cases have been described in which the pathology has clear elements of each clinical entity (Mori et al., 1994, 1996; Takahashi et al., 1996).

THE DIAGNOSTIC SPECIFICITY OF CBD

Recently, CBD has been reviewed by Litvan and colleagues (1997) concerning issues of diagnostic sensitivity and specificity. This study investigated how accurately three movement disorder specialists and three less experienced neurological clinicians could make the correct diagnosis of CBD from narrative descriptions of clinical history and examination. Ten cases of pathologically proven CBD were intermingled with cases of other neurodegenerative disorders that presented parkinsonian features, other types of movement disorder, or cognitive decline. The CBD patients, with a mean age of 62 ± 3 years, had symptoms for a mean period of 34 ± 8 months. Their brain pathology in each instance was typical of CBD. The sensitivity in recognizing the diagnosis of CBD was quite low, although the diagnostic specificity was 100%. False-negative misdiagnosis occurred in two-thirds of the cases, most commonly with progressive supranuclear palsy. Other misdiagnoses occurred with cases of vascular parkinsonism, Parkinson's disease, multiple system atrophy, Pick's disease, and Alzheimer's disease with extrapyramidal features. Among the false-positive misdiagnoses, most occurred with progressive supranuclear palsy, Alzheimer's disease with extrapyramidal features, and multiple system atrophy. A factor analysis for clinical features of predictive value found that the best overall predictors of a correct diagnosis included the presence of asymmetric limb dystonia and the absence of gait disorder, imbalance, ideomotor apraxia, early onset of cognitive impairment, and focal myoclonus.

This study indicates how difficult the clinical recognition of CBD can be. It is clear that disorders like Alzheimer's disease (Ceccaldi et al., 1995; Eberhard et al., 1996; Riley, 1996), parkinsonism with dystonia (Ford et al., 1996), and striatonigral degeneration may closely resemble the CBD syndrome, especially in early stages of their development. In its early stages, the hemiparkinsonism-hemiatrophy syndrome can mimic CBD (Giladi and Fahn, 1992). Other movement disorders that can be confused with CBD can have unilateral or asymmetrical involvement, limb dystonia, and unresponsiveness to levodopa. This is illustrated in a case of progressive supranuclear palsy reported by Kurihara and colleagues (1974) in which there were also findings of a dystonic arm, bilateral Babinski signs, and action myoclonus involving both limbs and the face. Other cases have illustrated the overlap of the typical syndrome of progressive supranuclear palsy with the pathology of CBD (Li et al., 1996). It is also possible that a rare patient might have the pathology of CBD and another neurodegenerative disorder such as Alzheimer's disease. Sometimes a detailed neuropsychological examination of cases with nondistinctive extrapyramidal disorders can offer the greatest chance to make a correct diagnosis of CBD (Rey et al., 1995). Ascertainment of this disorder may require careful testing for ideomotor apraxia, stimulus–responsive myoclonus, and evidence of cortical sensory deficits.

ACKNOWLEDGMENTS

This study was supported in part by a grant from the National Parkinson Foundation (Center of Excellence).

REFERENCES

Abe K, Hashimoto T, Tamaru F, Ueno E, Yanagisawa N (1995): Analysis of gait disturbance in a patient with corticobasal degeneration (in Japanese). Rinsho Shinkeigaku [Clin Neurol] 35:153–157.

Akelaitis AJ (1944): Atrophy of the basal ganglia in Pick's disease. Arch Neurol Psychiatry 51:27–34.

Baeck E (1996): Was Maurice Ravel's illness a corticobasal degeneration? Clin Neurol Neurosurg 98:57–61.

Ball JA, Lantos PL, Jackson M, Marsden CD, Scadding JW, Rossor MN (1993): Alien hand sign in association with Alzheimer's histopathology. J Neurol Neurosurg Psychiatry 56:1020–1023.

Bergeron C, Pollanen MS, Weyer L, Black SE, Lang AE (1996): Unusual clinical presentations of cortical-basal ganglionic degeneration. Ann Neurol 40:893–900.

Blin J, Vidhailet M-J, Pillon B, Dubois B, Feve JR, Agid Y (1991): Corticobasal degeneration: Decreased and asymmetrical glucose consumption as studied with PET. Mov Disord 7:348–354.

Boeve BF, Maraganore DM, Parisi JE, Ahlskog JE, Muenter M, Graff-Radford N, Caselli RJ, Petersen RC, Kokmen E, Berg L, McKeel D (1996a): Disorders mimicking the "classical" clinical syndrome of cortical-basal ganglionic degeneration: Report of nine cases. Mov Disord 11:351.

Boeve BF, Maraganore DM, Parisi JE, Ahlskog JE (1996a): A case presenting clinically as cortical-basal ganglionic degeneration without neuronal achromasia. Mov Disord 11:356–357.

Boeve BF, Maraganore DM, Parisi JE, Ahlskog JE, Graff-Radford N, Muenter M, Caselli RJ, Petersen RC (1996b): Clinical heterogeneity in patients with pathologically diagnosed cortical-basal ganglionic degeneration. Mov Disord 11:351–352.

Brown J, Lantos PL, Roques P, Fidani L, Rossor MN (1996): Familial dementia with swollen achromatic neurons and corticobasal inclusion bodies: A clinical and pathological study. J Neurol Sci 135:21–30.

Brunt ER, van Weerden TW, Pruim J, Lakke JW (1995): Unique myoclonic pattern in corticobasal degeneration. Mov Disord 10:132–142.

Cambier J, Masson M, Dairou R, Henin D (1981): Etude anatomo-clinique d'une forme parietale de maladie de Pick. Rev Neurol 137:33–38.

Carella F, Sciaoli V, Franceschetti S, Girotti F, Giovanni P, Ciano C, Caraceni T (1991): Focal reflex myoclonus in corticobasal degeneration. Funct Neurol 6:165–170.

Caselli RJ, Stelmach GE, Timman D, Tadikonda S (1996): Kinematic studies of upper limb apraxia in patients with cortical-basal ganglionic degeneration: Is apraxia a motor programming disorder? Mov Disord 11:354.

Castellani R, Smith MA, Richey PL, Kalaria R, Gambetti P, Perry G (1995): Evidence for oxidative stress in Pick disease and corticobasal degeneration. Brain Res 696:268–271.

Ceccaldi M, Poncet M, Gambarelli D, Guinot H, Bille J (1995): Apraxie unilaterale gauche d'aggravation progressive dans deux cas de maladie d'Alzheimer. Rev Neurol 151:240–246.

Chen R, Ashby P, Lang AE (1992): Stimulus-sensitive myoclonus in akinetic-rigid syndromes. Brain 115:1875–1888.

Clark AW, Manz HJ, White CL 3rd, Lehmann J, Miller D, Coyle JT (1986): Cortical degeneration with swollen chromatolytic neurons: Its relationship to Pick's disease. J Neuropathol Exp Neurol 45:268–284.

Constantinidis J, Richard J, Tissot R (1974): Pick's disease. Histological and clinical correlations. Eur Neurol 11:208–217.

Doody RS, Jankovic J (1992): The alien hand and related signs. J Neurol Neurosurg Psychiatry 55:806–810.

Eberhard DA, Lopes MB, Trugman JM, Brashear HR (1996): Alzheimer's disease in a case of cortical basal ganglionic degeneration with severe dementia. J Neurol Neurosurg Psychiatry 60:109–110.

Eidelberg D, Dhawan V, Moeller JR, Sidtis JJ, Ginos JZ, Strother SC, Cederbaum J, Greene P, Fahn S, Powers JM, Rottenberg DA (1991): The metabolic landscape of cortico-basal ganglionic degeneration: Regional asymmetries studied with positron emission tomography. J Neurol Neurosurg Psychiatry 54:856–862.

Factor SA, Molho ES, Dollar JD (1996): Alzheimer-like pathology in a patient with clinical features of corticobasal ganglionic degeneration. Mov Disord 11:355.

Feany MB, Mattiace LA, Dickson DW (1996): Neuropathologic overlap of progressive supranuclear palsy, Pick's disease, and corticobasal degeneration. J Neuropathol Exp Neurol 55:52–67.

Feifel E, Brenner M, Teiwes R, Lücking CH, Deuschl G (1994): Kortiko-basale Degeneration. Die Bedeutung klinischer Kriterien zur Diagnosestellung. Nervenarzt 65:653–659.

Ford B, Fahn S (1996): 78 year-old woman with tremors, Parkinsonism, and dementia. Mov Disord 11:355.

Ford B, Greene P, Fahn S (1996): 60 year-old woman with Parkinsonism and unilateral dystonia. Mov Disord 11:355–356.

Frisoni GB, Pizzolato G, Zanetti O, Bianchetti A, Chierichetti F, Trabucchi M (1995): Corticobasal degeneration: Neuropsychological assessment and dopamine D2 receptor SPECT analysis. Eur Neurol 35:50–54.

Gibb WRG, Luthert PJ, Marsden CB (1989): Corticobasal degeneration. Brain 112:1171–1192.

Giladi N, Fahn S (1992): Hemiparkinsonism-hemiatrophy syndrome may mimic early-stage cortical-basal ganglionic degeneration. Mov Disord 7:384–385.

Gimenez-Roldan S, Mateo D, Benito C, Grandas F, Perez-Gilabert Y (1994): Progressive supranuclear palsy and corticobasal ganglionic degeneration: Differentiation by clinical features and neuroimaging techniques. J Neural Transm 42(Suppl):79–90.

Greene PE, Fahn S, Lang AE, Watts RL, Eidelberg D, Powers JM (1990): What is it? Case 1, 1990: Progressive unilateral rigidity, bradykinesia, tremulousness and apraxia, leading to fixed postural deformity of the affected limb. Mov Disord 5:341–351.

Halliday GM, Davies L, MacRitchie DA, Cartwright H, Pamphlett RF, Morris JG (1995): Ubiquitin-positive achromatic neurons in corticobasal degeneration. Acta Neuropathol 90:68–75.

Hughes AJ, Daniel SE, Kilford L, Lees AJ (1992): The accuracy of clinical diagnosis of idiopathic Parkinson's disease: A clinicopathological study. J Neurol Neuropathol Psychiatry 55:181–184.

Ikeda K, Akiyama H, Iritani S, Kase K, Arai T, Niizato K, Kuroki N, Kosaka K (1996): Corticobasal degeneration with primary progressive aphasia and accentuated cortical lesion in superior temporal gyrus. Acta Neuropathol 92:534–539.

Jendroska K, Rossor MN, Mathias CJ, Daniel SE (1995): Morphological overlap between corticobasal degeneration and Pick's disease: A clinicopathological report. Mov Disord 10:111–114.

Kato M, Fukusako T, Negoro L, Nogaki H, Morimatsu M (1994): A study of transcranial magnetic stimulation in clinically diagnosed corticobasal degeneration. Mov Disord 9(Suppl 1):79.

Kawasaki K, Iwanaga K, Wakabayashi K, Yamada M, Nagai H, Idezuka J, Homma Y, Ikuta F (1996): Corticobasal degeneration with neither argyrophilic inclusions nor tau abnormalities: A new subgroup? Acts Neuropathol 9:140–144.

Kurihara T, Landau WM, Torack RM (1974): Progressive supranuclear palsy with action myoclonus. Neurology 24:219–223.

Lang AE, Bergeron C, Pollanen MS, Ashby P (1994): Parietal Pick's disease mimicking cortical-basal ganglionic degeneration. Neurology 44:1436–1440.

Lang AE, Riley DE, Bergeron C (1993): Cortical-basal ganglionic degeneration. In Calne DB (ed): Neurodegenerative Diseases. Philadelphia: WB Saunders, pp 877–894.

Leiguarda R, Lees AJ, Merello M, Starkstein S, Marsden CD (1994): The nature of apraxia in corticobasal degeneration. J Neurol Neurosurg Psychiatry 57:455–459.

Lerner A, Friedland R, Riley D, Whitehouse P, Lanska D, Vick N, Cochran E, Tresser N, Cohen M, Gambetti P (1992): Dementia with pathological findings of cortical-basal ganglionic degeneration. Ann Neurol 32:271.

LeWitt P, Friedman J, Nutt J, Korczyn A, Brogna C, Truong D (1989): Progressive dystonia with apraxia: The variety of clinical and pathological features. Neurology 39(Suppl 1):140.

Li F, Iseki E, Kosaka K, Nishimura T, Akiyama H, Kato M (1996): Progressive supranuclear palsy with frontal atrophy and various tau-positive abnormal structures. Clin Neuropathol 15:319–323.

Lindholm KM, Shannon KM, Stebbins GT (1996): A comparison of apraxia in PSP and cortical-basal ganglionic degeneration. Mov Disord 11:353.

Lippa CF, Smith TW, Fontneau N (1990): Corticonigral degeneration with neuronal achromasia. A clinicopathological study of two cases. J Neurol Sci 98:301–310.

Litvan I, Agid Y, Goetz C, Jankovic J, Wenning GK, Brandel JP, Lai EC, Verny M, Ray-Chaudhuri K, McKee A, Jellinger K, Pearce RKB, Bartko JJ (1997): Accuracy of the clinical diagnosis of corticobasal degeneration: A clinicopathologic study. Neurology 48:119–125.

Maraganore DM, Ahlskog JE, Petersen RG (1992): Progressive asymmetric rigidity with apraxia: A distinctive clinical entity. Mov Disord 7(Suppl 1):80.

Markus HS, Lees AJ, Lennox G, Marsden CD, Costa DC (1995): Patterns of regional blood flow studied in corticobasal degeneration studied with HMPAO SPECT: Comparison with Parkinson's disease and normal controls. Mov Disord 10:179–187.

Marti M, Carrera N (1994): Degeneration corticobasal gangliònica: a propòsito de siete obervaciones diagnosticadas clinicamente. Neurologia 9:115–120.

Massman PJ, Kreiter KT, Jankovic J, Doody RS (1996): Neuropsychological functioning in cortical-basal ganglionic degeneration: Differentiation from Alzheimer's disease. Neurology 46:720–726.

Mitani K, Uchihara T, Tamaru F, Endo K, Tsukagoshi H (1993): Corticobasal degeneration: Clinico-pathological studies on two cases (in Japanese). Rinsho Shinkeigaku [Clin Neurol] 33:155–161.

Miwa H, Mori H, Abe K, Hoshino I, Mizuno Y (1996): Corticobasal degeneration and progressive supranuclear palsy—differentiation by somatosensory-evoked potentials (in Japanese). No to Sinkei [Brain and Nerve] 48:253–257.

Mizuno Y, Yokochi F, Ohta S, Mori H, Takubo H (1996): A 65-year-old man with Parkinsonism, gaze palsy, and dementia (clinical conference) (in Japanese). No to Shinkei [Brain and Nerve] 48:381–393.

Mori H, Nishimura M, Namba Y, Oda M (1994): Corticobasal degeneration: A disease with widespread appearance of abnormal tau and neurofibrillary tangles, and its relation to progressive supranuclear palsy. Acta Neuropathol 88:113–121.

Mori H, Oda M, Mizuno Y (1996): Cortical ballooned neurons in progressive supranuclear palsy. Neurosci Lett 209:109–112.

Movement Disorder Society Symposium on Cortical-Basal Ganglionic Degeneration (CBGD) and Its Relationship to Other Asymmetrical Cortical Degeneration Syndromes (ACDs) Washington, D.C., October 25–26, 1995 (1996): Mov Disord 11:346–357.

Muhiddin KA, Hardie RJ, Pearce VR, Kirby BJ (1994): Corticobasal degeneration: A report of three cases. J R Soc Med 87:359–360.

Nagasawa H, Tanji H, Nomura H, Saito H, Itoyama Y, Kimura I, Tuji S, Iwata R, Itoh M, Ido T (1996): PET study of cerebral glucose metabolism and fluorodopa uptake in patients with corticobasal degeneration. J Neurol Sci 139:210–217.

Oda T, Ikeda K, Akamatsu W, Iwabuchi K, Akiyama H, Kondo H, Seta K, Kato Y, Kogure T, Hori K (1995): An autopsy case of corticobasal degeneration clinically misdiagnosed as Pick's disease (in Japanese). Seishin Shinkeigaku Zasshi [Psychiatrica Neurol Jap] 97:757–769.

Okuda B, Tachibana H, Kawabata K, Takeda M, Sugita M (1992): Slowly progressive limb-kinetic apraxia with a decrease in unilateral cerebral blood flow. Acta Neurol Scand 86:76–81.

Parashos SA, Matsumoto JY, McManis PG, Reeves AL, Ahlskog JE (1996): Action myoclonus resembling orthostatic tremor in a patient with Rebeiz's syndrome. Mov Disord 11:352.

Pillon B, Blin J, Vidhailhet M, DeWeer B, Sirigu A, Dubois B, Agid Y (1995): The neuropsychological pattern of corticobasal degeneration: Comparison with progressive supranuclear palsy and Alzheimer disease. Neurology 45:1477–1483.

Rajput A (1996): Cortical-basal ganglionic degeneration-like expression of Pick's disease. Mov Disord 11:356.

Rebeiz JJ, Kolodny EH, Richardson EP Jr (1967): Corticodentatonigral degeneration with neuronal achromasia: A progressive disorder of late adult life. Trans Am Neurol Assoc 92:23–26.

Rebeiz JJ, Kolodny EH, Richardson EP Jr (1968): Corticodentatonigral degeneration with neuronal achromasia. Arch Neurol 18:20–33.

Rey GJ, Tomer R, Levin BE, Sanchez-Ramos J, Bowen B, Bruce JH (1995): Psychiatric symptoms, atypical dementia, and left visual field inattention in corticobasal ganglionic degeneration. Mov Disord 10:106–110.

Riley DE (1996): Alzheimer's disease (AD) with a clinical presentation mimicking cortical-basal ganglionic degeneration. Mov Disord 11:357.

Riley DE, Lang AE, Lewis A, Resch L, Ashby P, Hornykiewicz O, Black S (1990): Cortical-basal ganglionic degeneration. Neurology 40:1203–1212.

Rinne JO, Lee MS, Thompson PD, Marsden CD (1994): Corticobasal degeneration: A clinical study of 36 cases. Brain 117:1183–1196.

Rosenfield DB, Bogatka CJ, Viswanath NS, Lang AE, Jankovic J (1991): Speech apraxia in cortical-basal ganglionic degeneration. Ann Neurol 30:296–297.

Rottach KG, Riley DE, DiScenna AO, Zivotofsky AZ, Leigh RJ (1996): Dynamic properties of horizontal and vertical eye movements in parkinsonian syndromes. Ann Neurol 39:368–377.

Saint-Hilaire M-H, Handler J, McKee AC, Feldman RG (1996): Clinical overlap between corticobasal gan-glionic degeneration and progressive supranuclear palsy. Mov Disord 11:356.

Sakurai Y, Hashida H, Uesugi H, Arima K, Murayama S, Bando M, Iwata M, Momose T, Sakuta M (1996): A clinical profile of corticobasal degeneration presenting as primary progressive aphasia. Eur Neurol 36:134–137.

Sawle GV, Brooks DJ, Marsden CD, Frackowiak RSJ (1991): Corticobasal degeneration. A unique pattern of regional cortical oxygen hypometabolism and striatal fluorodopa uptake demonstrated by positron emission tomography. Brain 114:541–556.

Scully RE, Mark EJ, McNeely BU (1985): Case records of the Massachusetts General Hospital. Case 38–1985. N Engl J Med 313:739–748.

Seal EC, Haight PL, Burns RS (1996): A formal study of speech and language changes in the syndrome of cortical-basal ganglionic degeneration: Is initial dominant hemisphere involvement a predictor of lan-guage impairment? Mov Disord 11:353–354.

Stark ME, Clark K, Grafman, Litvan I (1996): Evidence for a multimodal disruption of space in cortical-basal ganglionic degeneration. Mov Disord 11:353.

Stell R, Bronstein AM (1994): Eye movement abnormalities in extrapyramidal diseases. In Marsden CD, Fahn S (eds): Movement Disorders 3. London: Butterworths, 1994, pp 88–113.

Takahashi T, Amano N, Hanihara T, Nagatomo H, Yagishita S, Itoh Y, Tamaoka K, Toda H, Tanabe T (1996): Corticobasal degeneration: Widespread argentophilic threads and glia in addition to neurofi-brillary tangles. Similarities of cytoskeletal abnormalities in corticobasal degeneration and progressive supranuclear palsy. J Neurol Sci 138:66–77.

Thompson PD (1995–1996): Myoclonus in corticobasal degeneration. Clin Neurosci 3:203–208.

Thompson PD, Day BL, Rothwell JC, Brown P, Britton TC, Marsden CD (1994): The myoclonus in cor-ticobasal degeneration. Evidence for two forms of cortical reflex myoclonus. Brain 17:1197–1207.

Thompson PD, Marsden CD (1992): Corticobasal degeneration. In Rossor MN (ed): Unusual Dementias. Balliere's Clinical Neurology, Vol 1, No 3. London: Balliere Tindall, pp 677–686.

Tokumaru AM, O'uchi T, Kuru Y, Makia T, Murayama S, Horichi T (1996): Corticobasal degeneration: MR with histopathologic comparison. Am J Neuroradiol 17:1849–1852.

van Bogaert L (1934): Syndrome extrapyramidal au cours d'une maladie de Pick. J Belge Neurol Psychi-atr 34:315–321.

van Husen T (1934): Über ein Fall von Pick'scher Krankheit. Allg Z Psychiatrie 101:381–396.

Vidailhet M, Rivaud S, Gouider-Khouja N, Pillon B, Bonnet A-M, Gaymard B, Agid Y, Pierrot-Deseil-ligny CP (1994): Eye movements in Parkinsonian syndromes. Ann Neurol 35:420–426.

von Braunmühl A (1930): Über Stammganglienveränderungen bei Pickscher Krankheit. Z gesamte Neu-rol Psychiatrie 124:214–223.

Watts RL, Williams RS, Growdon JD, Young RR, Haley EC Jr, Beal MF (1985): Corticobasal ganglionic degeneration. Neurology 35(Suppl 1):178.

Watts RL, Mirra SS, Young RR, Burger PC, Villier JA, Heyman A (1989): Corticobasal ganglionic de-generation (CBGD) with neuronal achromasia: Clinical-pathological study of two cases. Neurology 39(Suppl 1):140.

Watts RL, Mirra SS, Richardson EP Jr (1994): Corticobasal ganglionic degeneration. In Marsden CD, Fahn S (eds): Movement Disorders 3, London: Butterworths, 1994, pp 282–299.

Wenning GK, Shephard B, Hawkes C, Petruckevitch A, Lees A, Quinn N (1995): Olfactory function in atypical parkinsonian syndromes. Acta Neurol Scand 91:247–250.

Westmoreland BF, Boeve BF, Maraganore DM, Ahlskog JE (1996): The EEG is cortical-basal ganglionic degeneration. Mov Disord 11:352.

Winkelman NW, Book MH (1948): Asymptomatic extrapyramidal involvement in Pick's disease. A clini-copathological study of two cases. J Neuropathol Exp Neurol 8:30–42.

CHAPTER 9

Cognitive Changes in Corticobasal Degeneration

ANDREW KERTESZ and PABLO MARTINEZ-LAGE

Department of Clinical Neurological Sciences (A.K.), St. Joseph's Health Centre, University of Western Ontario, London, Ontario Canada, N6A 4V2, and Faculty of Medicine (P.M.-L.), University of Navarra, Navarra, Spain

INTRODUCTION

After being neglected for up to 20 years, corticodentatonigral degeneration (Rebeiz et al., 1968) became widely recognized when several new cases were described as corticobasal ganglionic degeneration (CBGD) (Watts et al., 1989; Riley et al., 1990) and corticobasal degeneration (CBD) by Gibb et al. (1989). The unusual apractic, extrapyramidal syndrome drew the attention of those interested in movement disorders, and a number of clinicopathological studies were subsequently published. From its initial description in 1968, CBD was compared with Pick's disease (PiD) pathologically since "the pallor and swelling of the nerve cells" were reminiscent of the neuronal changes of the latter (Rebeiz et al., 1968). Some case reports describe patients presenting clinically as CBD with the pathological findings of PiD with Pick bodies (Brion et al., 1991; Lang et al., 1994; Jendroska et al., 1995; Fukui et al., 1996). Other cases of pathologically defined CBD have frontal-type dementia or aphasia clinically (Riley et al., 1990; Sakurai et al., 1996). While it is true that extrapyramidal features were not part of the original description of PiD, numerous subsequent cases published show this association (Löwenberg, 1935; Akelaitis, 1944; Winkleman and Book, 1944; Brion et al., 1991). The occurrence of extrapyramidal features is also recognized in frontotemporal dementia (FTD) (Lund and Manchester Groups, 1994). A substantial proportion (78%) of autopsied cases of PiD had striatopallidonigral degeneration (Kosaka et al., 1991). Another study showed selective loss of pigmented neurons from the substantia nigra in PiD (Uchihara et al., 1990).

The rather focused interest in the extrapyramidal syndrome led to the general idea that behavioral changes are rare and dementia occurs only in a minority of cases of CBD (Rinne et al., 1994). When the publications are specifically reviewed, however, cognitive decline, especially dysexecutive syndrome, language disturbances, and personality changes suggestive of

Pick's Disease and Pick Complex, Edited by Andrew Kertesz and David G. Munoz
ISBN 0-471-17792-X ©1998 Wiley-Liss, Inc.

frontal and temporal lobe involvement, seem to be frequent features, accompanying the extra-pyramidal manifestations, during the course of the disease. In this chapter, we focus on the clinical manifestations, behavioral changes, and cognitive alterations of CBD. The movement disorder of CBD and the pathology are discussed elsewhere in this volume.

BEHAVIORAL AND COGNITIVE CHANGES IN CBD

The first patient reported in the seminal article by Rebeiz et al. (1968) started to show personality changes 1 year after her initial motor symptoms appeared. She became "quiet and appeared depressed." Two years later, she became "fretful, querulous, and progressively withdrawn," although she had been a very social person. At that time she started to present some paraphasias ("misused a word at times") but not anomia. However, after 1 year her language had worsened, and "she spoke less and less, only occasionally answering questions in monosyllables." A pneumoencephalographic study showed frontal horn enlargement. The second patient showed "normal memory and judgement" during the early stages of his disease, which at that time was characterized by stiffness and involuntary movements of his left limbs. However, he had become "mentally slower," "was undertaking less [sic] activities than previously," and seemed to have lost the ability to solve new difficult problems. Neuropsychological testing 5 years after the onset of the disease showed intellectual decline "beyond that expected for his age," mainly in tasks requiring visuospatial organization. He was slow when facing new tasks. The third patient had noticed that her memory was "less reliable" and her "thought processes were becoming slower." However, "no abnormalities" were found on her mental state examination 1 year after the onset of her disease.

Twenty-one years later, Gibb et al. (1989) reported on three additional patients with pathology, renaming the disease *corticobasal degeneration.* Their first patient, a 67-year-old man whose clinical picture started with "tremor" in his right arm, with jerking, involuntary movements, showed average intellectual functioning on formal neuropsychological testing after 2 years. Six months later, however, his full-scale IQ had dropped 11 points. Abstract thinking had deteriorated, digit span scores were below average, and "delayed recall of logical memory passage and 12 pictured objects was very poor." Interestingly, "verbal fluency had deteriorated from 12 words/min to 4/min," and "there was some evidence of perseveration." After 6 months, "the nominal dysphasia had increased" and his intellectual decline had progressed. His language disturbances continued to worsen, and 3.5 years after disease onset he was "apathetic," with poor orientation in time and "very poor short-term memory." Neuropsychological features were apparently prominent in the second patient as well. After a 2-year history of slurred speech, unsteady gait, and akinetic rigid syndrome, "she was unable to do the WAIS, and the results of memory and learning tests suggested an impairment of intellectual function." At her first assessment, she was emotionally labile and tended to "answer yes to almost any question." The third patient was seen only once after 3.5 years of disease evolution. "Intellectual function was considered normal and verbal responses were not delayed."

Among the 15 cases (13 with a clinical diagnosis and 2 histologically proven) reported by Riley et al. (1990) 4 were demented, 3 showed aphasia, and 9 had "frontal lobe reflexes." A detailed description of the clinical picture is given for four patients. Patient 2 had a "normal mental status examination" 4 years after his first symptoms appeared. Two years later, he was emotionally incontinent and "his mental function begun to deteriorate." Patient 10 showed personality change with aggressiveness in the early stages of his disease. Neurological examination 2 years later showed "impaired repetition, right–left confusion, perseveration, [and] prominent apraxia." Later in the course of the disease, the patient started to show "literal and verbal paraphasias." His repetition continued to be impaired, but his verbal comprehension was preserved. His delayed recall of three objects was poor. No mention of the mental status is made for patients 5 and 1; the latter showed prominent bilateral grasp reflexes.

Rey et al. (1995) reported a case in which the diagnosis was based on the presence of some achromatic neurons in the striatum but not in the cerebral cortex, with moderate neuronal loss and depigmentation in the substantia nigra and locus coeruleus. This patient presented at the age of 67 with "mental and physical fatigue," loss of memory, and incoordination and weakness in the left limbs. Formal neuropsychological testing 2 years after disease onset showed impairment of "complex attention, conceptual reasoning, word fluency, verbal learning, and programming of repetitive motor sequences." He continued to be depressed, had severe left hemispatial inattention, and had an "unusual motor behavior characterized by a tendency to grab and touch objects in his immediate environment" (utilization behavior). Two autopsied patients were reported by Lippa et al. (1990) showing ballooned neurons in the neocortex and severe degeneration of the substantia nigra. In the first patient, a diagnosis of primary progressive aphasia (PPA) is applicable. The clinical picture started with difficulty finding words, followed 1 year later by a right-sided parkinsonian syndrome. Three years later, he developed a nonfluent aphasia with "reduced speech output, frequent literal paraphasias, [and] errors in repetition, comprehension and writing." He progressed to a severe global aphasia. In patient 2, memory loss and difficulty with concentration were the most striking initial symptoms, along with parkinsonian gait that did not respond to anticholinergic or dopaminergic treatment. Later, he became socially withdrawn and depressed. Neuropsychological testing showed "diffuse cerebral dysfunction. Verbal and visual memory as well as visuospatial abilities were most severely impaired."

Jendroska et al. (1995) reported a patient clinically diagnosed as having probable Steele-Richardson-Olszewski syndrome. The neuropathological examination showed ballooned, achromatic neurons in the frontal cortex, loss of pigmented cells, and the presence of swollen neurons with basophilic inclusions and argyrophilic inclusions "indistinguishable from Pick bodies" in the pyramidal neurons of the hippocampus, as well as in the amygdala, claustrum, and olfactory nucleus. The patient's mental status was considered normal at the beginning of the disease.

The largest clinical series of CBD cases published (Rinne et al., 1994) to date includes 36 patients, 6 of whom had neuropathologically proven diagnoses. Thirty of these patients were followed for a mean period of 5.2 years, and cognitive deficits were detected in nine of them. Two of these patients showed frontal lobe dysfunction in formal neuropsychological testing, and a third patient had "prominent personality and behavioral changes with impulsiveness and excessive eating and drinking." The authors admitted that "sometimes formal testing was difficult because of dysarthria, apraxia and loss of function of the dominant hand."

A neuropathologically selected series of CBD patients all had cortical involvement, and four of them had behavioral or language problems (Schneider et al., 1997). This very recent study supports our contention that FLD, PPA and CBD are related entities, and that patients with CBD have either significant behavioral and language deficits at the beginning or develop such symptoms later in the course of their illness. Therefore, CBD not only is related pathologically to PiD but also shows a major clinical overlap sooner or later in the course of the illness, with the common clinical manifestations of PiD.

We have now seen 22 patients with prominent corticobasal degeneration syndrome (CBDS) characterized by extrapyramidal symptoms of apraxia, alien hand, gaze palsies, and reflex myoclonus in various combinations. Nine of them have presented with motor disorder, eight with PPA, and five with personality and behavioral changes. Even among the nine patients with primarily motor presentation, seven had significantly reduced language output or documented aphasia, and the other two had personality and behavior changes suggesting significant frontal or anterior temporal involvement. A case illustrating the typical clinical features is presented:

Case Report

A 68-year-old retired factory worker was referred for decreased speech output. At the time of the initial visit, he complained of numbness of the left arm and leg of undetermined onset lasting for several months. He showed a cognitive deficit of impaired delayed recall, digit span backward, mental reversal, and impaired general knowledge of recent events on a short mental status examination. Further neuropsychological testing showed deficits in verbal memory and paired associates learning, as well as delayed visual reproduction in the WMS-R. His Mattis Dementia Rating Scale (MDRS) score of 113 fell into the range of mild dementia. On the Western Aphasia Battery (WAB) he was considered to have mild anomic aphasia. He was not apractic for gestural movements, but he had difficulty drawing. Arithmetic ability was impaired except for simple division. A magnetic resonance imaging (MRI) scan at that time revealed an area of atrophy of the anterior and medial aspects of the left temporal lobe (Figure 9.1).

Three months later, the patient started to complain of muscle aching in both arms and legs, relieved by getting up and walking around. His wife noticed that his memory had deteriorated, and his writing was much poorer. His right hand was slow and somewhat stiff. On examination he was apractic and agraphic. Over the following year, he showed progressive difficulties performing motor tasks like eating and dressing himself to the point when his right arm became completely useless. On examination, cogwheel rigidity in both arms, more marked in the right, was detected. His gait was slow, with absent arm swinging on the right hand. A trial of Amantadine (200 mg/day) first, and L-dopa (300 mg/day) afterward, provided no benefit.

Eighteen months after the initial examination, neuropsychological testing showed decreased memory performance. His verbal memory index and attention/concentration indices has dropped 16 points and 12 points, respectively. His performance on the verbal paired associates task was significantly worse. Spontaneous speech was hesitant, and the content was impaired. Word fluency was very low. Simple calculation was intact for addition but impaired for subtraction, multiplication, and divisions. On an extended apraxia battery, he showed mild orofacial apraxia and severe impairment for all transitive and intransitive movements with both arms. Performance was much worse on the right side, compounded by action tremor in his right hand. Comprehension of hand gestures was good. The (MDRS) score had fallen from 113 to 93. At this time of the evolution, a brain (HMPAO-SPECT) showed significantly decreased uptake over the left frontal, parietal, and temporal lobes.

Two years after disease onset, his verbal IQ (VIQ) of 78 had dropped 9 points from his initial evaluation and fell in the 7th percentile. His performance on the WAB remained stable, but his apraxia had significantly worsened. The MDRS score had dropped to 79. He developed gait difficulties and had an untriggered fall breaking his right arm.

Three years after disease onset, further neuropsychological testing showed evident decline in all areas, with the MDRS score falling to 69 and much poorer performance on the extended apraxia battery. Impairment of buccofacial praxis was noticed. His language had significantly deteriorated, and he showed problems with comprehension and naming. Word fluency remained very low at 3/20 expected words. His aphasia quotient (AQ) (Kertesz, 1982) had dropped from 91 to 81. Arithmetic performance was impaired for all tasks.

Four years after disease onset, his gait difficulty had worsened. He required assistance to stand and walk. His gait was described as "magnetic" and shuffling, with small steps. His language had declined further. He continued to show word-finding difficulties, and his sentences

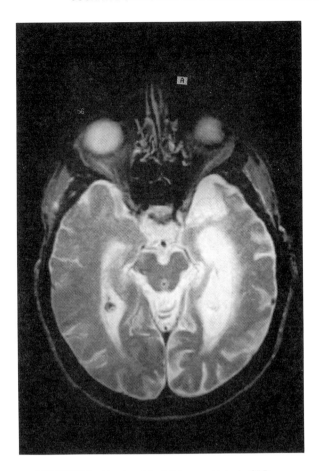

FIGURE 9.1. Atrophy of the left temporal lobe in CBD.

on conversational questioning were very simplified. He had problems with auditory word recognition tasks. Comprehension and repetition of complex material were poorer. His naming had deteriorated, and he was not able to produce a single word in a fluency task. His AQ was still fairly high (72.7) due to good comprehension.

Six years after the onset of his disease, in a nursing home, he was severely hypomimic, and he hardly spoke unless repeatedly prompted. On examination he showed vertical and horizontal gaze palsy. He was bound to his wheelchair and held his right hand in a clenched position in his lap. When asked to show or point to his right hand, he was unable to locate it. Persistent reflex myoclonus could be elicited on both hands, especially on the right.

CONCLUSION

In the literature, one can find several (nine by the latest count) patients with pathologically diagnosed CBD presenting as frontal lobe dementia (FLD) or FTD without extrapyramidal symptoms (Clark et al., 1986; Paulus and Selim, 1990; Lennox et al., 1994; Rinne et al., 1994; Rey et al., 1995; Frisoni et al., 1995). Moreover, frontal lobe dysfunction with behavioral disturbances, poor performance on frontal lobe tests, or both is described in 50% of the 57 patients with CBD for whom case reports were available in the literature (Rebeiz et al., 1968; Anonymous, 1985; Clark et al., 1986; Gibb et al., 1989; Eidelberg et al., 1990; Riley et al., 1990; Greene et al., 1990; Paulus and Lippa et al., 1990; Selim, 1990; Sawle et al., 1991; Ikuda et al., 1992; Lerner et al., 1992; Leiguarda et al., 1994; Horoupian and Chu, 1994; Lennox et al., 1994; Muhiddin et al., 1994; Frisoni et al., 1995; Rey et al., 1995). Hence, it is not surprising that two prospective studies have reported significantly low frontal scores in patients with CBD compared to controls (Vidailhet et al., 1994; Pillon et al., 1995). Similarly, CBD can present with a clinical picture of PPA (Lippa et al., 1990, 1991; Dobato et al., 1993; Marti-Masso et al., 1993; Kertesz et al., 1994).

The clinical overlap between PPA, CBD, and PiD is becoming increasingly recognized. PiD with Pick bodies usually manifests as FTD, but it can also present clinically as CBD (Cambier et al., 1981; Lang et al., 1994; Jendroska et al., 1995) or PPA (Graff-Radford et al., 1990). Symptomatic or asymptomatic extrapyramidal involvement in PiD is not infrequent (Akelaitis, 1994; Constantinidis et al., 1974; Munoz-Garcia and Ludwin, 1984). This condition was formerly called the *Akelaitis variety of PiD*. Rinne et al. (1994) suggested that patients belonging to groups B and C2 of Tissot et al. (1985) might well have CBD. The neuropathological overlap between PiD and CBD initially suggested by Rebeiz et al. (1968) has been repeatedly demonstrated and goes far beyond the mere presence of focal atrophy and ballooned neurons. White matter involvement, tau-positive astrocytic inclusions, oligodendroglial microtubular masses (Yamada et al., 1990; Ikeda et al., 1994; Feany et al., 1996), and argyrophilic grains (Ikeda et al., 1994) are the other, more recently characterized features of CBD, which to some extent distinguish this disease from PiD. However, it seems reasonable to postulate, on the basis of the commonalities of the pathological and clinical features of these variants of Pick complex, that they are essentially related.

From the literature and from our experience, it is evident that the behavioral and cognitive symptoms of CBD are the rule rather than the exception. Even in cases where CBD presents with the extrapyramidal/apraxic syndrome, progressive aphasia and disinhibition-apathy of the frontal lobe type supervene. In some cases, the typical CBD syndrome develops only after PPA and FLD run their course for several years. Longitudinal follow-up is needed to recognize the overlap of these syndromes. In the past, the cognitive changes were often overlooked when attention was focused on the movement disorder. However, when patients are examined systematically for cognitive deficits, these are almost invariable uncovered. Although CBDS is the least frequent variety of Pick complex as a primary presentation, it often supervenes in cases where the language disorder or the behavioral syndrome appears primarily.

REFERENCES

Akelaitis AJ (1944): Atrophy of basal ganglia in Pick's disease. Arch Neurol Psychiatry 51:27–34.

Brion S, Plas J, Jeaunea A (1991): Pick's disease. Rev Neurol 147:693–704.

Cambier JJ, Masson M, Dairou R, Henin D (1981): Etude anatomoclinique d'une forme parietale de maladie de Pick. Rev Neurol 137:33–38.

Case records of the Massachusetts General Hospital (1985): Weekly clinicopathological exercises. Case 38–1985. N Engl J Med 313:739–748.

Clark AW, Manz HJ, White CL III, Lehman J, Miller D, Coyle JT (1986): Cortical degeneration with swollen chromatolytic neurons: Its relationship to Pick's disease. J Neuropathol Exp Neurol 45:268–284.

Constantinidis J, Richard J, Tissot R (1974): Pick's disease: Histological and clinical correlations. Eur Neurol 11:208–217.

Dobato JL, Mateo D, de Andres C, Gimenez-Roldan S (1993): Degeneracion ganglionica corticobasal presentandose como un sindrome de afasia progresiva primaria. Neurologia 8:141.

Eidelberg D, Dhawan V, Moeller JR, Sidtis JJ, Ginos JZ, Strother SC, Cederbaum J, Greene P, Fahn S, Powers JM, Rottemberg DA (1991): The metabolic landscape of corticobasal ganglionic degeneration: Regional asymmetries studied with positron emission tomography. N Engl J Med 54:854–862.

Feany MB, Mattiace LA, Dickson DW (1996): Neuropathologic overlap of progressive supranuclear palsy, Pick's disease and corticobasal degeneration. J Neuropathol Exp Neurol 55:53–67.

Frisoni GB, Pizzolato G, Zanetti O, Bianchetti A, Chierichetti F, Trabucchi M (1995): Corticobasal degeneration: Neuropsychological assessment and dopamine D2 receptor SPECT analysis. Eur Neurol 35:50–54.

Fukui T, Sugita K, Kawamura M, Shiota J, Nakano I (1996): Primary progressive apraxia in Pick's disease: A clinicopathologic study. Neurology 47:467–473.

Gibb WRG, Luthert PJ, Marsden CD (1989): Corticobasal degeneration. Brain 112:1171–1192.

Graff-Radford NR, Damasio AR, Hyman BT, Hart MN, Tranel D, Damasio H, Van Hoesen GW, Rezai K (1990): Progressive aphasia in a patient with Pick's disease: A neuropsychological, radiologic, and anatomic study. Neurology 40:620–626.

Greene PE, Fahn S, Lang AE, Watts RL, Eidelberg E, Powers JM (1990): Progressive unilateral rigidity, bradykinesia, tremulousness, and apraxia leading to fixed postural deformity of the involved limb. Mov Disord 5:341–351.

Horoupian D, Chu PL (1994): Unusual case of corticobasal degeneration with tau/Gallyas-positive neuronal and glial tangles. Acta Neuropathol 88:592–598.

Ikeda K, Akiyama H, Haga C, Kondo H, Arima K, Oda T (1994): Argyrophilic thread-like structure in corticobasal degeneration and supranuclear palsy. Neurosci Lett 174:157–159.

Jendroska K, Rossor MN, Mathias CJ, Daniel SE (1995): Morphological overlap between corticobasal degeneration and Pick's disease: A clinicopathological report. Mov Disord 10:111–114.

Kertesz A (1982): The Western Aphasia Battery. New York: Psychological Corp.

Kertesz A, Hudson L, Mackenzie IRA, Munoz DG (1994): The pathology and nosology of primary progressive aphasia. Neurology 44:2065–2072.

Kosaka K, Ikeda K, Kobayashi K, Mehraein P (1991): Striatopallidonigral degeneration in Pick's disease: A clinicopathological study of 41 cases. J Neurol 238:151–160.

Lang AE, Bergeron C, Pollanen MS, Ashby P (1994): Parietal Pick's disease mimicking cortical-basal ganglionic degeneration. Neurology 44:1436–1440.

Leiguarda R, Lees AJ, Merello M, Starkstein S, Marsden CD (1994): The nature of apraxia in corticobasal degeneration. J Neurol Neurosurg Psychiatry 57:455–459.

Lennox G, Jackson M, Lowe J (1994): Corticobasal degeneration manifesting as frontal lobe dementia (abstract). Ann Neurol 36:273–274.

Lerner A, Friedland R, Riley D, Whitehouse P, Lanska D, Vick N, Cochran E, Tresser N, Cohen N, Gambetti P (1992): Dementia with pathological findings of corticobasal ganglionic degeneration (abstract). Ann Neurol 32:271.

Lippa CF, Cohen R, Smith TW, Drachman DA (1991): Primary progressive aphasia with focal neuronal achromasia. Neurology 41:882–886.

Lippa CF, Smith TW, Fontneau N (1990): Corticonigral degeneration with neuronal achromasia. A clinicopathological study of two cases. J Neurol Sci 98:301–310.

Löwenberg K (1935): Pick's disease—a clinicopathologic contribution. Arch Neurol Psychiatry 36:68–789.

The Lund and Manchester Groups (1994): Clinical and neuropathological criteria for frontotemporal dementia. J Neurol Neurosurg Psychiatry 57:416–418.

Marti-Masso JF, Lopez de Muniain A, Poza JJ, Urtasun M, Carrera N (1993): Degeneracion corticobasal ganglionica: A proposito de siete observaciones diagnosticada clinicamente. Neurologia 9:115–120.

Muhiddin KA, Hardie RJ, Pearce VR, Kirby BJ (1994): Corticobasal degeneration: A report of three cases. J R Soc Med 87:359–360.

Munoz-Garcia D, Ludwin SK (1984): Classic and generalized variants of Pick's disease: A clinicopathological, ultrastructural and immunocytochemical study. Ann Neurol 16:467–480.

Paulus W, Selim M (1990): Corticonigral degeneration with neuronal achromasia and basal neurofibrillary tangles. Acta Neuropathol 81:89–94.

Pillon B, Blin J, Vidailhet M, Deweer B, Sirigu A, Dubois B, Agid Y (1995): The neuropsychological pattern of corticobasal degeneration: Comparison with progressive supranuclear palsy and Alzheimer's disease. Neurology 45:1477–1483.

Rebeiz JJ, Kolodny EH, Richardson EP (1968): Corticodentatonigral degeneration with neuronal achromasia. Arch Neurol 18:20–33.

Rey GJ, Tower R, Levin BE, Sanchez-Ramos J, Bowen B, Bruce JH (1995): Psychiatric symptoms, atypical dementia, and left visual field inattention in corticobasal ganglionic degeneration. Mov Disord 10:106–110.

Riley DE, Lang AE, Lewis A, Resch L, Ashby P, Horneykiewicz O, Black SI (1990): Cortical-basal ganglionic degeneration. Neurology 40:1203–1212.

Rinne JO, Lee MS, Thompson PD, Marsden CD (1994): Corticobasal degeneration—A clinical study of 36 cases. Brain 117:1183–1196.

Sakurai Y, Hashida H, Uesugi H, Arima K, Murayama S, Bando M, Iwata M, Momose T, Sakuta M (1996): A clinical profile of corticobasal degeneration presenting as primary progressive aphasia. Eur Neurol 36:134–137.

Sawle GV, Brooks DJ, Marsden CD, Frackowiak RSJ (1990): Corticobasal degeneration. A unique pattern of regional cortical oxygen hypometabolism and striatal fluorodopa uptake demonstrated by positron emission tomography. Brain 114:541–556.

Schneider JA, Watts RL, Gearing M, Brewer RP, Mirra SS (1997): Corticobasal degeneration: Neuropathologic and clinical heterogeneity. Neurology 48:959–969.

Tissot R, Constantinidis J, Richard J (1985): Pick's disease. In Frederiks JAM (ed): Handbook of Clinical Neurology, Vol. 2 (46): Neurobehavioural Disorders. Amsterdam: Elsevier, pp 233–246.

Uchihara T, Tsychiya K, Kosaka K (1990): Selective loss of nigral neurones in Pick's disease. Acta Neuropathol 81:155–161.

Vidailhet M, Rivaud S, Goudier-Khouja N, Pillon B, Bonnet AM, Gaymard B, Agid Y, Pierrot-Deseilligny C (1994): Eye movements in Parkinsonian syndromes. Ann Neurol 35:420–426.

Watts RL, Mirra SS, Young RR, Burger PC, Villier JA, Heyman A (1989): Corticobasal ganglionic degeneration (CBGD) with neuronal achromasia: Clinical-pathological study of two cases. Neurology 39(Suppl 1):140 (abstract).

Winkelman NW, Book MH (1944): Asymptomatic extrapyramidal involvement in Pick's disease. Arch Neurol Psychiatry 8:30–42.

Yamada T, McGeer PL (1990): Oligodendroglial microtubular masses: An abnormality observed in some human neurodegenerative diseases. Neurosci Lett 120:163–166.

CHAPTER 10

Apraxia in the Syndromes of Pick Complex

RAMÓN LEIGUARDA, and SERGIO E. STARKSTEIN

Departments of Clinical Neurology (R.L., S.E.S.) and Neuropsychiatry (S.E.S.), Raúl Carrea Institute of Neurological Research-FLENI, Montañeses 2325, Buenos Aires, Argentia

INTRODUCTION

In 1905, Arnold Pick reported apraxia in a 43-year-old cavalry guard who Pick believed had a localized cortical atrophy. The patient became taciturn and apathetic at the end of 1902 and developed progressive naming difficulties. In November 1903 he showed nonfluent language and verbal comprehension deficits and was admitted to the Prague Hospital in April 1904. Pick gave the following examples of this patient's apraxia: "The patient is given a pipe and brings it correctly to his mouth, then expertly reaches for the tobacco pouch and takes a match from the box, but when asked to light it, sticks the head of the match into the mouth piece and puts the other end in his mouth as if to smoke it" . . . "the patient is requested to light a candle in its holder. He takes a match, holds it with both hands without doing anything further with it. When asked again, he takes the match upside down in his hand and tries to bore it into the candle" . . . "He puts a letter in an envelope correctly on request. He is asked to seal it and does so by pressing on the gummed edge as if it had already been moistened and he wanted to seal it" (see Brown, 1988, pp. 105) These descriptions not only demonstrate the clinical insight of Arnold Pick, but also suggest that apraxia may be an important manifestation of specific types of focal brain atrophies.

In this chapter, we will address our current knowledge of limb praxic disorders and examine the prevalence, type, and kinematic features of limb apraxia in patients with frontal lobe dementia (FLD), corticobasal degeneration (CBD), and primary progressive aphasia (PPA), recently grouped under the term *Pick complex* (Kertesz, 1996).

Praxic disturbances may involve specific parts of the body (e.g., limb apraxia, axial apraxia, buccolingual apraxia) (Kertesz and Ferro, 1984), may characterize the abnormal execution of a sequence (e.g., lighting a candle), or may be restricted to specific motor acts (e.g., dressing apraxia). While there are discrepancies about the nosological concept of apraxia, praxis

Pick's Disease and Pick Complex, Edited by Andrew Kertesz and David G. Munoz
ISBN 0-471-17792-X   ©1998 Wiley-Liss, Inc.

processing may be mediated by a two-part system involving both conceptual aspects and production of movements (Roy and Square, 1985). The praxis production system may consist of a sensorimotor component of action knowledge (i.e., information contained in motor programs), and disruption of this system may produce *ideomotor apraxia* (*IMA*), which is defined as "an impairment in the timing, sequencing, and spatial organization of gestural movements" (Rothi et al., 1991). The praxis conceptual system may be divided into three kinds of knowledge: (1) knowledge of those functions subserved by tools and objects, (2) knowledge of actions without tools, and (3) knowledge about the organization of single steps into a sequence. Disruption of this system is considered to produce the syndrome of *ideational apraxia* (*IA*) (Rothi et al., 1991).

Several authors described specific patterns of movement errors in IMA and IA, such as temporal, spatial, and content errors. *Temporal errors* may present as an abnormal speed of the pantomime (i.e., timing errors), a delay in the initiation of the movement (i.e., delay errors), errors in the specific sequence of a pantomime (i.e., sequencing errors), and subtractions or additions of movement cycles (i.e., occurrence errors). *Spatial errors* may present as the substitution of a body part for an object (e.g., use of fingers to simulate a comb), abnormalities in the required posture of the fingers or hand in relation to the target tool (i.e., internal configuration errors), abnormal orientation of the finger, hand, or arm in relation to the object receiving the action or in placing the object in space (i.e., external configuration-orientation errors), abnormalities of a movement when acting with a tool on an object due to improper joint stabilization and motion (i.e., movement or spatial trajectory errors), and variations in the amplitude of a pantomime (i.e., amplitude errors). Finally, *content errors* include the repetition and the substitution of all or part of a pantomime (i.e., perseverative errors) (Rothi et al., 1988).

IMA is characterized by tempororspatial errors. Patients with IMA make more errors when requested to pantomime transitive (i.e., using an object) than intransitive movements, and usually improve on imitation and when handling the target object. Although the target movement may be spatially and/or temporally incorrect, the intent of the act is usually recognizable. While these deficits may be clearly observed in the testing session, they are rarely present in real-life situations. On the other hand, patients with IA may show deficits in both settings. These patients often use inappropriately objects that can otherwise be correctly recognized and named. Patients with IA usually substitute one tool for another (e.g., using a toothbrush for a comb) and select actions inappropriately. The disorder is more evident when IA patients are requested to carry out a sequence of movements (e.g., to mail a letter) (Pick, 1905; Liepmann, 1920; Poeck, 1983), and the assessment of knowledge of tool function and action usually shows deficits (Ochipa et al., 1989, 1992).

IMA is most frequent among patients with damage to the dominant parietal association area (mainly the inferior parietal lobe), the premotor cortex (mainly the supplementary motor area), and the corpus callosum or intrahemispheric white matter bundles such as the arcuate and superior occipitofrontal tracts (Kertesz and Ferro, 1984; Faglioni and Basso, 1985; Heilman and Rothi, 1985). While patients with lesions of the dominant frontal lobe or association pathways from parietal to frontal lobes usually show bilateral IMA and normal comprehension and discrimination of gestures, patients with lesions to the left parietal lobe (which may disrupt visuokinesthetic motor engrams [Heilman et al., 1982; Kertesz and Ferro, 1984]) may also show comprehension/discrimination deficits (Heilman and Rothi, 1985; Watson et al., 1986). When damage involves the corpus callosum and interrupts the outflow from the left to the right premotor regions, apraxia is present only in the left limb. On the other hand, IA is usually found after widespread brain damage (such as in Alzheimer's disease) or after the development of focal lesions involving the left parietotemporal region (De Renzi and Lucchelli, 1988; Ochipa et al., 1992).

The nosological position of melo or *limb-kinetic apraxia* (LKA) is still under debate. First proposed by Kleist in 1907 (see Brown, 1988) and considered by Liepmann (1920) a type of limb apraxia, it has not been assessed with enough accuracy to deserve widespread acceptance. Patients with LKA show clumsiness, awkwardness, and decomposition of fine distal movements of the hand contralateral to the brain lesion (which usually involves the primary sensorimotor and premotor areas). All types of movements are affected, whether symbolic (intransitive or transitive) or asymbolic. Whereas in LKA distal limb movements may lack precision, the spatial and temporal errors characteristic of IMA are not found. Several authors do not acknowledge LKA as a true apraxia, suggesting that it may be a mild corticospinal deficit (Heilman and Rothi, 1985), LKA most likely results from dysfunction of more complex motor processes.

Limb apraxia may be assessed both qualitatively and quantitatively. We will briefly review the testing paradigms most frequently used.

Transitive movements: Patients are asked to perform learned movements, pretending they are using a tool (e.g., "show me how you use a hammer"). Patients are also asked to imitate the examiner and to perform the movement with the target tool.

Intransitive movements: Patients are asked to perform learned movements that do not require a tool. These movements may be either representational (e.g., "wave good-bye") or nonrepresentational (e.g., "touch your nose"). Imitation of intransitive movements is also assessed.

Recognition and discrimination of learned skilled movements: Patients are shown videotapes of actors performing different types of transitive movements, as well as correct and incorrect transitive movements. Patients have to identify the movements and discriminate correct from incorrect ones.

Movement imitation test: Patients are asked to imitate finger and hand postures (symbolic and nonsymbolic) and finger and hand sequences.

Sequencing tasks: Patients are asked to perform specific tasks that usually require several steps and different objects (e.g., when patients are asked to mail a letter, they have to fold the paper, put the paper into an envelope, close the envelope, and glue the stamp to the envelope).

Conceptual knowledge of tool function and action: This is an assessment of tool function knowledge (e.g., identifying tools from verbal functional descriptions, tool function identification, and tool selection) and knowledge of action (i.e., the verbal description of actions required for tool use and the selection of tools required to complete a specific task) (Ochipa et al., 1989, 1992).

Three-dimensional computergraphic analysis of transitive movements: This assessment usually requires three optoelectric cameras that sense the positions of infrared emitting diodes secured to the patient's arms, shoulders, elbows, wrists, and hands. The patient is asked to carry out a learned movement (e.g., to slice a loaf of bread), and kinematic measurements are obtained on the trajectories of the wrist and angular motions of the upper limb joints. The following kinematic measurements of wrist trajectories are obtained: *spatial accuracy:* measurements of amplitude, linearity, plane of motion, and planarity; *temporal attributes:* measurements of acceleration and velocity; and *spatiotemporal relationships:* measurements of velocity–curvature decoupling and kinematic measurements of interjoint coordination (Poizner et al., 1990, 1995; Clark et al., 1994).

APRAXIA IN PRIMARY PROGRESSIVE APHASIA (PPA)

PPA is a progressive language disturbance in the absence of other cognitive deficits characterized by either nonfluent, anomic speech with normal language comprehension or fluent output with reduced comprehension and poor repetition. Associated neurological abnormalities may include dysphagia, hyperreflexia, unilateral or bilateral limb rigidity, bradykinesia, gegenhalten, and primitive reflexes. Acalculia, loss of analytical musical skills, loss of semantic memory, and buccofacial and limb apraxia may also develop (Mesulam, 1982; Kempler et al., 1990; Northen et al., 1990; Tyrrel et al., 1991; Beland and Ska, 1992; Caselli et al., 1992; Mesulam and Weintraub, 1992; Cohen et al., 1993; Karbe et al., 1993; Polk and Kertesz, 1993; Breedin et al., 1994; Fuh et al., 1994; Hodges et al., 1994; Kertesz et al., 1994).

Few studies have assessed apraxia in patients with PPA. Kempler et al. (1990) examined three patients with PPA with the apraxia subtests of the Western Aphasia Battery (WAB). All three had mild limb apraxia at the initial evaluation, and at follow-up two of them showed progression of their praxic deficits. Karbe et al. (1993) assessed 10 PPA patients with the WAB and found mild apraxia in most of them. Among patients with PPA, orofacial apraxia may be more frequent than limb apraxia. Tyrrell et al. (1991) reported 3 patients with progressive loss of speech output and orofacial apraxia, 1 of whom also had limb apraxia, and Caselli et al. (1992) found that 7 out of 10 patients with nonfluent PPA had orofacial but not limb apraxia. Recently, Bianchetti et al. (1996) found orofacial apraxia in three out of seven patients with PPA, and Arima et al. (1994) reported a patient with PPA and dysarthria who also showed orofacial apraxia.

While the above studies were the first to demonstrate apraxia in PPA, most of them lacked a comprehensive evaluation of apraxia, and none of them used kinematic measurements. We recently studied four patients who met the Mesulam-Weintraub (1992) criteria of at least 2 years of aphasia in the absence of neuropsychological deficits. All four were right-handed females, with an average age at onset of the disease of 74 years (range, 64–83 years) and a 2-year duration of language deficits at the time of the initial evaluation. Patients 1, 2 and 3 had nonfluent aphasia, and patient 4 had fluent aphasia. Associated neurological findings at initial examination were mild rigidity of the right upper limb, hyperreflexia, and clumsiness of fine finger movements in two patients. Magnetic resonance imaging (MRI) showed left perisylvian atrophy in patients 1 and 2, left perisylvian plus bilateral parietal atrophy in patient 3, and diffuse but asymmetric (left > right) cerebral atrophy in patient 4. Single photon emission computed tomography (SPECT) studies with 99-technetium hexamethyl propylene-amine oxime (HMPAO) showed left frontotemporal hypoperfusion in patient 1 with extension into the parietal region in patient 3; bitemporal perfusion deficits in patient 2; and bilateral temporoparietal perfusion deficits in patient 4.

All four patients had bilateral IMA, two had orofacial apraxia, and one patient (case 4) also had IA. All four patients showed deficits on the movement imitation test. IMA was mild to moderate, and transitive movements were more affected than intransitive movements. Performance improved on imitation and when using the target objects. Spatial errors were more frequent than temporal errors. Among spatial errors, external configuration (orientation) and trajectory errors were most frequently observed. Temporal errors (mainly timing and occurrence) and sequence errors were rarely observed. Discrimination/comprehension of pantomimes was normal in two patients (patients 1 and 2), a mild deficit was shown by patient 3, and a moderate deficit was shown by patient 4. This patient also showed deficits on the multiple-steps task (perplexity, omission, mislocation, and sequencing errors) and in the tool-object action and tool-object association tests (mostly content errors).

While 2 years after the initial evaluation patients 1 and 2 only showed progression of their language deficit, patient 3 developed an asymmetric akineto-rigid syndrome with myoclonus (probably CBD), and patient 4 showed progression of her language and praxic deficits together with other cognitive impairments, meeting the criteria for probable Alzheimer's disease.

In conclusion, both IMA and orofacial apraxia are common findings in patients with nonfluent PPA, whereas patients with fluent PPA may also show IA. While in most PPA patients IMA is mild and slowly progressing, PPA patients with more severe IMA may develop a motor disorder resembling CBD. Finally, the presence of IA may indicate further progression of the cognitive impairments.

APRAXIA IN CORTICOBASAL DEGENERATION (CBD)

CBD is a slowly progressive disorder characterized by an asymmetric akinetic-rigid syndrome, limb dystonia, myoclonus, limb and orofacial apraxia, cortical sensory loss, and alien limb behavior. Supranuclear gaze palsy, eyelid apraxia, and signs of corticospinal tract dysfunction are less common. Cognitive decline may develop at a later stage, and language disturbances are absent or mild (Rebeiz et al., 1968; Gibb et al., 1989; Watts et al., 1989; Riley et al., 1990; Rinne et al., 1994). Less frequently, patients may present with progressive aphasia, orofacial apraxia, and progressive loss of speech output (Cambier et al., 1981; Lippa, et al., 1991; Lang 1992; Arima et al., 1994; Rinne et al., 1994).

The whole spectrum of praxic disorders has been described in patients with CBD (Cambier et al., 1981; Riley et al., 1990; Leiguarda et al., 1994; Okuda and Tachibana, 1994; Rinne et al., 1994; Jacobs et al., 1995). Jacobs et al. (1995) found IMA with intact gesture recognition in six patients with CBD and suggested that apraxia may result from dysfunction of the supplementary motor area. On the other hand, Okuda and Tachibana (1994) reported four CBD patients who showed an asymmetric LKA, more severe on the side of greater clumsiness, as well as difficulties in pantomiming gestures with or without handling the target objects.

In a recent study, we examined the prevalence and clinical correlates of apraxia in a series of 10 patients with CBD (Leiguarda et al., 1994). To minimize the confounding effects of akinesia, rigidity, and involuntary movements, praxis was assessed in the less affected limb. We found that 7 of 10 CBD patients showed deficits on tests of IMA and movement imitation, but none had orofacial apraxia. Four of the seven patients with IMA could correctly recognize and discriminate gestures performed by the examiner, whereas the remaining three patients had comprehension/discrimination deficits. These three patients also showed deficits on the multiple-steps task.

The most frequent praxic errors found in our CBD patients were those of internal and external configuration, sequencing, body part as object, and trajectory. Conceptual deficits included perplexity, absent or unrecognizable response, omissions, mislocations, and sequence errors. IMA was significantly more frequent in patients with onset of motor symptoms on the right side, and the alien limb behavior was present only in apraxic patients. We also found a significant correlation between IMA and scores on frontal lobe tasks.

In conclusion, IMA is the most frequent type of apraxia in CBD and may be secondary to dysfunction of the supplementary motor area. A subgroup of CBD patients may show severe apraxia (both IMA and IA), which may result from additional parietal or diffuse cortical involvement.

APRAXIA IN FRONTAL LOBE DEMENTIA (FLD)

FLD is a chronic, progressive disease characterized by early loss of personal and social awareness, disinhibition signs (e.g., unrestrained sexuality and violence, moria, joking, and exhibitionism), apathy and inertia, and lack of drive and initiative. Behavior is inflexible and perseverative. Stereotypic features and hyperorality are common, and utilization behavior may also be observed. Affective symptoms (i.e., depression, hypochondria, emotional unconcern and emotional lability are also frequent and may herald the beginning of the illness (Brun et al., 1994; Neary and Snowden, 1996).

Motor examination usually demonstrates primitive reflexes such as grasping, palmomental response and sucking, extensor plantar responses, and parkinsonian signs (e.g., rigidity, bradykinesia, and tremor). A minority of patients may develop signs of motor neuron disease with predominance of bulbar over limb involvement. While motor perseveration and poor performance of sequential motor acts are commonly observed, the presence of apraxia has not been systematically examined.

We recently examined eight male patients with FLD for the presence of apraxia. Mean age at onset of the disease was 73 years (range, 61–85 years), and mean duration of the disease at the time of praxis assessment was 6 years (range, 2–15 years). Two of the 8 patients showed mild to moderate bilateral IMA (mainly for transitive movements) and deficits on the movement imitation test. The most frequent temporal errors were those of hesitation, timing, and occurrence, whereas the most frequent spatial errors were those of external and internal configuration, body part as object, and amplitude errors. None of the patients showed abnormalities on the multiple-steps task, the tool-object action and tool-object association test, or the comprehension/discrimination of movements. Both patients with apraxia had a long duration of illness (>10 years) and prominent primitive reflexes, and mild parkinsonism was present in one. However, no specific neurological signs were present in apraxic compared to nonapraxic patients.

In conclusion, IMA with normal comprehension/discrimination of movements may be found in some patients with FLD. The presence of apraxia in FLD may result from pathological changes in specific areas of the frontal lobe, with further involvement of the striatum and parietal cortex.

Three-Dimensional Computergraphic Analysis of Transitive Movements

We carried out kinematic analysis of the gesture of slicing a loaf of bread in two patients with PPA (both with IMA), two patients with CBD (both with IMA), and two patients with FLD (1 with and 1 without IMA). Patients with PPA and CBD and the apraxic patient with FLD showed kinematic deficits in spatial accuracy, timing, spatiotemporal coupling, and interjoint coordination. We will briefly illustrate the most relevant aspects of the kinematic analysis.

Spatial Accuracy   Figure 10.1 shows a lateral view of the reconstructed trajectories of the limb segments during the slicing gesture performed by a normal control (10.1a) and by patients with PPA (10.1b), CBD (10.1c), or FLD (10.1d). Stick figure representations of the arm, forearm, and hand show successive limb positions at 20-msec intervals. When produced by a normal control, the gesture consisted of a stereotyped sequence of forward and backward movements of the hand (Figure 10.1a). The trajectory paths of the wrist were located perpendicular to the object, with minimal horizontal and vertical displacement, and were aligned in the sagittal plane. The PPA patient showed an abnormal pattern due to more shoulder and less elbow displacement than the control, and the wrist and hand paths exhibited marked vertical and hor-

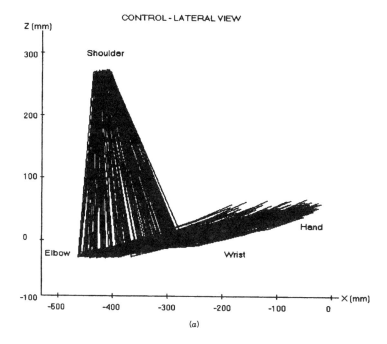

CONTROL - LATERAL VIEW

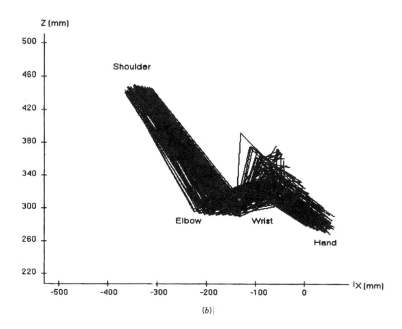

PPA PATIENT - LATERAL VIEW

FIGURE 10.1. Lateral view of shoulder, elbow, and wrist paths in a normal control (a) and in PPA (b), CBD (c), and FLD (d) patients. Stick figures represent successive limb positions at 20-msec intervals. Note the abnormal vertical and horizontal motion of the wrist in the PPA patient, the marked and irregular anterior-posterior motion of the elbow and horizontal motion of the wrist in the CBD patient, and the chop-like character of the movement in the FLD patient.

CBD PATIENT

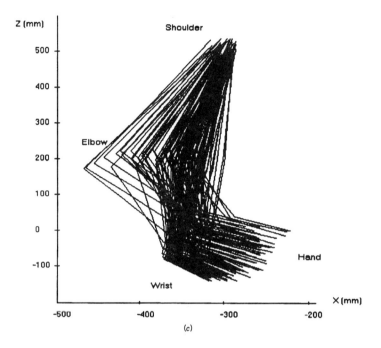

(c)

FLD PATIENT - LATERAL VIEW

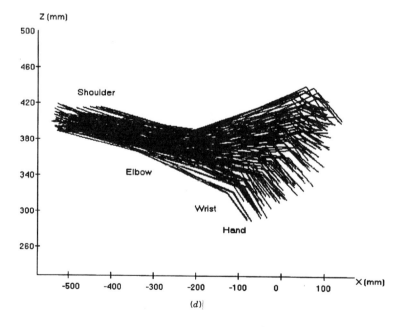

(d)|

FIGURE 10.1. (*continued*)

izontal displacement (Figure 10.1b). The patient with CBD showed the greatest distortion in the spatial pattern of motion. The elbow moved excessively and irregularly in the anterior-posterior direction, and the wrist was displaced in all directions (Figure 10.1c). Finally, the patient with FLD and apraxia showed an incorrect orientation of the movement axis, with marked vertical displacement of the hand and wrist, which moved in a chop-like fashion (Figure 10.1d).

Spatiotemporal Relationships   Complex trajectories are planned through the proportional control of speed and spatial path of the movement, which is expressed as a strong correspondence between velocity of movement and radius of curvature. Time differences approaching zero indicate tight spatiotemporal coupling (normal control, Figure 10.2a), whereas larger time differences reflect spatiotemporal decoupling (Figure 10.2b–d).

Interjoint Coordination   The kinematic abnormalities of the wrist in our apraxic patients may reflect deficits in interjoint coordination, since the trajectory of the wrist results from the combined motion of the shoulder and elbow joints. Our kinematic studies in control subjects demonstrated a smooth linear relationship between elbow flexion/extension and upper arm yaw (Figure 10.3a). This normal relationship helps to keep the wrist in the sagittal plane. In contrast, patients with PPA, CBD, or FLD showed a distorted angle/angle relationship due to dissimilar elbow/flexion extension and upper arm yaw movements (Figure 10.3b–d). Moreover,

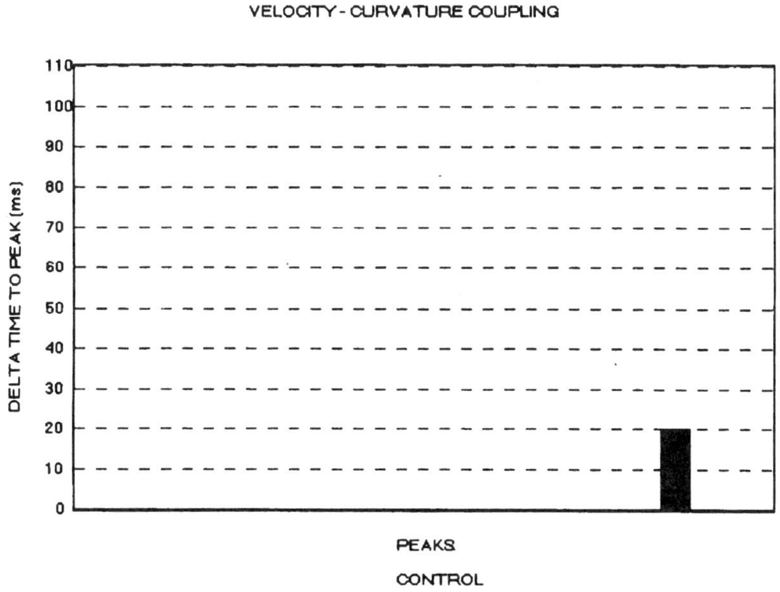

VELOCITY - CURVATURE COUPLING

PEAKS

CONTROL

(a)

FIGURE 10.2.   Time correspondence between velocity minima and radius of curvature minima. Normally, the time difference between each minimum wrist tangential velocity and the minimum radius of curvature approaches zero, indicating tight spatiotemporal coupling (Figure 10.2a). On the other hand, all three patients showed greater than zero time differences, demonstrating important velocity-curvature decoupling (Figure 10.2b–d).

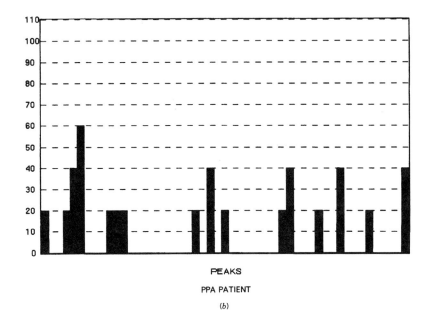

PPA PATIENT

(b)

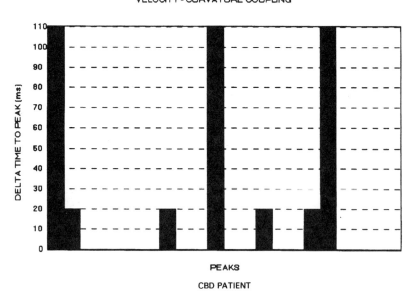

CBD PATIENT

(c)

FIGURE 10.2. (*continued*)

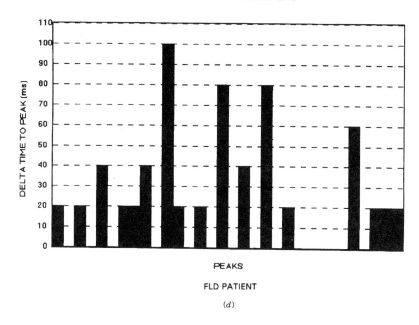

FIGURE 10.2. (*continued*)

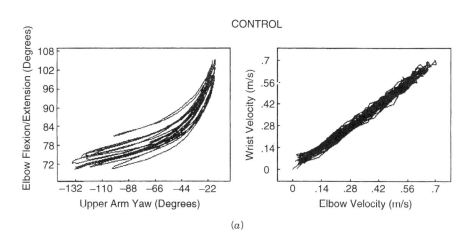

FIGURE 10.3. Kinematic relationships between elbow flexion/extension and upper arm yaw, and wrist and elbow speeds, in a normal control (a) and in patients with PPA (b), CBD (c), or FLD (d). While the normal control produced a smooth linear relationship between elbow flexion/extension and upper arm yaw, all three patients showed a significantly distorted angle/angle relationship, and asynchronous intersegmental joint velocities.

PPA PATIENT

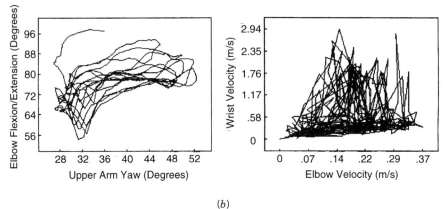

(b)

CBD PATIENT

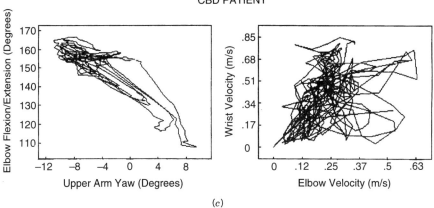

(c)

FLD PATIENT

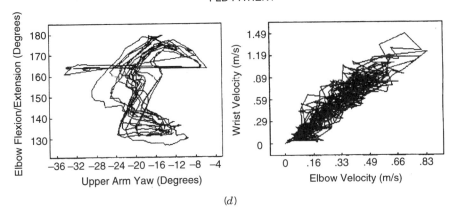

(d)

FIGURE 10.3. (*continued*)

while in the control subject there was a strong linear association between speed at the wrist and speed at the elbow, all three patients showed asynchronous intersegmental joint velocities.

In conclusion, the kinematic abnormalities observed in the orientation of movement, shape of the wrist trajectory, timing, spatiotemporal relationships and disruption of interjoint coordination during the performance of a transitive movement constitute objective parameters underlying spatial and temporal errors observed on clinical examination.

CONCLUSIONS

Apraxia is a frequent finding among patients with PPA or CBD, but it is rarely found in patients with FLD. The whole spectrum of praxic disorders may be present in CBD. While IMA is the most frequent type, IA and LKA may also be found. Orofacial apraxia and IMA are the most frequent types of apraxia in nonfluent PPA. Whereas severe IMA may herald the onset of CBD, the presence of IA may indicate progression toward a full-blown dementia. In FLD apraxia is not a frequent finding, although some patients may show IMA in the late stages of the disease.

ACKNOWLEDGMENTS

This work was partially supported by grants from the Raúl Carrea Institute of Neurological Research and the Fundación Pérez Companc. We thank Marcelo Merello, M.D.: Erán Chemerinski, M.D.; and Jorge Balej, Ph.D. for providing data for the present chapter.

REFERENCES

Arima K, Uesugi H, Fujita Y, Sakkurai Y, Oyanagi S, Andoh S, Izumiyama Y, Inose T (1994): Corticonigral degeneration with neuronal achromasia presenting with primary progressive aphasia: Ultrastructural and immunocytochemical studies. J Neurol Sci 127:186–197.

Beland R, Ska B (1992): Interaction between verbal and gestural language in progressive aphasia: A longitudinal study. Brain Lang 43:355–385.

Bianchetti A, Frisoni GB, Trabucchi M (1996): Primary progressive aphasia and frontal lobe involvement. Neurology 46:289–290.

Breedin SD, Saffran EM, Coslett HB (1994): Reversal of the concreteness effect in a patient with semantic dementia. Cogn Neuropsychol 11:617–660.

Brown JW (1988): Agnosia and Apraxia: Selected Papers of Liepmann, Lange, and Pötzl. Hillsdale, NJ: Lawrence Erlbaum.

Brun A, Englund B, Gustafson L, Passant U, Mann DMA, Neary D, Snowden JS (1994): Clinical and neuropathological criteria for frontotemporal dementia. J Neurol Neurosurg Psychiatry 57:416–418.

Cambier J, Masson M, Dairou R, Henin D (1981): Etude anatomo-clinique d'une forme parietale e maladie de Pick. Rev Neurol 137:33–38.

Caselli RJ, Jack C Jr, Peterson R, Wahner H, Yanagihara T (1993): Slowly progressive aphasia. Neurology 43:1858–1860.

Caselli RJ, Jack J, Peterson R, Wahner H, Yanagihara T (1992): Asymmetrical cortical degenerative syndromes: Clinical and radiologic correlations. Neurology 42:1462–1468.

Clark MA, Merians AS, Kothari A, Poizner H, Macauley B, Gonzalez Rothi LJ, Heilman KM (1994): Spatial planning deficits in limb apraxia. Brain 117:1093–1106.

Cohen L, Benoit N, Van Eeckhout P, Ducarne B, Brunet P (1993): Pure progressive aphemia. J Neurol Neurosurg Psychiatry 56:923–924.

De Renzi E, Lucchelli F (1988): Ideational apraxia. Brain 111:1173–1185.

Faglioni P, Basso A (1985): Historical perspectives of neuroanatomical correlates of limb apraxia. In Roy EA (ed): Advances in Psychology: Neuropsychological Studies of Apraxia and Related Disorders, Vol 23. Amsterdam: North Holland, pp 3–44.

Fuh JL, Liao KK, Wang SJ, Lin KN (1994): Swallowing difficulty in primary progressive aphasia: A case report. Cortex 30:701–705.

Gibb WR, Luthert PJ, Marsden CD (1989): Corticobasal degeneration. Brain 112:1171–1192.

Heilman KM, Rothi LJG (1985): Apraxia. In Heilman KM, Valenstein E (eds): Clinical Neuropsychology. New York: Oxford University Press, pp 131–150.

Heilman KM, Rothi LJG, Valenstein E (1982): Two forms of ideomotor apraxia. Neurology 32:342–346.

Hodges J, Patterson K, Tyler L (1994): Loss of semantic memory: Implications for the modularity of mind. Cogn Neuropsychol 11:505–542.

Jacobs DH, Boston MA, Adair JC, Macauley BL, Gold M, Gonzalez Rothi LJ, Heilman KM (1995): Apraxia in corticobasal degeneration (CBD). Neurology 45(Suppl 4): A266–A267.

Karbe H, Kertesz A, Polk M (1993): Profiles of language impairment in primary progressive aphasia. Arch Neurol 50:193–201.

Kempler D, Metter EJ, Riege WH, Jackson CA, Benson DF, Hanson WR (1990): Slowly progressive aphasia: Three cases with language, memory, CT and PET data. J Neurol Neurosurg Psychiatry 53:987–993.

Kertesz A (1996): Pick complex and Pick's disease. Eur J Neurol 3:280–282.

Kertesz A, Appell J, Fisman M (1994): The pathology and nosology of primary progressive aphasia. Neurology 44:2065–2072.

Kertesz A, Ferro JM (1984): Lesion size and location in ideomotor apraxia. Brain 107:921–933.

Lang AE (1992): Cortical basal ganglionic degeneration presenting with progressive loss of speech output and orofacial dyspraxia. J Neurol Neurosurg Psychiatry 55:1101.

Leiguarda R, Lees AJ, Merello M, Starkstein S, Marsden CD (1994): The nature of apraxia in corticobasal degeneration. J Neurol Neurosurg Psychiatry 57:455–459.

Liepmann H (1920): Apraxie. Ergeb Gesamten Med 1:516–543.

Lippa CF, Cohen R, Smith TW, Drachman DA (1991): Primary progressive aphasia with focal neuronal achromasia. Neurology 41:882–886.

Mesulam MM (1982): Slowly progressive aphasia without generalized dementia. Ann Neurol 11:592–598.

Mesulam MM, Weintraub S (1992): Heterogeneity in Alzheimer's disease. In Boller F, Focette F, Khachaturian Z, Poncet M, Christen Y (eds): Primary Progressive Aphasia: Sharping the Focus on a Clinical Syndrome. Berlin: Springer-Verlag, pp 43–66.

Neary D, Snowden J (1996): Fronto-temporal dementia: Nosology, neuropsychology, and neuropathology. Brain Cogn 31:176–187.

Northen B, Hopcutt B, Griffiths H (1990)· Progressive aphasia without generalized dementia. Aphasiology 4:55–65.

Ochipa C, Rothi LJG, Heilman KM (1989): Ideational apraxia: A deficit in tool selection and use. Ann Neurol 25:190–193.

Ochipa C, Rothi LJG, Heilman KM (1992): Conceptual apraxia in Alzheimer's disease. Brain 115:1061–1071.

Okuda B, Tachibana H (1994): The nature of apraxia in corticobasal degeneration (letter). J Neurol Neurosurg Psychiatry 57:1548–1549.

Pick A (1905): Studien über Motorische Apraxie und ihr Nahestehende Erscheinungen, ihre Bedeutung in der Symptomatologie Psychopathischer Symptomen-Komplexe. Leipzig: Deuticke.

Poeck K (1983): Ideational apraxia. J Neurol 230:1–5.

Poizner H, Clark MA, Merians AS, Macauley B, Gonzalez Rothi LJ, Heilman KM (1995): Joint coordination deficits in limb apraxia. Brain 118:227–242.

Poizner H, Mack L, Verfaellie M, Gonzalez Rothi LJ, Heilman KM (1990): Three-dimensional computer-graphic analysis of apraxia: Neural representations of learned movement. Brain 113:85–101.

Polk M, Kertesz A (1993): Music and language in degenerative disease of the brain. Brain Cogn 22:98–117.

Rebeiz JJ, Kolodny EH, Richardson EP (1968): Corticodentatonigral degeneration with neuronal achromasia. Arch Neurol 18:20–33.

Riley DE, Lang AE, Lewis A, Resch L, Asby P, Horykiewicz O, Black S (1990): Corticobasal ganglionic degeneration. Neurology 40:1203–1212.

Rinne J, Lee M, Thompson P, Marsden C (1994): Corticobasal degeneration: A clinical study of 36 cases. Brain 117:1183–1196.

Rothi LJG, Mack L, Verfaille M, Brown P, Heilman KM (1988): Ideomotor apraxia: Error pattern analysis. Aphasiology 2:381–388.

Rothi LJG, Ochipa C, Heilman KM (1991): A cognitive neuropsychological model of praxis. Cogn Neuropsychol 8:443–458.

Roy EA, Square PA (1985): Common considerations in the study of limb, verbal and oral apraxia. In Roy EA (ed): Advances in Psychology: Neuropsychological Studies of Apraxia and Related Disorders, Vol 23. Amsterdam: North Holland, pp 111–161.

Tyrrel PJ, Kartsounis LD, Frackowiak RSJ, Findley LJ, Rossor MS (1991): Progressive loss of speech output and orofacial dyspraxia associated with frontal lobe hypometabolism. J Neurol Neurosurg Psychiatry 54:351–357.

Watson R, Fleet S, Gonzalez Rothi LJ, Heilman KM (1986): Apraxia and the supplementary motor area. Arch Neurol 43:787–792.

Watts RL, Mirra SS, Young RR, Burger PC, Villier JA, Heyman A (1989): A cortico-basal ganglionic degeneration. Neurology 35(Suppl 1):140.

CHAPTER 11

Frontotemporal Dementia with Motor Neuron Disease

DAVID NEARY, DAVID M.A. MANN, and JULIE S. SNOWDEN

Department of Neurology (D.N. and J.S.), Manchester Royal Infirmary, Manchester M13 9WL, United Kingdom, and Department of Pathological Sciences (D.M.), University of Manchester, Manchester M13 9PT, United Kingdom

INTRODUCTION

A clinical syndrome in which progressive dementia occurs in association with motor neuron disease (MND) has been recognized since the early part of the century. First documented in 1929 (Meyer, 1929), the syndrome has since been the subject of a number of reports from different parts of the world (Mitsuyama and Takamiya, 1979; Hudson, 1981; Salazar et al., 1983; Mitsuyama, 1984; Clark et al., 1986; Morita et al., 1987). The designation *amyotrophic lateral sclerosis* (ALS) *dementia syndrome* has been adopted by some authors. These studies, although emphasizing the presence of dementia, were not primarily concerned with characterization of the pattern of mental change. Nevertheless, the available clinical information typically suggests a quality indicative of frontal lobe dysfunction. There are references, for example, to breakdown in personality and conduct, to social disinhibition, to progressive reduction in speech output and echolalia, and to altered eating habits, all features associated with frontal lobe pathology. There are, moreover, references that suggest an absence of more posterior cortical symptomatology: patients have been reported to show no signs of visual agnosia or apraxia.

A decade ago, Gustafson (1987) and Neary et al. (1988) drew attention to a form of dementia, clinically and pathologically distinct from Alzheimer's disease (AD), associated with circumscribed atrophy of the frontal and temporal lobes. The designation *frontotemporal dementia* (*FTD*) has since been adopted (Brun et al., 1994). In 1990 an explicit link was made between FTD and MND (Neary et al., 1990). A group of patients who had presented with a form of dementia indistinguishable from that of FTD developed over the ensuing months the amyotrophic form of MND. At autopsy, the pathological changes were those seen in FTD. The findings have since been confirmed in further cases (Snowden et al., 1996). Physical signs of

Pick's Disease and Pick Complex, Edited by Andrew Kertesz and David G. Munoz
ISBN 0-471-17792-X   ©1998 Wiley-Liss, Inc.

145

fasciculation have been noted, moreover, in other series of patients with FTD (Gustafson, 1987), reinforcing the link between FTD and MND. The similarities in clinical characteristics, neurological signs, and demographic features between FTD with MND (FTD/MND) and earlier reports of "ALS dementia" suggest that they represent a common clinical condition. Indeed, recent independent reports of dementia with MND have emphasized the "frontal-type" quality of the dementia (Gunnarsson et al., 1991; Peavy et al., 1992; Chang et al., 1995). That FTD/MND and ALS dementia refer to a single entity is reinforced, moreover, by striking similarities in the pathological findings of patients with FTD/MND (Neary et al., 1990; Snowden et al., 1996; Mann and Neary, in press) and those reported in earlier series of patients with dementia and MND (Morita et al., 1987). In summary, FTD/MND is a rapidly progressive condition in which the clinical features of FTD are combined with the amyotrophic form of MND. This chapter summarizes its clinical and demographic features, describes the pathological alterations underlying the disorder, and examines the relationship between FTD/MND and both FTD and the classical form of MND.

DEMOGRAPHIC FEATURES

The age of onset of FTD/MND is similar to that both for FTD alone and for classical MND. The disorder most commonly begins between 50 and 60 years of age, although ages ranging from 30 to 70 years have been reported (Hudson, 1981; Salazar et al., 1983; Mitsuyama, 1984; Morita et al., 1987). The duration of the illness is typically 2–3 years, substantially shorter than that for FTD alone. Death is usually from respiratory failure resulting from the bulbar palsy. The disorder appears to be more common in men than in women. A male:female ratio of approximately 2:1 has been most commonly reported (Hudson, 1981; Salazar et al., 1983; Horoupian et al., 1984; Morita et al., 1987; Gilbert et al., 1988; Ferrer et al., 1991; Okamoto et al., 1992; Wightman et al., 1992), similar to that seen in classical MND (Hudson, 1981). Although rare, the disorder appears to be present worldwide, with cases reported from North America, Europe, and Japan.

In most instances, the disease appears sporadic (Mitsuyama, 1984; Morita et al., 1987; Neary et al., 1990), although occasionally familial cases occur (Robertson, 1953; Yvonneau et al., 1971; Finlayson et al., 1973; Pinsky et al., 1975; Constantinidis, 1987; Neary et al., 1990; Gunnarsson et al., 1991). Familial cases have been estimated by some authors (Salazar et al., 1983) to account for about 18% of cases. The mother of one patient with FTD/MND (Neary et al., 1990) was reported to have suffered from dementia of the frontotemporal type but showed no physical signs of MND, reinforcing the link between FTD and FTD/MND. Familial and sporadic cases do not appear to differ with respect to sex ratio, age of onset, or duration of disease.

CLINICAL FEATURES

Several recent reports have described the clinical features of FTD/MND (Neary et al., 1990; Gunnarsson et al., 1991; Peavy et al., 1992; Yoshida et al., 1992, Snowden et al., 1996). The salient characteristics are outlined below and outlined in Table 11.1.

Presenting Characteristics

Alterations in mental function typically precede the development of symptoms and signs of MND, although occasionally mental and physical changes occur simultaneously. The present-

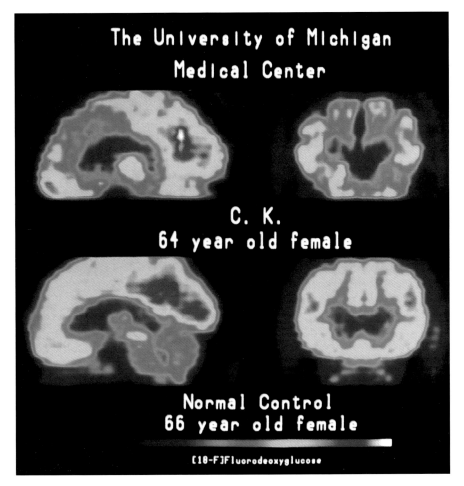

The University of Michigan Medical Center

C. K.
64 year old female

Normal Control
66 year old female

[18-F]Fluorodeoxyglucose

COLOR FIGURE 14.1. Positron emission tomography demonstrating decreased glucose metabolism in the frontal lobes and cingulate gyrus (III-35). (Permission to publish this image was kindly given by Norman Foster M.D, Department of Neurology, University of Michigan Medical Center).

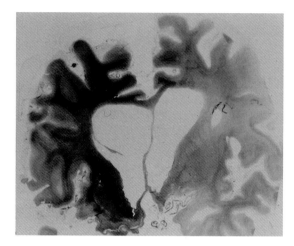

COLOR FIGURE 14.3. Neuropathological coronal section (III-53) demonstrating severe temporal and frontal atrophy. (Permission to publish this image was kindly given by K. Keohane FRCPath, Department of Neuropathology, Cork University Hospital, Cork, Ireland).

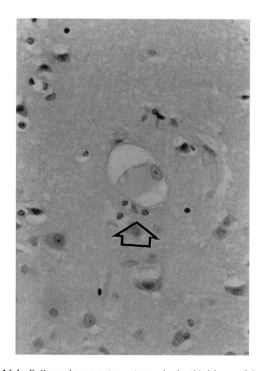

COLOR FIGURE 14.4. Ballooned neuron (arrow) seen in the third layer of the frontal cortex (H&E stain). (Permission by R. Defendini M.D., Department of Neuropathology, Columbia-Presbyterian Medical Center, New York).

COLOR FIGURES

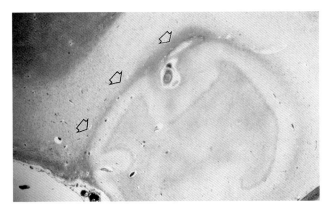

COLOR FIGURE 14.5. Deafferentiation of the hippocampus from the entorhinal cortex, as judged by a severely gliotic perforant pathway (arrows) (PTH stain). (Permission by A.A.F. Sima M.D., P.R.D., Department of Pathology and Neurology, Wayne State University and Detroit Medical Center).

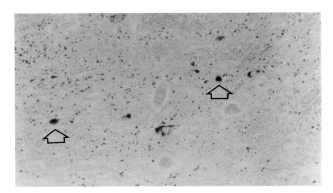

COLOR FIGURE 14.6. Neuronal loss with extracellular pigment (arrows) in the substantia nigra (Bielschowsky stain). (Permission by A.A.F. Sima M.D., P.R.D., Department of Pathology and Neurology, Wayne State University and Detroit Medical Center).

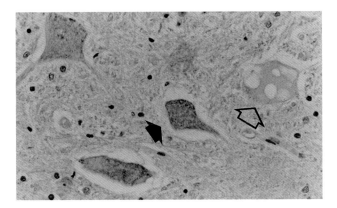

COLOR FIGURE 14.7. Abnormal shrunken cervical anterior horn cells (closed arrow) with vacuolation in another anterior horn cell (open arrow) (H&E stain). (Permission by R. Defendini M.D., Department of Neuropathology, Columbia-Presbyterian Medical Center, New York).

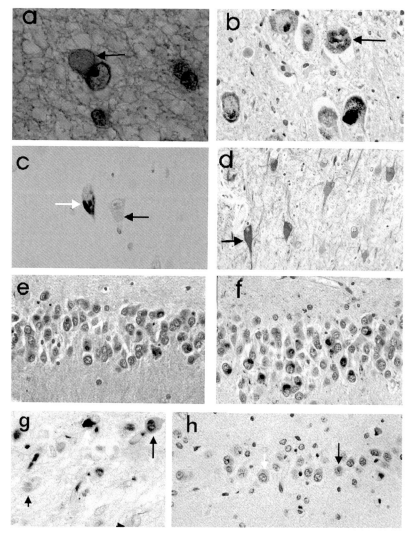

COLOR FIGURE 15.1. Pick bodies (type R-1) inclusions). **(a)** A Pick body (arrow) in the cytoplasm of a neocortical neuron. Note the slight basophilia and the distinct ring of darker, more eosinophilic staining. H & E. **(b)** Pick bodies in the locus ceruleus are often multilobed (arrow). Tau-2 immunostain. **(c)** The absence of tau immunoreactivity in the Pick body (black arrow) in this hippocampal neurons contrast with its presence in the adjacent neurofibrillary tangle (NT-1) (white arrow). Tau-2 immunostain. **(d)** The microtubule associated protein MAP-2 labels Pick bodies (arrow), but with the same intensity as the rest of the cytoplasm. Hippocampus. **(e)** Pick bodies in the dentate gyrus are labeled by ubiquitin antibodies. **(f)** Intense expression of chromogranin A in Pick bodies in the dentate gyrus. Note also the abundant abnormal neurites among the cell bodies. **(g)** Pick bodies in the temporal neocortex demonstrate marked divergence in their argyrophilia as demonstrated in the Gallyas stain. Three round bodies range from unstained (shortest black arrow) to moderately dark (longest black arrow). An irregularly shaped body (neurofibrillary tangle?) is intensely argyrophilic (white arrow). **(h)** Variation in antigenic expression of Pick bodies is obvious even in such homogeneous neuronal population as the dentate granular cells. Some Pick bodies show intense tau-2 immunoreactivity (black arrow), contrasting with others where expression is absent (white arrow) or weak.

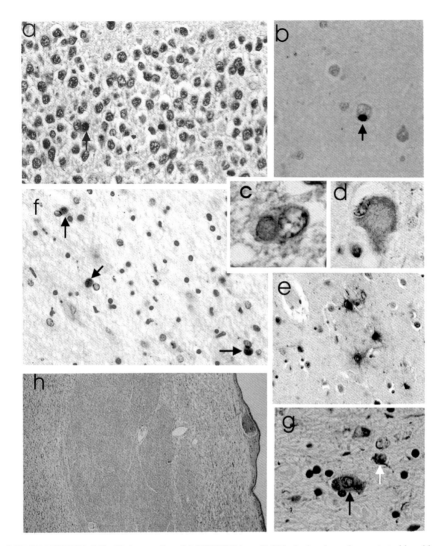

COLOR FIGURE 15.2. Pick complex (a) UTNNEI (type R-II inclusions) are demonstrated by ubiquitin in scattered neurons in the dentate gyrus. One is indicated by an arrow. (b) UTNNEI (arrow) are considerably rarer in neocortical neurons. Layer III, middle temporal gyrus. Ubiquitin immunostain. (c) A basophilic inclusion body (type R-III inclusion) in a neuron in the periaqueductal grey. H&E. (d) A ballooned neuron (type DP-I lesion) in the frontal cortex of a patient with corticobasal degeneration demonstrating diffuse perikaryal tau immunoreactivity. (e) Radiating pattern of the processes of type A-II astrocytes ("glial plaque") in the putamen of a patient with corticobasal degeneration. Tau-2 immunostain. (f) Several rounded tau-immunoreactive inclusions (type A-III, arrows) in the white matter of a patient with dementia lacking distinctive histopathology. (g) The appearance of oligodendrocytes demonstrating tau immunoreactivity (O-I) is pleomorpic, and includes diffuse expression in a swollen perikaryon (black arrow) and coiled bodies (white arrow). (h) The severe atrophy of the caudate and putamen in cases of basophilic inclusion body disease is evident in this solochrome-H&E.

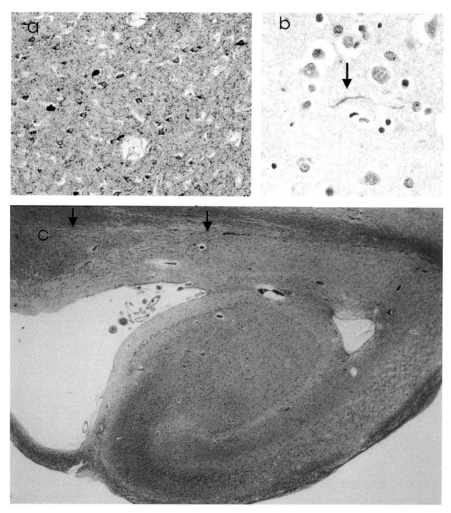

COLOR FIGURE 15.3. Pick complex (a) Numerous neurons in the subiculum show dispersed tau immunoreactivity (DP-II type lesions) in a patient with cortico-basal degeneration. Tau-2 immunostain. **(b)** Ubiquitin-immunoreactive elongated neurites (type N-III lesions) are often found in the deep cortical layers in dementia with UTNNEI. **(c)** The atrophy of the subiculum (between arrows) illustrated here is common to all forms of Pick complex. This patient with Pick Body Dementia additionally demonstrated atrophy of the dentate gyrus and CA1 sector. Solochrome-H&E.

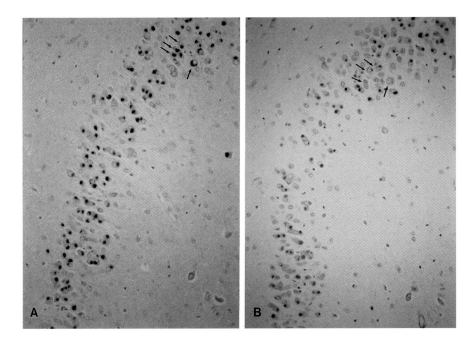

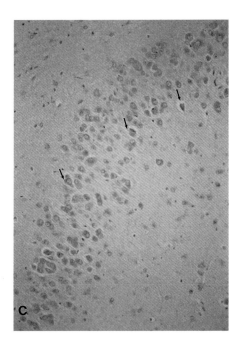

COLOR FIGURE 16.6. Dentate gyrus, PiD brain. **(a)** Exon 2 antibody reveals strongly immunolabeled PB within most granule cells. **(b)** Exon 3 shows less affinity for PB at the same dilution (1/1000), although fewer PB are marked compared with the exon 2 antibody (arrows in A and B). **(c)** Exon 10 displayed no PB, but rare fine intracytoplasmic elongated profiles (arrows) consistent with the neurofibrillary tangles were moderately immunolabeled (A–C X 300).

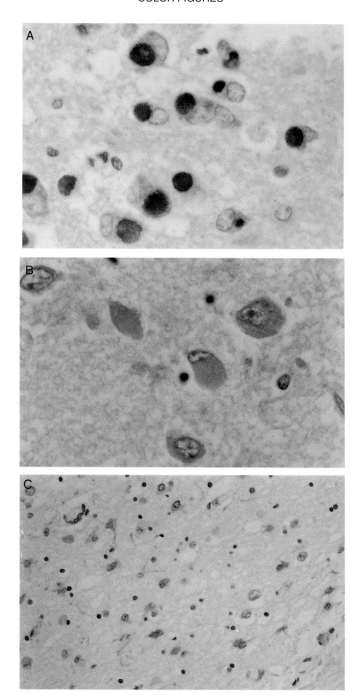

COLOR FIGURE 17.3. Immunodetection of complement on neurons and astrocytes in Pick's disease brains. Tissues sections were immunostained according to the protocol described by Singhrao et al. (1996). **(a)** immunostaining for tau. **(b)** immunostaining of ballooned neurons for complement C3. **(c)** staining of astrocytes for complement C3. All magnification (x 1200).

TABLE 11.1   Clinical Characteristics of FTD/MND

Presents with character change and altered social conduct. Physical signs typically emerge later.

Cognitive impairment indicative of frontal lobe dysfunction. Primary perceptual and spatial functions intact.

Adynamic language disorder, with economy of speech, concreteness, stereotypies, echolalia, and perseveration.

Physical signs of limb weakness, wasting, and fasciculation, with bulbar palsy leading to respiratory death. Late or absent akinesia and rigidity.

Electrophysiology confirms anterior horn cell disease.

Electroencephalogram normal.

Functional imaging (single proton emission computed tomography) reveals abnormalities in anterior cerebral hemispheres.

ing symptoms are indistinguishable from those of FTD (Gustafson, 1987; Neary et al., 1988; Snowden et al., 1996). Character change is typically the most striking feature. Patients become unconcerned, lacking in initiative, judgment and foresight, and they neglect personal appearance and hygiene, as well as domestic and occupational responsibilities. Tasks are carried out in a perfunctory manner, without concern for accuracy. Some patients become inert and avolitional, and if left to their own devices would be totally inactive, spending the day in bed or sitting in front of the television. However, many patients display purposeless overactivity. They become restless and may wander, typically following a fixed route. They are impulsive, distractible, and disinhibited. Stereotypic and ritualistic behaviors may be present, such as repetitive limb movements, stereotyped use of a word or phrase, or more complex hoarding and toileting behaviors. Gluttony and an altered preference for sweet foods may occur.

Alteration in language may represent an early presenting feature. Typically, this constitutes a diminution in spontaneous speech output rather than a frank aphasia, paralleling the findings in FTD (Snowden et al., 1996). It is worth noting, however, that MND may occur rarely in association with progressive aphasia (Caselli et al., 1993), a clinical variant of non-Alzheimer frontotemporal lobar degeneration (Snowden et al., 1996).

Changes in Affect

Patients show emotional blunting. Affect is bland and fatuous, and there is a loss of feelings of sympathy for and empathy with others, so that patients are often described by relatives as thoughtless, selfish, and callous. Patients show a total loss of insight into the change in their own mental state and express no signs of anxiety or concern.

Changes in Cognition

Language   As noted above, language typically has an adynamic rather than an aphasic quality. Patients produce little speech spontaneously, and responses to questions are economical and unelaborated. Nevertheless, what little speech is produced is fluent (unless compromised by bulbar palsy) and free from grammatical or phonological errors. There is frequently evidence of concreteness of thought. Perseveration, echolalia, and stereotypic use of words and phrases are common, increasingly providing a substitute for novel propositional content. The paucity of propositional speech contrasts with the relative preservation of "automatic" speech: patients have no difficulty reciting highly rehearsed verbal material, such as the months of the year or common nursery rhymes. The reduction in propositional speech becomes progressively more marked over the course of the disease until mutism supervenes. In patients with FTD/MND, unlike those with FTD alone, dysarthria occurs, relating to the development of bulbar palsy.

Word-finding difficulty is not a notable feature of patients' general conversation precisely because of patients' economy of mental effort: stereotyped responses and perseverations replace active, effortful word search. Formal naming tasks typically yield poor scores. These are particularly evident in open-ended verbal fluency tasks: generating members of a category or words beginning with a specified letter, suggesting that executive deficits such as failure to adopt active retrieval strategies and failure of information retrieval account in large part for the impaired performance. Semantic errors in naming are common. In some instances, these may reflect a loss of lexical-semantic knowledge and may be associated with pathological involvement of temporal lobe structures. However, patients' perfunctory mode of responding without checking, their lack of concern for accuracy, and the variability in their performance across repeated tests suggest that some semantic errors may be construed as secondary consequences of impaired regulatory executive functions.

Phonological errors are rare in FTD/MND. It has been noted above, however, that MND has occasionally been observed in association with progressive aphasia (Caselli et al., 1993), another clinical manifestation of frontotemporal lobar degeneration. In such patients, a nonfluent aphasia with phonemic paraphasias may dominate the clinical picture.

Perceptuospatial skills.   Spatial navigational skills in patients with FTD/MND are strikingly preserved, as indicated by patients' ability to localize and orient objects and to negotiate their environment without becoming lost. Performance on formal tests of spatial function is also often well preserved, although, as for all other cognitive tasks, scores are potentially compromised by patients' perfunctory performance: tasks are embarked on impulsively and abandoned rapidly, with minimal expenditure of mental effort and little concern for accuracy of responses. Constructional tasks tend to be performed poorly, but for reasons of poor organization and lack of strategy rather than spatial disorder. Drawings and block constructions show preserved spatial relationships between elements. Primary visual perceptual and praxic skills are typically preserved. However, motor performance may be compromised by perseverations.

Memory.   Patients typically remain oriented for time and place and can provide an adequate account of current autobiographical events. Nevertheless, in common with patients with FTD, performance on formal memory tests is poor, reflecting poor attention, organizational skills, and use of active retrieval strategies. Typically, some benefit to performance is derived from the use of directed rather than open-ended memory probes and cued recall compared to free recall paradigms, suggesting a frontal rather than a limbic form of amnesia.

Attention.   Attentional deficits may be evident clinically. Patients may show poor maintenance of attention on tasks and distractibility from irrelevant environmental stimuli. On formal assessment, deficits are typically elicited in the realm of selective attention and attentional shifting, and may sometimes also be demonstrated in sustained attention.

Frontal executive skills.   As in FTD, patients' most profound cognitive difficulties lie in the realm of regulation of mental function: in abstraction, planning, and organizational and strategic skills. Such deficits are manifested by profoundly impaired performance across a wide range of traditional tests sensitive to frontal lobe dysfunction. Perseverative errors, temporal sequencing failures, and difficulties in shifting mental set are common.

Neurological Features

At the time of presentation of their dementia, patients and their carers are typically unaware of any physical disability. However, in a proportion of patients, fasciculations of the limb muscles are evident on initial neurological examination. Within weeks or months, all patients develop weakness and wasting of limb muscles together with progressive bulbar palsy leading to dysarthria and dysphagia with wasting and fasciculation of the tongue. The respiratory complications of the bulbar palsy are invariably the cause of death, which occurs within 3 years of symptom onset.

This "amyotrophic" picture contrasts with the relative absence of severe spasticity of the limbs, although the tendon reflexes are invariably exaggerated and the plantar responses extensor. Grasp reflexes are elicitable early in the course of the disease. Extrapyramidal signs of akinesia, rigidity, or tremor may be absent, although they have been reported in some series (Salazar et al., 1983) and in particular in patients with a longer duration of illness (Morita et al., 1987).

Neurophysiology and Neuroimaging

The electroencephalogram remains normal until the emergence of terminal metabolic complications. Electrophysiological studies of neuromuscular function reveal normal nerve conduction studies, multifocal muscular fasciculations, reduced muscle firing rates, and giant motor units compatible with widespread muscular denervation due to anterior horn cell death.

On computed tomography prominent atrophy may be noted in the frontal and temporal lobes, although often appearances are nonspecific or normal. Circumscribed atrophy of the frontal and temporal lobes is more evident on magnetic resonance imaging. Functional imaging using single photon emission tomography reveals bilaterally reduced uptake in the anterior regions, with preservation of the posterior hemispheres.

PATHOLOGICAL FEATURES

Gross Changes

The characteristic features have been described by Neary et al. (1990). At autopsy, brain weight is reduced, although typically less than in FTD. Atrophy, although mild, is well circumscribed, affecting bilaterally the frontal lobes, frontoparietal cortex, and anterior temporal lobe (Figure 11.1), a distribution paralleling that seen in FTD. The remaining cortical regions, including the hippocampus and amygdala, appear superficially normal. When sliced coronally, mild to moderate dilatation of the lateral ventricles is seen (Figure 11.1), accompanied by a thinning of the corpus callosum, especially anteriorly. There is loss of both gray and white matter from atrophic cortical regions (Figure 11.1), although the white matter loss is more marked. The substantia nigra is typically underpigmented, although the locus ceruleus appears normal (Neary

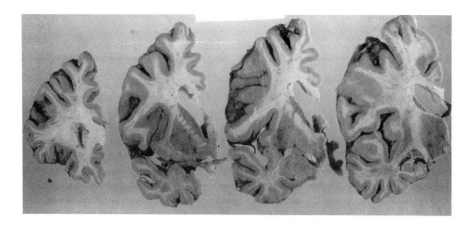

FIGURE 11.1 Coronal sections of brain showing mild frontotemporal atrophy and ventricular enlargement.

et al., 1990). The cerebellum and spinal cord are superficially normal and show no obvious changes on slicing.

Histopathological Changes

Two histological patterns are encountered, as found in FTD (Brun et al., 1994). These are characterized, respectively, by pronounced microvacuolar change with relatively mild gliosis and an absence of swollen cells and neuronal inclusions (frontal lobe degeneration [FLD] type) and by severe gliosis, with or without Pick cells and bodies (Pick type). In the majority of cases, histology conforms to the former pattern (see Neary et al., 1990). Atrophied areas of the frontal and temporal cortices show a microvacuolar degeneration of the outer laminae (Figure 11.2a). There is loss of layer III pryamidal cells, while those of layers V and VI are shrunken rather than lost. Occasional surviving nerve cells, mostly in layers II and III, also show ubiquitinated inclusions (Figure 11.3a) that, like those in spinal and other motor neurons, are not immunoreactive with any other antisera, nor are they apparent on silver staining. A mild astrocytosis within subpial regions is seen, but a pronounced reaction is usually present at the gray/white matter interface and within the white matter itself. The hippocampus appears normal, apart from a mild astrocytosis of the end folium and subiculum. However, on immunostaining (Figure 11.3b), ubiquitinated inclusions are present in the granule cells of the dentate gyrus. The basal ganglia and cerebellum are histologically normal. The main subcortical nuclei are unaffected, except for the substantia nigra, which shows severe nerve cell loss and profound astrocytosis (Figure 11.2b), though no inclusions are present.

FTD/MND in association with Pick-type histology has been reported less commonly, both in familial and in sporadic cases. Constantinidis (1987) described four members of two generations of a family who developed a typical frontotemporal form of dementia and later MND. In two autopsied cases, there was frontotemporal atrophy, asymmetrically favoring the left hemisphere, and histological findings of gliosis, nerve cell loss, and swollen (ballooned) neurons, but without inclusion bodies. Brion et al. (1980) reported sporadic cases of dementia and MND with a gliotic rather than a microvacuolar pathology, and Sam et al. (1991) described a

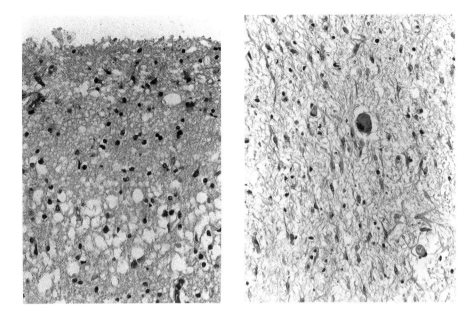

FIGURE 11.2 (a) Microvacuolar degeneration of superficial laminae of the frontal cortex. (b) Severe nerve cell loss and gliosis of substantia nigra.

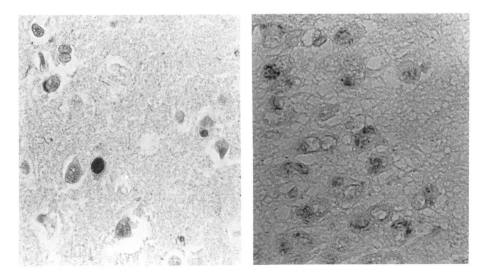

FIGURE 11.3 Ubiquitin-immunoreactive inclusions in (a) the frontal cortex and (b) hippocampal granular cells.

case in which swollen neurons, inclusion bodies, and gliosis were present in the cerebral cortex.

The brainstem and spinal cord in patients with FTD/MND show histological changes typical of classical MND, though often to a lesser degree (Neary et al., 1990). There is a loss of anterior horn cells from the spinal cord, this being more severe medially than laterally and affecting the cervical more than the lumbar levels; in this latter region, many cells are preserved. Surviving anterior horn cells may contain ubiquitinated inclusion bodies similar to those seen in classical (nondemented) cases of MND. Such inclusions appear as large, rounded, globular or solid entities or (more commonly) as loosely "woven" skeins of material and are not apparent on silver staining or immunostaining for cytoskeletal proteins. A loss of nerve cells from the hypoglossus and trigeminal motor nuclei occurs in many instances, and surviving cells can also contain the same kinds of inclusion found in neurons of the spinal cord. The Betz cells of the precentral gyrus are often shrunken and again, as in classical MND, contain inclusions, though no overt loss of cells is usually seen. While some cells containing such inclusions seem otherwise normal histologically, most show a loss of basophilia and fragmentation of the nuclear chromatin, eventually appearing as "ghost cells." Following cell death and breakdown of the external cell membrane, the ubiquitinated material is left behind in the extracelluar space. Despite the loss of anterior horn cells, the long white matter tracts within the spinal cord and brainstem remain well myelinated, and no overt loss of axons is seen.

COMPARISON OF PATHOLOGY IN FTD/MND AND FTD

The distribution of gross pathology in FTD/MND, with involvement principally of the frontal and anterior temporal regions, is similar to that seen in FTD (Brun, 1987; Mann and South, 1993; Mann et al., 1993) (Table 11.2). FTD/MND pathology is, however, less severe, reflecting the shorter duration of illness, resulting from the early death from respiratory failure due to the bulbar palsy. There is, as in FTD, atrophy of basal ganglia: the absence of reported extrapyramidal signs in many patients with FTD/MND (contrasting with the late onset of extrapyramidal signs in FTD) is probably a reflection of the patients' premature death before extrapyramidal signs have time to emerge.

The histological changes found in FTD/MND show marked similarities to those reported in FTD alone (Brun, 1987; Englund and Brun, 1987; Mann et al., 1993). Nevertheless, there are also differences: in FTD nigral cell degeneration and gliosis are not prominent features (Table 11.2). A further distinction is the presence of inclusion bodies within the cerebral cortex and hippocampus in FTD/MND. Although not apparent in hematoxylin and eosin- or silver-stained sections, pyramidal neurons within layers II (mostly), III, and occasionally V and VI of the frontal, temporal, and (sometimes) entorhinal cortex also contain ubiquitinated inclusions. These appear as rounded, elongated, or irregular filamentous structures. They are not present in other cortical regions, nor are they seen in basal ganglia or cerebellum. Similar inclusions are present in the granule cells of the hippocampal dentate gyrus, but not in neurons of the pyramidal cell layer. These dentate gyrus inclusions form a rod or crescent shape or a circular pattern around the nucleus of affected cells, which otherwise appear normal; up to 15% of cells can be affected in this way. The ubiquitinated filamentous deposits within motor neurons are composed of bundles of 10- to 15-nm filaments (Migheli et al., 1990; Okamoto et al., 1991; Schiffer et al., 1991). However, cortical and motor neuron inclusions alike do not stain with silver impregnation methods and, although ubiquitin positive, they are not immunoreactive with antisera to any other cytoskeletal protein, or indeed to any noncytoskeletal protein, so far investigated (Mather et al., 1993). Hence although they are apparently not immunoreac-

TABLE 11.2   Comparison of Pathological Changes in FTD/MND and FTD

	Atrophy				Neuronal Inclusions (Ubiquitin)			Nigral Cell Loss
	Frontal cortex	Temporal cortex	Hippocampus Amygdala	Striatum	Cortex	Hippocampus	Brainstem motor neurones	
FTD/MND	+	+	−	−	+++	+++	+++	+++
FTD	+++	+++	+/++	+/++	−	−	−	−/+

Symbols: −, no change (relative to normal controls); +, mild; ++, moderate; +++, severe.

Note: The histological changes shown for FTD apply to the majority of cases—those with microvacuolar change (FLD type; Brun et al., 1994)—but not to the minority of cases with Pick-type histology.

tive with antibodies directed against neurofilament protein, it is still possible that the structures are derived from neurofilaments that have been altered by ubiquitination, causing a masking of neurofilament epitopes, or that they represent abnormally formed neurofilaments that cannot be recognized by antibodies raised against normal neurofilaments or neurofilament protein subunits. These "cortical" deposits, like the ubiquitinated structures within motor neurons, are not immunoreactive with antisera against tau proteins or antineurofilament antibodies; this clearly sets them apart from the tau- and ubiquitin-positive inclusions of Pick's disease.

FTD/MND AND CLASSICAL MND

Classical MND has traditionally been considered to spare cognitive function, and evidence continues to accumulate in support of this view (Capitani et al., 1994). Nevertheless, a number of recent neuropsychological studies have identified in some patients mild cognitive changes consistent with frontal lobe dysfunction (David and Gillham, 1986; Montgomery and Erickson, 1987; Gallassi et al., 1989; Iwasaki et al., 1990; Talbot et al., 1995). In the study by Talbot et al. (1995), a series of patients with classical MND entered into a therapeutic trial on the basis of having no overt cognitive impairment were studied by semiquantitative single proton emission computed tomography imaging and neuropsychological testing. Despite the absence of overt behavioral disorder, one-third of the patients had evidence of orbital frontal lobe deficits on imaging. Moreover, mild abnormalities were detected on cognitive tests suggestive of frontal lobe dysfunction. These findings were interpreted as lending support to the notion of a clinical continuum between MND and FTD. The possibility exists that behavioral changes in classical MND are typically submerged by the severe clinical motor deficits or are preempted in their development by the rapidly fatal effects of generalized weakness and wasting. The argument for linking classical MND with FTD is further supported by family studies. In a family described by Gunnarsson et al. (1991), in which 13 members from four generations were affected, three of the four affected individuals from the fourth generation were said to have MND with only mild cognitive deficits, whereas other affected individuals had a clear frontal-lobe type of dementia. In a family reported by Snowden et al.(1996), one man had FTD, but without evidence of MND, while his brother had classical MND, with only minimal evidence of frontal executive deficits demonstrated on neuropsychological testing.

From the pathological perspective, the ubiquitinated inclusions present in spinal anterior horn cells, motor neurons of the brainstem nuclei, and Betz cells in FTD/MND are identical to those seen in classical MND (Leigh et al., 1988; Lowe et al., 1988, 1989; Wightman et al., 1992) and presumably have the same etiopathogenetic origins. The histological changes in the brainstem and spinal cord in FTD/MND are essentially those of classical MND. Evidence for a continuum of the same pathological process is suggested, moreover, by the finding of hippocampal and neocortical inclusions in some cases of typical MND (Okamoto et al., 1991) and the loss of neurons from the substantia nigra in others (Burrow and Blumbergs, 1992). Nonetheless, the pathological changes of microvacuolation and neuronal loss seen in FTD/MND have not been demonstrated in an unselected sample of patients with classical MND (Cooper et al., 1995).

RELATIONSHIP TO ALZHEIMER'S, LEWY BODY, AND PARKINSON'S DISEASE

In FTD/MND, the predominant pathological change is degeneration of the frontotemporal cortex, accompanied, in most instances, by damage to the substantia nigra. There is no evidence that the dementia is due to a concurrent AD; the minority of reported patients, in whom minor degrees of AD-type pathological change are present (plaques, β-amyloid, tangles) are elderly and probably reflect age-related alterations. Similarly, the absence of Lewy bodies in the cortex or nigra argues against Parkinson's disease, or against cortical Lewy body disease as a concomitant or even a principal disorder.

The clinical dementia relates to the disruption and disconnection of cortical processing due to damage in the outer laminae, which leads to loss of nerve cells and fibers that make up corticocortical pathways. The pathological substrate underlying this damage appears to involve the presence of ubiquitinated inclusions within affected cells; the presence of similar immunoreactive material within hippocampal dentate gyrus cells and cortical, spinal, and brainstem motor neurons implies a common pathogenetic mechanism.

RELATIONSHIP TO CREUTZFELDT-JAKOB DISEASE (CJD)

Early reports of dementia and MND suggested that it represented an amyotrophic form of CJD (Allen et al., 1971; Sherratt, 1974) because of the superficial resemblance of the spongiform (microvacuolar) changes within the outer cortical laminae to the cortical spongiosus of CJD. It is now clear that neither FTD/MND nor FTD represents a form or variant of CJD. The deposition in the brain of an abnormal isoform of the prion protein (PrP), characteristic of CJD, does not occur in FTD/MND or FTD, either as immunohistochemically detectable "prion plaques" or in immunoblotting or Western blotting of PrP (Owen et al., 1993). Likewise, no abnormality of the prion gene has been detected in FTD/MND or FTD.

PATHOGENESIS AND ETIOLOGY

The occurrence of a positive family history in about 50% of the cases of patients with FTD (Gustafson, 1987; Neary et al., 1988) and in some cases of FTD/MND (Neary et al., 1990; Gunnarsson et al., 1991) suggests that genetic factors play an important role in the determination of the disease, although these remain to be identified. Linkage to chromosome 17 has been reported in one family with a similar clinical phenotype (Lynch et al., 1994). In the series of patients studied by the present authors, abnormalities in the prion gene have been excluded (Owen et al., 1993), as have excessive CAG repeats in the IT15 gene, as found in Huntington's disease. Also absent are the codon 717 mutations in the APP gene, as found in familial AD, and mutations in exons of the superoxide dismutase gene, as in familial MND. Nor has an association been found with unusual allelic variations of the apolipoprotein E gene, as in late-onset AD (Pickering-Brown et al., 1995). Comparable findings have been reported by other authors (Brun and Gustafson, in press).

CONCLUDING REMARKS

FTD can coexist with MND, giving rise to the syndrome of FTD/MND. The form of dementia in FTD/MND is identical to that seen in FTD alone and is associated with a common distribution of pathology within the frontal and temporal lobes. It is likely that FTD and FTD/MND are different phenotypic variations of a common non-AD pathology. In most instances of FTD/MND, as in FTD, histological changes are of a spongiform type involving microvacuolation of the outer cortical laminae, as well as loss of large cortical nerve cells from layer III with minimal gliosis, whereas in a minority of cases a Pick-type form of histology is present, with inclusion bodies and swollen neurons. Microvacuolar degeneration and Pick-type changes may be different stages within, or different phenotypic expressions of, a common pathological process, which in view of the high familial incidence surrounding these disorders may be driven by a particular genetic disturbance or by different alterations within a related pool of genes. The task for future studies will be to determine the nature of the differing pathologies behind these forms of lobar atrophy and to find a molecular biological basis that might explain them. Once precise molecular markers become available, it will be possible to specify the exact nosological relationship between FTD/MND and FTD and between FTD/MND and classical MND, and to establish whether they do indeed represent phenotypic variants of a common genotype or whether the clinical associations found between FTD/MND and classical MND are merely fortuitous.

REFERENCES

Allen IV, Dermott E, Connolly JH, Hurwitz LJ (1971): A study of a patient with the amyotrophic form of Creutzfeldt-Jakob disease. Brain 94:715–724.

Brion S, Psimaras A, Chevalier JF (1980): L'association maladie de Pick et sclérose latérale amyotrophique. Etude d'un cas anatomo-clinique et revue de la litterature. Encephale 6:250–286.

Brun A (1987): Frontal lobe degeneration of non-Alzheimer-type. I Neuropathology. Arch Gerontol Geriatr 6:193–207.

Brun A, Englund B, Gustafson L, Passant U, Mann DMA, Neary D, Snowden JS (1994): Consensus Statement. Clinical and neuropathological criteria for fronto-temporal dementia. J Neurol Neurosurg Psychiatry 4:416–418.

Brun A, Gustafson L (in press): Frontal lobe degeneration of non-Alzheimer type. In Clark AW, Dickson DW (eds): Primary Degenerative Dementias Other Than Alzheimer's Disease. Durham, NC: Carolina Academic Press.

Burrow JNC, Blumbergs PC (1992): Substantia nigra degeneration in motor neurone disease. A quantitative study. Aust NZ J Med 22:469–472.

Capitani E, Della Sala S, Marchetti C (1994): Is there a cognitive impairment in MND? A survey with longitudinal data. Schweiz Arch Neurol Psychiatr 145:11–13.

Caselli RJ, Windebank AJ, Petersen RC, Komori T, Parisi JE, Okazaki H, Kokmen E, Iverson R, Dinapoli RP, Graff-Radford NR, Stein SD (1993): Rapidly progressive aphasic dementia and motor neuron disease. Ann Neurol 33:200–207.

Chang L, Cornford M, Miller BL, Itabashi H, Mena I (1995): Neuronal ultrastructural abnormalities in a patient with frontotemporal dementia and motor neuron disease. Dementia 6:1–8.

Clark AW, White CL, Manz HJ, Parhad IM, Curry B, Whitehouse PJ, Lehmann J, Coyle JT (1986): Primary degenerative dementia without Alzheimer pathology. Can J Neurol Sci 13:462–470.

Constantinidis J (1987): Syndrome familial: Association de Maladie de Pick et sclérose latérale amyotrophique. Encephale 13:285–293.

Cooper PN, Siddons MA, Mann DMA (1995): Normal cortex histology and immunohistochemistry in patients with motor neurone disease. (letter) J Neurol Neurosurg Psychiatry 59:644.

David AS, Gillham RA (1986): Neuropsychological study of motor neurone disease. Psychosomatics 27:441–445.

Englund E, Brun A (1987): Frontal lobe degeneration of non-Alzheimer type. IV. White matter changes. Arch Gerontol Geriatr 6:235–243.

Ferrer I, Roig C, Espino A, Peiro G, Matias Guiu X (1991): Dementia of frontal lobe type and motor neuron disease. A golgi study of the frontal cortex. J Neurol Neurosurg Psychiatry 54:932–934.

Finlayson MH, Guberman A, Martin JB (1973): Cerebral lesions in familial amyotrophic lateral sclerosis and dementia. Acta Neuropathol 26:237–246.

Gallassi R, Montagna P, Morreale A, Lorusso S, Tinuper P, Daidone R, Lugaresi E (1989): Neuropsychological, electroencephalogram and brain computed tomography findings in motor neuron disease. Eur Neurol 29:115–120.

Gilbert JJ, Kish SJ, Chang L-J, Morito C, Shannak K, Hornykiewicz O (1988): Dementia, Parkinsonism and motor neuron disease: Neurochemical and neuropathological correlates. Ann Neurol 24:688–691.

Gunnarsson LG, Dahlbom K, Strandman E (1991): Motor neuron disease and dementia reported among 13 members of a single family. Acta Neurol Scand 84:429–433.

Gustafson L (1987): Frontal lobe degeneration of non-Alzheimer-type. II Clinical picture and differential diagnosis. Acta Gerontol Geriatr 6:209–223.

Horoupian DS, Thal L, Katzman R, Terry RD, Davies P, Hirano A, De Teresa R, Fuld PA, Petito C, Blass J, Ellis JM (1984): Dementia and motor neuron disease: Morphometric, biochemical and golgi studies. Ann Neurol 16:305–313.

Hudson AJ (1981): Amyotrophic lateral sclerosis and its association with dementia, Parkinsonism and other neurological disorders: A review. Brain 104:217–247.

Iwasaki Y, Kinoshita M, Ikeda K, Takamiya K, Shiojima T (1990): Cognitive impairment in amyotrophic lateral sclerosis and its relation to motor disabilities. Acta Neurol Scand 81:141–143.

Leigh PN, Anderton BH, Dodson A, Gallo J-M, Swash M, Power DM (1988): Ubiquitin deposits in anterior horn cells in motor neurone disease. Neurosci Lett 93:197–203.

Lowe JS, Aldridge F, Lennox G, Doherty F, Jefferson D, Landon M, Mayer RJ (1989): Inclusion bodies in motor cortex and brainstem of patients with motor neurone disease detected by immunocytochemical localization of ubiquitin. Neurosci Lett 105:7–13.

Lowe JS, Lennox G, Jefferson D, Morrell K, McQuire D, Gray T, Landon M, Doherty FJ, Mayer RJ (1988): A filamentous inclusion body within anterior horn neurones in motor neurone disease defined by immunocytochemical localization of ubiquitin. Neurosci Lett 94:203–210.

Lynch T, Sano M, Marder KS, Bell KL, Foster NL, Defendini RF, Sima AAF, Keohane C, Nygaard TG, Fahn S, Mayeux R, Rowland LP, Wilhelmsen UC (1994): Clinical characteristics of a family with chromosome 17-linked disinhibition-dementia-parkinsonism-amyotrophy complex. Neurology 44:1878–1884.

Mann DMA, Neary D (in press): Dementia and motor neurone disease. In Clark AW, Dickson DW (eds): Primary Degenerative Dementias Other Than Alzheimer's Disease. Durham, NC: Carolina Academic Press.

Mann DMA, South PW (1993): The topographic distribution of brain atrophy in frontal lobe dementia. Acta Neuropathol 85:335–340.

Mann DMA, South PW, Snowden JS, Neary D (1993): Dementia of frontal lobe type; neuropathology and immunohistochemistry. J Neurol Neurosurg Psychiatry 56:605–614.

Mather V, Martin JE, Swash M, Vowles G, Brown, A, Leigh PN (1993): Histochemical and immunocytochemical study of ubiquitinated neuronal inclusions in amyotrophic lateral sclerosis. Neuropathol Appl Neurobiol 19:141–145.

Meyer A (1929): Uber eine der amyotrophischen Lateralsklerose nahestende Erkrankung mit psychischen Storungen. Z Gesamte Neurol Psychiatrie 121:107–128.

Migheli A, Autilio-Gambetti L, Gambetti P, Mocellini C, Vigliani MC, Schiffer D (1990): Ubiquitinated filamentous inclusions in spinal cord of patients with motor neuron disease. Neurosci Lett 114:5–10.

Mitsuyama Y (1984): Presenile dementia with motor neuron disease in Japan: Clinico-pathological review of 26 cases. J Neurol Neurosurg Psychiatry 47:953–959.

Mitsuyama Y, Takamiya S (1979): Presenile dementia with motor neuron disease. Arch Neurol 36: 592–593.

Montgomery GK, Erickson LM (1987): Neuropsychological perspectives in amyotrophic lateral sclerosis. Neurol Clin 5:61–81.

Morita K, Kaiya H, Ikeda T, Namba M (1987): Presenile dementia combined with amyotrophy: A review of 34 Japanese cases. Arch Gerontol Geriatr 6:263–277.

Neary D, Snowden JS, Mann DMA, Northern B, Goulding PJ, Macdermott N (1990): Frontal lobe dementia and motor neuron disease. J Neurol Neurosurg Psychiatry 53:23–32.

Neary D, Snowden JS, Northern B, Goulding PJ (1988): Dementia of frontal lobe type. J Neurol Neurosurg Psychiatry 51:353–361.

Okamoto K, Hirai S, Yamazaki T, Sun X, Nakazato Y (1991): New ubiquitin-positive intraneuronal inclusions in the extramotor cortices in patients with amyotrophic lateral sclerosis. Neurosci Lett 129:233–236.

Okamoto K, Murakami N, Kusaka H, Yoshida M, Hashizume Y, Nakazato Y, Matsubara E, Hirai S (1992): Ubiquitin-positive intraneuronal inclusions in the extramotor cortices of presenile dementia patients with motor neuron disease. J Neurol 239:426–430.

Owen F, Cooper PN, Pickering-Brown S, McAndrew C, Mann DMA, Neary D (1993): The lobar atrophies are not prion encephalopathies. Neurodegeneration 2:195–199.

Peavy GM, Herzog AG, Rubin NP, Mesulam M-M (1992): Neuropsychological aspects of dementia of motor neurone disease. A report of two cases. Neurology 42:1004–1008.

Pickering-Brown S, Siddons M, Mann DMA, Owen F, Neary D, Snowden JS (1995): Apolipoprotein E allelic frequencies in lobar atrophy. Neurosci Lett 188:105–207.

Pinsky L, Finlayson MH, Libman I, Scott BH (1975): Familial amyotrophic lateral sclerosis with dementia; a second Canadian family. Clin Genet 7:186–191.

Robertson EE (1953): Progressive bulbar paralysis showing heredo-familial incidence and intellectual impairment. Arch Neurol Psychiatry 69:197–207.

Salazar AM, Masters CL, Gajdusek DC, Gibbs CJ (1983): Syndromes of amyotrophic lateral sclerosis and dementia: Relation to transmissible Creutzfeldt-Jakob disease. Ann Neurol 14:17–26.

Sam M, Gutmann L, Schochet SS, Doshi H (1991): Pick's disease: A case clinically resembling amyotrophic lateral sclerosis. Neurology 41:1831–1833.

Schiffer D, Autilio-Gambetti L, Chio A, Gambetti P, Giordana MT, Gullotta F, Migheli A, Vigliani MC (1991): Ubiquitin in motor neuron disease: Study at the light and electron microscope. J Neuropathol Exp Neurol 50:463–473.

Sherratt RM (1974): Motor neurone disease and dementia: Probably Creutzfeldt-Jakob disease. Proc R Soc Med 67:1063–1064.

Snowden JS, Neary D, Mann DMA (1996): Fronto-Temporal Lobar Degeneration: Fronto-temporal Dementia, Progressive Aphasia, Semantic Dementia. London: Churchill Livingstone.

Talbot PR, Goulding PJ, Lloyd JJ, Snowden JS, Neary D, Testa HJ (1995): The inter-relationship between "classical" motor neurone disease and fronto-temporal dementia: A neuropsychological and single photon emission tomographic study. J Neurol Neurosurg Psychiatry 58:541–547.

Wightman G, Anderson VER, Martin J, Swash M, Anderton BH, Neary D, Mann DMA, Luthert P, Leigh PN (1992): Hippocampal and neocortical ubiquitin immunoreactive inclusions in amyotrophic lateral sclerosis with dementia. Neurosci Lett 139:269–274.

Yoshida M, Murakami N, Hashizume Y, Takahashi A (1992): A clinicopathological study on 13 cases of motor neuron disease with dementia (Japanese). Rinsho Shinkeigaku 32:1193–1202.

Yvonneau M, Vital C, Belly C, Coquet M (1971): Syndrome familiar de Sclérose latérale amyotrophique avec démence. Encephale 60:449–462.

CHAPTER 12

Dementia and Amyotrophic Lateral Sclerosis

MICHAEL J. STRONG and GLORIA M. GRACE

Department of Clinical Neurological Sciences (M.J.S.) and Department of Psychology (G.M.G.), The University of Western Ontario, London, Ontario, N6A 5A5 Canada

INTRODUCTION

Traditionally, amyotrophic lateral sclerosis (ALS) has been considered a progressive adult-onset neurodegenerative process restricted to the motor neurons, the clinical manifestation of which is a fatal muscle atrophy and weakness. Clinical or neuropathological evidence of non-motor system involvement, with few exceptions, has been held to be either rare or restricted to less common variants of the disorder (e.g., the Western Pacific variant). However, as reviewed by previous authors (see Chapter 11, this volume; Strong et al., 1996), the contemporary view of ALS encompasses both motor and non-motor system degeneration. Although the cognitive impairments in ALS most consistently reflect frontal lobe dysfunction, some patients develop a more widespread abnormality with a florid dementia, with rare patients even developing the Klüver-Bucy syndrome (Dickson et al., 1986). Whether this co-occurrence of ALS with altered cognition represents a continuum of a single disease process, or overlapping but discrete syndromes, remains to be determined.

Unfortunately, the pathogenesis of ALS remains an enigma, impeding our understanding of these interrelationships. This holds true not only for our understanding of ALS and dementia, but also in regard to the relationship of the dementia of ALS to other disease processes that present with a frontotemporal dementia. As will be discussed, similarity of the clinical phenomenology may not imply biological homogeneity—a principle well established in disorders of the motor system (Strong and Garruto, 1994).

CLINICAL PHENOMENOLOGY IN THE DEMENTIA OF ALS

The characterization of the dementia in ALS has been diverse, including a form of Creutzfeldt-Jakob disease, a form of Alzheimer's or Pick's disease, or the so-called subcortical dementia.

Pick's Disease and Pick Complex, Edited by Andrew Kertesz and David G. Munoz
ISBN 0-471-17792-X ©1998 Wiley-Liss, Inc.

More recently, the dementia of ALS has been categorized as a frontotemporal dementia, key clinical manifestations of which include an insidiously progressive behavioral disorder, affective symptoms, speech disorder, and failure on neuropsychological testing reflective of frontal lobe dysfunction (Brun et al., 1994; Levy et al., 1996). The frequency with which ALS patients are afflicted with this process is unknown, with estimates ranging from rare (Poloni et al., 1986; Lishman, 1987; Montgomery and Erickson, 1987) to common (Canter, 1963; Hudson, 1981; Gallassi et al., 1985, 1989; Ludolph et al., 1992). In the absence of a formal prospective study of a consecutive series of ALS patients, the true incidence of ALS with dementia will remain unknown. Several studies do, however, suggest that the extent of the problem may be underappreciated.

In a review of 52 patients with ALS, 24 of whom had clinical features suggestive of frontal lobe involvement, Abrahams et al. (1995a, 1995b) found that all ALS patients, regardless of the presence of a dementia, were impaired on verbal fluency testing ($p = 0.027$) and that those with bulbar dysfunction were more impaired than those without it ($p = 0.041$). ALS patients as a group performed less well in word recognition testing and demonstrated a tendency toward greater difficulty with card sorting. Detailed neuropsychological studies of ALS patients in the absence of an overt dementia have also demonstrated a variety of deficiencies, including impairments in mental flexibility, fluency, and abstract reasoning (Gallassi et al., 1985); reduced verbal and nonverbal fluency and picture recall times (Ludolph et al., 1992), reduced verbal fluency and picture recall (Kew et al., 1993); and lower scores on mini mental status (MMS) and on immediate and delayed logical memory testing (Iwasaki et al., 1990a, 1990b). Significantly lower scores on tests of memory and learning in ALS patients compared to controls have also been demonstrated by David and Gillham (1986) and Peterson et al. (1990). In addition, individual case reports support the presence of frontal lobe dysfunction as a frequent occurrence in ALS (Montgomery and Erickson, 1987; Neary et al., 1990; Peavy et al., 1992; Caselli et al., 1993; Tanaka et al., 1993).

Language deficits in ALS also suggest frontal lobe dysfunction. Deficits such as word-finding difficulties, lexical disorganization, and reliance on stereotypic sentences (Gallassi et al., 1985, 1989; Iwasaki et al., 1990a; Ludolph et al., 1992) are reminiscent of Pick's disease (Montgomery and Erickson, 1987), in which a deterioration in formal syntactic elements of language with auditory agnosia and excessive use of verbal stereotypes can be an early manifestation (Cummings and Duchen, 1981; Cummings, 1982; Holland et al., 1985).

It is clear that a subpopulation of ALS patients will develop changes in cognitive functioning ranging from isolated cognitive impairment of one or two areas of function to a full-blown syndrome recognized as a frontotemporal dementia. The exact frequency of these changes in cognition awaits detailed prospective studies, both clinically and neuropathologically.

THE NEUROANATOMICAL SUBSTRATE OF ALS/DEMENTIA

Neuroimaging

Both neuroimaging and neuropathological studies have been utilized to define the neuroanatomical substrate of the dementia of ALS. Although neuropsychological testing consistently indicates frontotemporal pathology, this is not always apparent using static neuroimaging techniques. In an analysis of 22 patients with sporadic ALS, 13 of whom developed a progressive supranuclear palsy and 3 of whom developed dementia, Kew et al. (1993a) observed cortical atrophy by computed tomography (CT) scanning initially involving the frontal and temporal lobes, followed by atrophy of the precentral gyrus and then of the postcentral gyrus, anterior cingulate gyrus, corpus callosum, and brainstem tegmentum. An increase in the magnetic resonance imaging (MRI) T2 signal in the precentral and adjacent gyri, frontal and temporal white matter, pyramidal tracts, globus pallidus, and thalamus was also observed, although insufficient cases were studied with this modality to provide a temporal analysis of these latter changes. In contrast, a study of 21 patients, of whom only 2 demonstrated cognitive dysfunction, failed to show significant structural deficits on CT scanning (Poloni et al., 1986). Gallossi et al. (1989) observed cognitive impairments consisting of impaired associative functions (e.g., word fluency, phrase construction, temporal rule induction, and analogies) in 22 of 35 ALS patients, in the absence of overt dementia, but found no evidence of CT changes.

Attempts to further define the anatomical substrate of cognitive dysfunction using functional neuroimaging techniques have included ^{123}I-N-isopropyl-p-iodoamphetamine (^{123}I-IMP) (Ludolph et al., 1989; Ohnishi et al., 1991) and [^{99m}Tc]-d,l-hexamethyl-propylene-amine-oxime (HMPAO) (Waldemar et al., 1992; Talbot et al., 1995) in single positron emission computed tomography (SPECT) studies. With both isotopes, reduced blood flow was observed in the frontal and temporal cortices of ALS patients, more prominently when dementia was also present.

Positron emission tomography (PET) has also been utilized to provide a map of the metabolic changes in ALS. Although deficits in cognition were not specifically assessed, Dalakas et al. (1987) demonstrated a 21% reduction in cortical and basal ganglia metabolism in 8/12 patients with PET scanning performed in a resting state. Tanaka et al. (1993) observed reduced regional cerebral blood flow (rCBF) in anterior cerebral hemispheres only when dementia was clinically evident. The dementia was characterized as a mild to moderate personality change, breakdown in social conduct, disinhibition, apathy, and an "economy of mental effort"—features suggestive of a frontotemporal dementia. In patients with reduced verbal fluency scores, Kew et al. (1993), observed reduced rCBF to the primary motor cortex, motor association cortex, and anterior cingulate gyrus. Ludolph et al. (1992) similarly observed a significant correlation between deficits on subtests of word fluency and both right thalamic ($p < 0.01$) and diffuse cortical reductions in glucose metabolism ($p < 0.05$) in 14 patients with ALS/dementia.

In one of the first attempts at functional neuroimaging, Abrahams et al. (1995b) observed reduced metabolism in the right dorsolateral prefrontal cortex (areas 46 and 9) and the left middle and superior temporal gyrus (areas 39 and 22) ($p < 0.001$) during a verbal fluency/word generation task with a PET activation program. This finding was observed only in the cognitively impaired ALS population, as defined by impaired word fluency (Abrahams et al., 1995a).

Neuropathology

The traditional neuropathological view of ALS is that of a progressive and selective loss of spinal motor neurons, degeneration of the corticospinal tracts, and variable loss of motor neurons in the precentral gyrus (Lawyer and Netsky, 1963; Brownell et al., 1970; Hirano, 1991). In the familial variant, degeneration of the posterior columns and of the spinocerebellar tracts is evident (Hirano et al., 1967), while neurofibrillary tangles are widespread in the western Pacific variant (Rodgers-Johnson et al., 1986). An ultrastructural hallmark of the neuronal degeneration in ALS is an accumulation of neurofilamentous material within the perikarya of the anterior horn cells and axonal processes (Carpenter, 1968; Averback, 1981; Delisle and Carpenter, 1984) and of both neurofilament and peripherin, a related intermediate filament, in neuroaxonal spheroids (Migheli et al., 1993). Utilizing ubiquitin immunoreactivity as a marker of neuronal degeneration, many of these intracytoplasmic neurofilamentous inclusions have been shown to be ubiquitin-conjugated (Chou, 1988; Martin et al., 1990). However, even in the absence of overt inclusion formation, degenerating motor neurons in ALS demonstrate both skeins and homogeneous patterns of ubiquitin immunoreactivity (Murayama et al., 1990; Leigh and Swash, 1991), suggesting that ubiquitin immunoreactivity can be utilized as a sensitive early marker of neuronal involvement in ALS. With immunoelectron microscopy, the ubiquitin immunoreactivity is seen to be associated with arrays of 10- to 15-nm filaments. The observation of this ubiquitin-immunoreactive material in neuronal populations distinct from the motor neuron pool in ALS has given rise to the concern that the pathogenesis of ALS may not be restricted to motor neurons alone (Aldridge et al., 1989; Okamato et al., 1991; Sasaki et al., 1992; Lowe, 1994).

In addition to these traditional findings in ALS, the neuropathological features of the dementia of ALS include a marked loss of neurons and spongiform changes restricted to cortical layers II and III, most pronounced in the posterior frontal lobes and precentral gyrus. This are similar to the pathology described in the Pick complex (see Chapter 15, this volume). However, it is the unique presence of intraneuronal inclusions in the dentate granule cells of the hippocampus, superficial layers of the frontal and temporal cortex, and entorhinal cortex that are immunoreactive for ubiquitin but not for the microtubule-associated protein tau or neurofilament that is the pathognomonic feature distinguishing the dementia of ALS from these other entities (Mitsuyama, 1984; Okamoto et al., 1992; Wightman et al., 1992; Anderson et al., 1995). Neuronal density is reduced in the cingulate gyrus but spared in the dentate gyrus (Soni et al., 1993). With immunoelectron microscopy, the ubiquitin-immunoreactive inclusions are seen to consist of loosely arranged 10- to 15-nm linear filaments coated with granular materials in the absence of a limiting membrane (Okamoto et al., 1991, 1992). This appearance is reminiscent of that described for the ubiquitinated inclusions in spinal motor neurons.

A troublesome issue is the observation of this neuronal pathology in the absence of clinical evidence of ALS and the nosology of such an entity. In an analysis of 50 patients with frontotemporal dementia, Cooper et al. (1995) found ubiquitin-positive, tau-negative, immunoreactive intraneuronal inclusions localized to hippocampal dentate granule cells in 12 patients. In addition, microvacuolation, variable neuronal loss and gliosis, rare or absent swollen neurons, and ubiquitinated inclusions in cortical layer II were observed. However, seven of these patients had no clinical evidence of weakness in life, while the spinal cord showed typical intraneuronal inclusions. Three of the five cases of frontotemporal dementia described by Tolnay and Probst (1995) demonstrated similar ubiquitinated inclusions in the absence of neuropathological abnormalities in spinal motor neurons. The possibility remains that the patients in each of these reports may have had incipient ALS, which would have become clinically evident had they survived for a sufficient period.

Support for such a concept comes from the analysis of three individuals in whom the dementia clearly antedated the development of amyotrophy (Horoupian et al., 1984). In two, amyotrophy remained restricted to the bulbar territory, while one patient developed classical ALS. Pathologically, these patients developed spongiform changes in the upper cortical layers and severe degeneration of the substantia nigra. Similar findings have been described in 11 cases of progressive frontotemporal dementia in the absence of ALS (Jackson et al., 1995). In these latter cases, the spinal cord was not available for a neuropathological assessment.

These observations do raise the possibility that the entity of ALS with dementia may belong to a spectrum of neurodegeneration that can ultimately evolve to a multisystem degeneration. The existence of such a spectrum is clearly evident in ventilator-dependent ALS patients with long-term survival (Hayashi and Kato, 1989; Mizutani et al., 1990; Hayashi et al., 1991). Pathologically, these patients develop neuronal loss and gliosis of the oculomotor nuclei, spinocerebellar tracts, substantia nigra, and inferior olives. Komachi et al. (1994) observed neuronal loss and spongiform degeneration in layer II of the frontal cortex, a moderate neuronal loss of neurons with gliosis in the substantia nigra and red nucleus, and chromatolytic oculomotor nuclei in a case of ALS with both dementia and ophthalmoplegia. Of note, none of the aforementioned cases contained neurofibrillary tangles, Lewy bodies, or Pick's bodies. Kishikawa et al. (1995) described a single case of ALS with long-term survival (9 years, no respiratory support) with a severe dementia in whom the pathology showed severe frontal lobe atrophy with "degenerative changes" in the frontal lobe, vacuolar changes in cortical layer II, and moderate to marked neuronal loss (particularly in the precentral gyrus). Although ubiquitin immunoreactivity was not assessed, tau-positive inclusions were not observed.

Neurochemistry

The neurochemical substrate of dementia in ALS is even less well understood and is largely restricted to small series of patients. In an analysis of nitric oxide synthase (NOS) immunoreactivity in 3 patients with ALS/dementia, 3 with sporadic ALS, and 19 controls, Kuljis and Schelper (1996) observed NOS/NADPH diaphorase-positive dystrophic neurites in sensory, motor, and limbic cortices affecting specific subgroups of neurons (smooth stellate and spiny neurons). In addition, masses of NADPH-diaphorase-positive material thought to be dying neurons were observed. No abnormalities were observed in either control or nondemented ALS cases. Kato et al. (1993b), in an analysis of 15 patients with ALS and 3 with ALS/dementia, observed a significant depletion of dopaminergic neurons in "frontal-lobe" dementing ALS patients and in patients with an supranuclear gaze palsy. A similar observation was made by Gilbert et al. (1988) in a patient with clinical evidence of dementia, parkinsonism, and ALS. However, the linkage to chromosome 17 of a similar disorder of disinhibition-dementia-parkinsonism-amyotrophy suggests that this may represent a discrete entity (Lynch et al., 1994). Ferrer et al. (1993), in an analysis of two patients with ALS/dementia, observed a significant depletion of calbindin D 23 K-immunoreactive neurons in upper cortical layers, while parvalbumin-immunoreactive neurons were preserved. In remaining calbindin-immunoreactive neurons, reduced dendritic arborization was observed. It is noteworthy that both patients demonstrated a fulminant, atypical disease course, with death after 2 and 4 months, respectively. These studies suggest a loss of corticocortical projecting pathways in ALS/dementia.

CONCLUSIONS

There is little doubt that classical ALS, traditionally viewed as a disorder primarily of the motor system, can be associated with a syndrome of progressive cognitive decline that may be best characterized as a frontotemporal dementia. Although initially thought to be a rare occurrence, both neuropsychological and neuroimaging studies suggest that a significant proportion of ALS patients may suffer from this cognitive impairment or dementia. The neuroanatomical substrate, in the absence of overt atrophy, is reflected by a regional deficit in both cerebral blood flow and metabolic activation within the inferior frontal regions, anterior cingulate gyrus, and middle and superior temporal gyri. The neuropathological hallmarks, in addition to the well-characterized motor system pathology, include mild to severe frontal atrophy, vacuolar degeneration of cortical layer II, and the presence of ubiquitin-positive, tau-negative inclusions in dentate granule cells and the amygdala.

The critical issue, however, remains our lack of understanding of the neurobiological substrate giving rise to these inclusions. Although of value in defining the topographic localization of the neuropathology, the presence of ubiquitin immunoreactivity itself cannot be taken as a marker of a pathogenic process.

The covalent linkage of multiple ubiquitin molecules in an ATP-dependent process targets protein for nonlysosomal proteolytic degradation into free amino acids (Ciechanover, 1993). Protein conjugation to ubiquitin has been shown to be important to a number of diverse processes, including the regulation of gene expression, responses to cellular injury and stress, the synthesis of ribosomes, DNA repair, and the uptake of protein precursors. Neuropathologically, there is a consistent association between intraneuronal cytoskeletal inclusions and their ubiquitinization (Lowe et al., 1993). As discussed by Lowe et al. (1993), the formation of ubiquitin-intermediate filament inclusions may represent a common cellular response to neuronal injury, although in several instances the substrate for the ubiquitin conjugation remains to be defined. Nonetheless, it is generally agreed that the accumulation of ubiquitinated materials reflects a common response to neuronal damage rather than a primary abnormality of the ubiquitin-mediated proteolytic pathway (Lowe et al., 1988; Manetto et al., 1988). In an experimental model of ALS bearing the histological features of ALS, including intermediate filament ubiquitinization, we have shown that the induction of the neurofilamentous aggregates clearly antedates the presence of ubiquitin-immunoreactive material (Strong et al., 1995). Hence, its presence in ALS likely reflects a reactive process.

Thus, until the fundamental composition of the intraneuronal inclusions, within both the degenerating motor neurons and the cortical neurons, is known, any attempt to develop an etiologic linkage between the intraneuronal inclusions of ALS and those of the ALS dementia complex remains speculative. One view of this process might hold that there are two parallel but independent processes in which the occurrence of ALS/dementia reflects the overlapping of these syndromes that can also occur independent of each other.

An alternate view includes the concept that the frontotemporal dementias are the primary manifestation of a continuum of a single disease process, from which arises a number of syndromes. However, as discussed in the introduction, the nervous system is limited in its ability to clinically express a disease state (concept of limited phenotypic expression). Thus it is not altogether surprising that a disease entity such as a frontal dementia can be derived from a number of distinct disease processes affecting a single region. Until more is learned about the pathogenesis of these disorders, including ALS, they are thus best considered as distinctive entities, and not necessarily as part of a biological continuum.

REFERENCES

Abrahams S, Goldstein LH, Lloyd CM, Brooks DJ, Leigh PN (1995a): Cognitive deficits in non-demented amyotrophic lateral sclerosis patients: A neuropsychological investigation. J Neurol Sci 129:54–55.

Abrahams S, Leigh PN, Kew JJM, Goldstein LH, Lloyd CML, Brooks DJ (1995b): A positron emission tomography study of frontal lobe function (verbal fluency) in amyotrophic lateral sclerosis. J Neurol Sci 129:44–46.

Aldridge JLF, Lennox G, Doherty F, Jefferson D, Landon M, Mayer RJ (1989): Inclusion bodies in motor cortex and brainstem of patients with motor neurone disease are detected by immunocytochemical localization of ubiquitin. Neurosci Lett 105:7–13.

Anderson VER, Cairns NJ, Leigh PN (1995): Involvement of the amygdala, dentate and hippocampus in motor neuron disease. J Neurol Sci 129:75–78.

Averback P (1981): Unusual particles in motor neuron disease. Arch Pathol Lab Med 105:490–493.

Brownell B, Oppenheimer DR, Hughes JT (1970): The central nervous system in motor neurone disease. J Neurol Neurosurg Psychiatry 33:338–357.

Brun A, England B, Gustafson L, Passant U, Mann DMA, Neary D, Snowden JS (1994): Clinical and neuropathological criteria for frontotemporal dementia. J Neurol Neurosurg Psychiatry 57:416–418.

Canter GJ (1963): Speech characteristics of patients with Parkinson's disease: I. Intensity, pitch and duration. J Speech Hear Dis 28:221–229.

Carpenter S (1968): Proximal axonal enlargement in motor neuron disease. Neurology 18:841–851.

Caselli RJ, Windebank AJ, Petersen RC, Komori T, Parisi JE, Okazaki E, Iverson R, Dinapoli RP, Graff-Radford NR, Stein SD (1993): Rapidly progressing aphasic dementia and motor neuron disease. Ann Neurol 33:200–207.

Chou SM (1988): Motor neuron inclusions in ALS are heavily ubiquitinated. J Neuropathol Exp Neurol 47:334.

Ciechanover A (1993): The ubiquitin-mediated proteolytic pathway. Brain Pathol 3:67–75.

Cooper PN, Jackson M, Lennox G, Lowe J, Mann DMA (1995): τ, ubiquitin, and αβ-crystallin immunohistochemistry define the principal causes of degenerative frontotemporal dementia. Arch Neurol 52:1011–1015.

Cummings J (1982): Cortical dementias. In Benson DF, Blumer D (eds): Psychiatric Aspects of Neurological Disease. New York: Grune and Stratton, pp 93–120.

Cummings J, Duchen L (1981): Klüver-Bucy syndrome in Pick's disease: Clinical and pathological correlates. Neurology 31:1415–1422.

Dalakas MC, Hatazawa J, Brooks RA, Di Chiro G (1987): Lowered cerebral glucose utilization in amyotrophic lateral sclerosis. Ann Neurol 22:580–586.

David AS, Gillham RA (1986): Neuropsychological study of motor neuron disease. Psychosomatics 27:441–445.

Delisle MB, Carpenter S (1984): Neurofibrillary axonal swellings and amyotrophic lateral sclerosis. J Neurol Sci 63:241–250.

Dickson DW, Horoupian DS, Thal LJ, Davies P, Walkley S, Terry RD (1986): Klüver-Bucy syndrome and amyotrophic lateral sclerosis: A case report with biochemistry, morphometrics, and Golgi study. Neurology 36:1323–1329.

Ferrer I, Tunon T, Serrano MT, Casas R, Alcantara S, Zujar MJ, Rivera RM (1993): Calbindin D-28k and parvalbumin immunoreactivity in the frontal cortex in patients with frontal lobe dementia of non-Alzheimer type associated with amyotrophic lateral sclerosis. J Neurol Neurosurg Psychiatry 56:257–261.

Gallassi R, Montagna P, Ciardulli C, Lorusso S, Mussato V, Stracciari A (1985): Cognitive impairment in motor neurone disease. Acta Neurol Scand 71:480–484.

Gallassi R, Montagna P, Morreale A, Lorusso S, Tinuper P, Daidone R, Lugaresi E (1989): Neuropsychological, electroencephalogram and brain computed tomography findings in motor neuron disease. Eur Neurol 29:115–120.

Gilbert JJ, Kish SJ, Chang L-J, Morito C, Shannak K, Hornykiewicz O (1988): Dementia, parkinsonism and motor neuron disease: Neurochemical and neuropathological correlates. Ann Neurol 24:688–691.

Hayashi H, Kato S (1989): Total manifestations of amyotrophic lateral sclerosis. J Neurol Sci 93:19–35.

Hayashi H, Kato S, Kawada A (1991): Amyotrophic lateral sclerosis patients living beyond respiratory failure. J Neurol Sci 105:73–78.

Hirano A (1991): Cytopathology of amyotrophic lateral sclerosis. In Rowland LP (ed): Amyotrophic Lateral Sclerosis and Other Motor Neuron Disorders. New York: Raven Press, pp 91–101.

Hirano A, Kurland LT, Sayre GP (1967): Familial amyotrophic lateral sclerosis. Arch Neurol 16:232–242.

Holland A, McBurney D, Mossy J, Reinmuth O (1985): The dissolution of language in Pick's disease with neurofibrillary tangles: A case study. Brain Lang 24:36–58.

Horoupian DS, Thal L, Katzman R, Terry RD, Davies P, Hirano A, DeTeresa R, Fuld PA, Petito C, Blass J, Ellis JM (1984): Dementia and motor neuron disease: Morphological, biochemical, and golgi studies. An Neurol 16:305–313.

Hudson A (1981): Amyotrophic lateral sclerosis and its association with dementia, parkinsonism and other neurological disorders: A review. Brain 194:217–247.

Iwasaki Y, Kinoshita M, Ikeda K, Takamiya K, Shiojima T (1990a): Neuropsychological dysfunctions in amyotrophic lateral sclerosis: Relation to motor disabilities. Int J Neurosci 54:191–195.

Iwasaki Y, Kinoshita M, Ikeda K, Takamiya K, Shiojima T (1990b): Cognitive impairment in amyotrophic lateral sclerosis and its relation to motor disabilities. Acta Neurol Scand 81:141–143.

Jackson M, Lennox G, Ward L, Lowe J (1995): Frontal dementia with MND inclusions without clinical ALS: Report of eleven cases. Neuropathol Appl Neurobiol 21:148–145.

Kato S, Hayashi H, Yagishita A (1993a): Involvement of the frontotemporal lobe and limbic system in amyotrophic lateral sclerosis: As assessed by serial computed tomography and magnetic resonance imaging. J Neurol Sci 116:52–58.

Kato S, Oda M, Tanabe H (1993b): Diminution of dopaminergic neurons in the substantia nigra of sporadic amyotrophic lateral sclerosis. Neuropathol Appl Neurobiol 19:300–304.

Kew JJM, Goldstein LH, Leigh PN, Abrahams S, Cosgrave N, Passingham RE, Frackowiak RSJ, Brooks DJ (1993): The relationship between abnormalities of cognitive function and cerebral activation in amyotrophic lateral sclerosis. Brain 116:1399–1423.

Kishikawa M, Nakamura T, Iseki M, Ikeda T, Shimokawa I, Tsujihata M, Nagasato K (1995): A long surviving case of amyotrophic lateral sclerosis with atrophy of the frontal lobe: A comparison with the Mitsuyama type. Acta Neuropathol 89:189–193.

Komachi H, Okeda R, Ishii N, Yanagisawa K, Yamada M, Miyatake T (1994): Motor neuron disease with dementia and ophthalmoplegia. A clinical and pathological study. J Neurol 241:592–596.

Kuljis RO, Schelper RL (1996): Alterations in nitrogen monoxide-synthesizing cortical neurons in amyotrophic lateral sclerosis with dementia. J Neuropathol Exp Neurol 55:25–35.

Lawyer T, Netsky MG (1963): Amyotrophic lateral sclerosis. Arch Neurol 8:117–127.

Leigh P, Swash M (1991): Cytoskeletal pathology in motor neuron disease. In Rowland LP (ed): Advances in Neurology. Amyotrophic Lateral Sclerosis and Other Motor Neuron Diseases. New York: Raven Press, pp 115–124.

Levy ML, Miller BL, Cummings JL, Fairbanks LA, Craig A (1996): Alzheimer disease and frontotemporal dementias. Arch Neurol 53:687–690.

Lishman WA (1987): Organic Psychiatry, 2nd ed. Oxford: Blackwell Scientific.

Lowe J (1994): New pathological findings in amyotrophic lateral sclerosis. J Neurol Sci 124:38–51.

Lowe J, Blanchard A, Morrell K, Lennox G, Reynolds L, Billett M, Landon M, Mayer RJ (1988): Ubiquitin is a common factor in intermediate filament inclusion bodies of diverse type in man, including those of Parkinson's disease, Pick's disease, and Alzheimer's disease, as well as Rosenthal fibres in cerebellar astrocytomas, cytoplasmic bodies in muscle, and mallory bodies in alcoholic liver disease. J Pathol 155:9–15.

Lowe J, Mayer RJ, Landon M (1993): Ubiquitin in neurodegenerative disease. Brain Pathol 3:55–65.

Ludolph AC, Elger CE, Böttger IW, Kuttig AG, Lottes G, Brune GG (1989): N-isopropyl-p-^{123}I-amphetamine single photon emission computed tomography in motor neuron disease. Eur Neurol 29:255–260.

Ludolph AC, Langen KJ, Regard M, Herzog H, Kemper B, Kuwert T, Bottger IG, Feinendegen L (1992): Frontal lobe function in amyotrophic lateral sclerosis: A neuropsychological and positron emission tomography study. Acta Neurol Scand 85:81–89.

Lynch T, Sano M, Marder KS, Bell KL, Foster NL, Defendini RF, Sima AAF, Keohane C, Nygaard TG, Fahn S, Mayeux R, Rowland LP, Wilhelmsen KC (1994): Clinical characteristics of a family with chromosome 17-linked disinhibition-dementia-parkinsonism-amyotrophy complex. Neurology 44:1878–1884.

Manetto V, Perry G, Tabaton M, Mulvihill P, Fried VA, Smith HT, Gambetti P, Autilio-Gambetti L (1988): Ubiquitin is associated with abnormal cytoplasmic filaments characteristic of neurodegenerative disease. Proc Natl Acad Sci USA 85:4501–4505.

Martin JE, Swash M, Schwartz MS (1990): New insights in motor neuron disease. Neuropathol Appl Neurobiol 16:97–110.

Migheli A, Pezzulo T, Attanasio A, Schiffer D (1993): Peripherin immunoreactive structures in amyotrophic lateral sclerosis. Lab Invest 68:185–191.

Mitsuyama Y (1984): Presenile dementia with motor neuron disease in Japan: Clinicopathological review of 26 cases. J Neurol Neurosurg Psychiatry 47:953–959.

Mizutani T, Aki A, Shiozawa R, Unakami M, Nozawa T, Yajima K, Tanabe H, Hara M (1990): Development of ophthalmoplegia in amyotrophic lateral sclerosis during long-term use of respirators. J Neurol Sci 99:311–319.

Montgomery GK, Erickson LM (1987): Neuropsychological perspectives in amyotrophic lateral sclerosis. Neurol Clin 5:61–81.

Murayama S, Mori H, Ihara Y, Bouldin W, Suzuki K, Tomonaga M (1990): Immunocytochemical and ultrastructural studies of lower motor neurons in amyotrophic lateral sclerosis. Ann Neurol 27:137–148.

Neary D, Snowden JS, Mann DMA, Northern B, Goulding PJ, MacDermott N (1990): Frontal lobe dementia and motor neuron disease. J Neurol Neurosurg Psychiatry 53:23–32.

Ohnishi T, Hoshi H, Nagamachi S, Futami S, Watanabe K, Mitsuyama Y (1991): Regional cerebral blood flow study with ^{123}I-IMP in patients with degenerative dementia. Am J Neuroradiol 12:513–520.

Okamato K, Hirai S, Yamazaki T, Sun X, Nakazato Y (1991): New ubiquitin-positive intraneuronal inclusions in the extra-motor cortices in patients with amyotrophic lateral sclerosis. Neurosci Lett 129:233–236.

Okamoto K, Murakami N, Kusaka H, Yoshida M, Hashizume Y, Nakazato Y, Matsubara E, Hirai S (1992): Ubiquitin-positive intraneuronal inclusions in the motor cortices of presenile dementia patients with motor neuron disease. J Neurol 239:426–430.

Peavy GM, Herzog AG, Rubin NP, Mesulam M (1992): Neuropsychological aspects of dementia of motor neuron disease. Neurology 42:1004–1008.

Peterson RC, Ivnik RJ, Litchy WJ, Windebank AJ, Daube JR (1990): Cognitive function in amyotrophic lateral sclerosis. Neurology 40:315.

Poloni M, Capitani E, Mazzini L, Ceroni M (1986): Neuropsychological measures in amyotrophic lateral sclerosis and their relationship with CT scan-assessed cerebral atrophy. Acta Neurol Scand 74:257–260.

Rodgers-Johnson P, Garruto RM, Yanigahara R, Chen KM, Gajdusek DC, Gibbs CJ Jr (1986): Amyotrophic lateral sclerosis and parkinsonism-dementia on Guam: A 30-year evaluation of clinical and neuropathological trends. Neurology 36:7–13.

Sasaki S, Tsutsumi Y, Yamane K, Sakuma H, Maruyama S (1992): Sporadic amyotrophic lateral sclerosis with extensive neurological involvement. Acta Neuropathol 84:211–215.

Soni W, Luthert PJ, Leigh PN, Mann DMA (1993): A morphometric study of the neuropathological substrate of dementia in patients with motor neuron disease. Neuropathol Appl Neurobiol 19:203.

Strong MJ, Garruto RM (1994): Experimental paradigms of motor neuron degeneration. In Woodruff ML Nonneman A (eds): Animal Models of Toxin-Induced Neurological Disorders. New York: Plenum Press, pp 39–88.

Strong MJ, Gaytan-Garcia S, Jakowec D (1995): Reversibility of neurofilamentous inclusion formation following repeated sublethal intracisternal inoculums of $AlCl_3$ in New Zealand white rabbits. Acta Neuropathol 90:57–67.

Strong MJ, Grace GM, Orange JB, Leeper HA (1996): Cognition, language and speech in amyotrophic lateral sclerosis: A review. J Clin Exp Neuropsychol 18:291–303.

Talbot PR, Goulding PJ, Lloyd JJ, Snowden JS, Neary D, Testa HJ (1995): Inter-relation between "classic" motor neuron disease and frontotemporal dementia: Neuropsychological and single photon emission computed tomography study. J Neurol Neurosurg Psychiatry 58:541–547.

Tanaka M, Kondo S, Hirai S, Sun X, Yamagishi T, Okamoto K (1993): Cerebral blood flow and oxygen metabolism in progressive dementia associated with amyotrophic laterals sclerosis. J Neurol Sci 120:22–28.

Tolnay M, Probst A (1995): Frontal lobe degeneration: Novel ubiquitin-immunoreactive neurites within frontotemporal cortex. Neuropathol Appl Neurobiol 21:492–497.

Waldemar G, Varstrup S, Jensen TS, Johnsen A, Boysen G (1992): Focal reductions in cerebral blood flow in amyotrophic lateral sclerosis: A [^{99m}Tc]-*d,l*-HMPAO SPECT study. J Neurol Sci 107:19–28.

Wightman G, Anderson VER, Martin J, Swash M, Anderton BH, Neary D, Mann D, Luthert P, Leigh PN (1992): Hippocampal and neocortical ubiquitin-immunoreactive inclusions in amyotrophic lateral sclerosis with dementia. Neurosci Lett 139:269–274.

CHAPTER 13

Dementias Lacking Distinctive Histology

DAVID S. KNOPMAN

Department of Neurology, University of Minnesota, Minneapolis, MN 55455

DEMENTIA LACKING DISTINCTIVE HISTOLOGY: DEFINING A DISEASE

Dementia lacking distinctive histology (*DLDH*) is a term that my colleagues and I (Knopman et al., 1990) coined to describe neuropathological findings common to a series of patients in a dementia brain bank. The brains of these patients were devoid of senile plaques, neurofibrillary tangles, Lewy bodies, Pick bodies, and swollen neurons. What was seen on microscopic examination had been considered to be nonspecific: neuronal dropout in cortical and subcortical regions, astrocytic proliferation that paralleled cell loss, and spongiform changes of the neocortex (Kim et al., 1981). Our report called attention to the many other cases with fundamentally similar pathology that had been reported as single cases or as families. They have been mentioned occasionally in the literature for many years. However, because of the combination of the lack of distinctive histology, the lack of appreciation of the distinctive clinical profile, and the inability to capitalize on the knowledge of the familial tendency of the disorders, they were largely ignored.

By calling attention to DLDH, it was as if we had proposed a new disorder, although we really only pointed out the commonality of the many previously reported cases. In making this synthesis from a collection of cases thought previously to be unrelated, it is appropriate to consider the assumptions underlying the "new" disease's construct. First, there should be a clinical syndrome associated with the disorder. Dementia was the common theme in our patients. There were other, noncognitive syndromes that our patients exhibited, including an extrapyramidal disorder and a motor neuron disorder. It turned out that the other cases in the literature often had more than a dementing disorder as well. Nonetheless, the shared clinical phenotype of our cases with DLDH was dementia. Usually but not always, the dementia was associated with prominent behavioral abnormalities and prominent frontal cognitive deficits (Gustafson, 1987, 1993; Neary et al., 1988; Neary and Snowden, 1991). A defined clinical syndrome is necessary to recognize commonality. Classification of the clinical syndromes of dementia is a use-

Pick's Disease and Pick Complex, Edited by Andrew Kertesz and David G. Munoz
ISBN 0-471-17792-X   ©1998 Wiley-Liss, Inc.

ful conceptual structure for practicing physicians, but it should not be construed as sufficient. Indeed, recognizing the dementia with prominent behavioral (and executive/frontal lobe-type) deficits leads to the next level of analysis, namely, the differential diagnosis of the underlying pathology. This syndrome could be due to Alzheimer's disease (AD), Pick body-positive Pick's disease (PiD), Pick body-negative but swollen, neuron-positive disease, DLDH, progressive subcortical gliosis, one of the leukodystrophies, vascular dementia, or other even rarer disorders.

A second feature of a defined disease is that there should be a set of neuropathological inclusion and exclusion criteria. In our patients to whom we applied the label DLDH, these were cell loss, gliosis, and spongiform changes in the frontal neocortex, temporal neocortex, hippocampal formation, and other subcortical regions and the lack of other distinctive histological features. Since specific histopathological markers such as neurofibrillary tangles, senile plaques, Pick bodies, swollen neurons, and Lewy bodies were diagnostic of other processes, we felt that their absence was necessary for case definition. Our neuropathological description of DLDH thus differentiates it from the other causes of fronto-temporal dementia (FTD), but the neuropathological phenotype of DLDH has nothing about it to indicate that it is homogeneous.

The location and intensity of the DLDH-like changes vary dramatically. The common neuropathology of the neocortex and the commonly associated subcortical changes across our patients led us to an inclusive definition of DLDH. It may be presumptuous of us to lump striatonigral degeneration (e.g., Adams et al., 1964), dementia with motor neuron disease (MND) (e.g., Morita et al., 1987; Neary et al., 1990), and the frontal lobe dementia (Brun, 1987, 1993; Neary et al., 1988) into a single entity. Surely, they cannot be all one disease, but the histopathology of these three conditions, plus others discussed below, share striking similarities. It may also be presumptuous to separate DLDH-like pathology from cases with Pick bodies and ballooned cells. Pick body-positive PiD and what we called DLDH may be part of the same disease. In the absence of a molecular genetic description, the boundaries of DLDH are fuzzy, and disease classification remains based on features that are detectable by histopathological examination. A phenotypic classification does not allow resolution of relationships between phenotypically related but mechanistically distinct disorders. Careful description of the phenotypic variation at the histological level will lead to greater insights into the molecular mechanisms. Until a better understanding of the molecular mechanisms of cell death in DLDH and other possibly related disorders is available, we must be content with a tentative neuropathological classification, with emphasis on "tentative."

Knowledge of the genetics of degenerative neurological diseases has begun to expand and to offer, potentially, the key to explicating the relationships of the DLDH-like disorders. In other diseases, molecular advances have shown us the limitations of phenotypic classification. In addition to the identification of genes involved in AD (e.g., see Hyman, 1996, for a succinct overview) and prion diseases (Collinge and Palmer, 1993; Prusiner and Hsiao, 1994), the past 2 years have also brought advances in other neurological disorders. In the ataxias, the apparent clinical and neuropathological similarities of the many variants did not imply a single genetic basis for all subtypes (Rosenberg, 1995). Although the clinical syndrome differentiates the ataxic disorders from other movement disorders, the overlap in pathology between apparently different subtypes of the ataxias led to much confusion in their classification. It was not until genetic markers appeared that attempts at neuropathological classification were abandoned in favor of genetic classification. In the case of Huntington's disease (Brandt et al., 1996; Furtado et al., 1996), the clinical and pathological features were sufficiently homogeneous that diagnosis and classification were rarely contentious. On the other hand, the heterogeneity in age of onset and neuropathological severity in Huntington's disease turned out to have a clear genetic basis, that is, it was related to the number of trinucleotide repeats.

Experience with other neurodegenerative diseases may thus provide some insights into how to think about DLDH. Although it is still premature to propose a molecular basis for the DLDH disorders, we can anticipate that these disorders will eventually be classified on molecular grounds. There are probably several molecular mechanisms that produce the DLDH phenotype, as turned out to be the case with AD. On the other hand, a broad view of the phenotype is also warranted at this stage. Considering the surprising relationship between prion diseases and thalamic degeneration (Petersen et al., 1992), phenotypic variation could turn out to be due to different mutations within the same gene.

This chapter will discuss the basis for identifying a phenotype of DLDH and how knowledge of that phenotype will inform the molecular biologists as they strive to understand the genetic basis of dementing disorders that lack distinctive histological features. Recognizing the existence of DLDH advanced the field, but the next, bigger steps are (1) to elucidate the phenotypic variations as thoroughly as possible and then (2) to discover the possible molecular mechanisms.

VARIANTS OF AND SYNONYMS FOR DLDH

Distinctive histological features are common in the dementias, although a rarity in other neurological diseases. As a consequence, the distinctive histological features created a context in which their presence formed the basis of disease classification. The existence of senile plaques, neurofibrillary tangles, Pick bodies, ballooned neurons, and Lewy bodies became the gold standards for diagnosis, forcing patients without those histological markers into a category of "other" or "unclassified." In the days when neuropathologists who examined the brains of dementia patients had little clinical information, or information only about the terminal illness, one can imagine that the "nonspecific" cases were thought to be uninteresting. Alternatively, if there was clinical information, and since the clinical picture of these DLDH cases sometimes resembled that of frontal dementias or extrapyramidal-like "Parkinson's plus" disease, the DLDH disorders sometimes ended up in classifications under PiD or striatonigral degeneration. As a consequence, DLDH-like pathology was reported under a variety of other names.

The most common place to find cases of DLDH prior to the latter 1980s was under the label of PiD. Constantinidis and coworkers (1974) called them *type C Pick's disease.* In this scheme, *type A Pick's disease* referred to cases with Pick bodies and *type B Pick's disease* denoted the cases with only ballooned neurons (*Pick's cells*). There was considerable empirical rationale, prior to a molecular genetic explanation, for such a grouping. Clinically, many of the patients with the DLDH pathology present with frontal lobe behavioral syndromes or progressive aphasia (Kim et al., 1981; Brun, 1987, 1993; Gustafson, 1987, 1993; Kirshner et al., 1987; Mehler et al., 1987; Neary et al., 1988, 1993; Snowden et al., 1992; Turner et al., 1996). The pathology of DLDH often includes considerable frontal and temporal atrophy. The degree of atrophy in DLDH is usually less than in Pick body-positive PiD, and the absence of Pick bodies is the other major distinguishing feature. North American neuropathologists have tended not to diagnose a case as PiD unless Pick bodies are present. We went along with that convention when we separated DLDH cases from the category of PiD. Because of the phenotypic similarity to Pick body-positive PiD, Kertesz and colleagues (1994) have taken a second look at the relationship between DLDH and Pick body-positive PiD. They have added the latter disorder to those without Pick bodies to create the category *Pick complex,* the organizing theme of this book. Until the molecular biology of the disorders is clarified, the relationship between cases with Pick bodies and those without them is unresolvable.

DLDH also included patients with prominent subcortical pathology. There are descriptions of a number of cases with DLDH-like pathology in which there is prominent involvement outside the neocortex in regions such as the striatum or thalamus (Adams et al., 1964; Masse et al., 1981; Torack and Morris, 1986; Moossy et al., 1987; Deymeer et al., 1989; Verity et al.,

1990), motor neurons (Caselli et al., 1993; Wilkstrom et al., 1982; Houropian et al., 1984; Morita et al., 1987; Gilbert et al., 1988; Neary et al., 1990; Peavy et al., 1992; Caselli et al., 1993), white matter (Neuman and Cohn, 1967), or, most commonly, combinations of these. They have been labeled *dementia with motor neuron disease, thalamic dementia, subcortical gliosis, striatonigral degeneration,* and *mesolimbic dementia,* among others. A number of the described cases have had some neocortical involvement. Whether these are part of one DLDH disease or representatives of several different molecular mechanisms awaits resolution.

Another diagnostic category that might include DLDH cases is hippocampal sclerosis (Dickson et al., 1994). We have observed some brains in which the only pathological feature is neuronal loss in the hippocampal formation. A problem arises when the examining neuropathologist assumes that such damage, if it tends to be limited to the CA1 region, must represent anoxic injury. The neuropathological diagnosis might be recorded as anoxic brain injury. It is only with thorough clinical documentation and clinical–pathological correlation that, in the absence of a history of cardiac arrest, a degenerative process rather than an ischemic process could be diagnosed. Still, without some independent means of establishing a degenerative pathogenesis, the status of hippocampal sclerosis remains up in the air.

One final disorder that may turn out to be related to DLDH is one described under the label of *dementia with argyrophilic grains* (Braak and Braak, 1989; Itagaki et al., 1989; Yamada et al., 1992). In their original description, the Braaks found that 20 of 80 brains of dementia patients had no distinctive histological features except cell loss and gliosis accompanied by argyrophilic grain pathology. They commented that the distribution of the argyrophilic material was similar to that in Pick body-positive PiD, but the degree of atrophy was less than in the latter disorder.

THE PREVALANCE AND DEMOGRAPHICS OF DLDH

Pathological series in the past 10–15 years have noted one or more of the DLDH-like disorders, usually under one of the synonyms mentioned in the previous section (Wade et al., 1987; Joachim et al., 1988; Boller et al., 1989; Risse et al., 1990; Galasko et al., 1994; Gearing et al., 1995). The prevalence and demographics of DLDH are very difficult to assess in a population since it is a pathological diagnosis. In our experience, patients with DLDH constituted 10% of individuals with dementia who were under age 70 years at death (Knopman et al., 1990). Including all autopsied patients in the brain bank, the proportion was only 3%, but because most DLDH patients are under 75, while most AD patients are over 75, looking at the younger age range may give a more clinically relevant view. Others have also found that DLDH patients tend to be younger (Brun, 1987, 1993; Giannakopoulos et al., 1995). Our autopsy series (representing autopsies performed by one neuropathologist from 1980 to 1986) applied consistent criteria for the diagnosis of AD. These criteria were the absence of AD-type changes, Pick cells, Pick bodies, or Lewy bodies. The cases had cortical vacuolation to some degree, gliosis of cortical or subcortical structures, and cell loss in affected regions. Some degree of cortical pathology was required for inclusion as a case of DLDH. Because of its diagnostic uncertainty, pure hippocampal sclerosis was not included under DLDH.

In the experience of A. Brun and colleagues in Lund, Sweden, patients with FTD without distinctive histology constituted 10% of their series of dementia patients (Brun, 1987, 1993). Giannakopoulos et al. (1995) found a similar proportion (9.3%) for DLDH among all dementia patients coming to autopsy at the Psychiatric Hospital of the University of Geneva.

Since DLDH is a pathological diagnosis, and since autopsy populations are far from representative of an epidemiologically defined population, the estimates of the incidence and prevalence of DLDH are biased. It is possible that the autopsy experience overestimates their prevalence because the distinctive clinical presentation leads to higher autopsy rates. Furthermore, the DLDH patients in our experience tend to be under age 70 at death, and these individuals are more likely to be autopsied than older patients. On the other hand, it is possible that DLDH is correctly estimated relative to AD. If DLDH patients actually have clinical presentations that are indistinguishable from those of AD to the vast majority of laypeople and practicing physicians, then they might be autopsied at a rate equal to that of AD patients. A third possibility is that DLDH could be undercounted if patients with minimal pathology were excluded. We have observed such an instance in a patient who happened to be the sister of one of our other patients who had had prominent DLDH-like pathology. The sister with the minimal pathology might have been excluded had she not had a sister who died previously with a typical picture of DLDH.

CLINICAL SPECTRUM

The clinical spectrum of DLDH may prove to be more homogeneous than we originally thought, since most of the patients in our series were not studied prospectively during life. Cases in our series (Knopman et al., 1990) were defined by the presence of dementia and by the neuropathological findings described above. Taking those two criteria as the starting point, the predominant clinical presentation of the DLDH cases in our experience was that of a FTD virtually indistinguishable from the clinical course of Pick body-positive PiD. The onset was almost always insidious. The initial presentation included loss of skills, personality changes, or the development of socially inappropriate behaviors. As our clinical experience broadened beyond our original series, patients who presented with language disturbances were also observed. The behavioral disturbance consisted of poor judgment, impulsive decision making, and socially inappropriate behavior. On mental status testing, judgment and concentration were more impaired than learning. The language disturbance consisted initially of word- and name-finding complaints. Reductions in fluency and impaired articulation invariably followed. Severe nonfluency and mutism occurred subsequently. In general, behavioral abnormalities were a regular feature of DLDH patients, but by the reports of caregivers, most of our patients with DLDH had memory impairment and might still have had AD as part of the differential diagnosis at some point in the illness. Memory complaints were sometimes prominent in our DLDH cases, making the clinical presentation of DLDH sometimes quite difficult to distinguish from that of AD. Perhaps the most consistent finding from the cognitive assessment was that visuospatial tasks such as block design were spared in the face of the other amnesic and executive deficits. The duration of the illness in our patients ranged from 2 years in two patients with associated MND to over 10 years. The dementia of DLDH invariably progressed to involve severe deficits in all areas of cognition and function, and as a result, the dementia was indistinguishable from AD in the latter stages of the disease.

The clinical syndrome of FTD in the patients we described with DLDH was usually unaccompanied by major abnormalities in motor function early in the illness. Later in the illness, rigidity, masked facies, gait disturbances, dysarthria, and dysphagia occurred.

PATHOLOGICAL FINDINGS

The pathological spectrum in our cases led us to group patients into three broad categories: a primarily cortical type, a striatal-thalamic type, and a motor neuron type (Knopman et al.,

1990). We did not include a fourth category of patients within our original series, but patients with gliosis of the subcortical white matter (progressive subcortical gliosis) could be considered as a fourth category (Knopman, 1993). We recognized that this classification probably has no etiological significance but is merely a convenient way to summarize the neuropathological findings. Giannakopoulos and colleagues (1995) have classified their large series of DLDH cases somewhat differently, although they also emphasized the distinction between primarily neocortical and primarily subcortical pathology. In both Knopman et al. (1990) and Giannakopoulos et al. (1995), case definition was primarily neuropathological, so that the case material from these two series may be broader (especially in terms of subcortical pathology) than that of authors who defined their cases clinically, such as the Manchester and Lund groups (Brun, 1987, 1993; Gustafson, 1987, 1993; Neary et al., 1988; Mann et al., 1993).

The cortical pathology consists of neuronal loss and gliosis of the neocortex. There is usually a concomitant vacuolation of the upper cortical layers (Figure 13.1). The degree of cell loss and gliosis can vary dramatically from case to case. The distribution of the neocortical changes is almost always frontal and temporal (Mann and South, 1993). In this dimension, DLDH-like cases resemble Pick body-positive PiD (Mann and South, 1993). Rarely, it has been reported as focal (e.g., Kirshner et al., 1987). In some cases, the parietal lobes are heavily involved. The insula is usually involved to the same extent that the frontal neocortex is affected.

The caudate nucleus is frequently affected. Grossly, the caudate head is shrunken. Neuronal loss and astrocytic proliferation are observed (Figure 13.2). The putamen is not usually as heav-

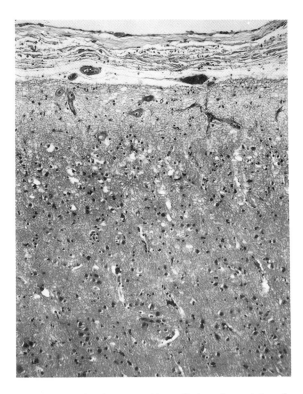

FIGURE 13.1. Frontal neocortex showing neuronal loss, gliosis, and vacuolation of upper cortical layers (Original magnification 120×).

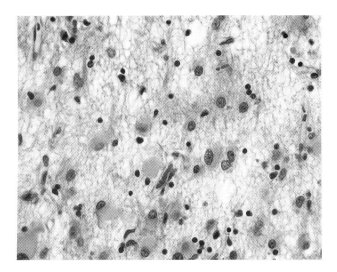

FIGURE 13.2 Histological changes in the caudate nucleus in a patient with thalamostriate dementia lacking distinctive histology. Neuronal cell loss and gliosis are especially prominent; virtually all neurons have disappeared from this representative field from the head of the caudate. Gross atrophy of the caudate was marked in this patient as well (Original magnification 480×).

ily lesioned, but in some cases it is drastically shrunken. The medial thalamus may be similarly affected.

In the hippocampus, areas of involvement with cell loss and gliosis include CA1, subiculum, and entorhinal cortex (Figure 13.3). The dentate gyrus and CA4, CA3 are usually unaffected. The amygdala is frequently severely affected, though in some patients it may be completely normal.

Other than the motor nuclei in the brainstem and spinal cord in a subset of patients, the only other area affected below the diencephalon is the substantia nigra. Loss of pigmented neurons may be striking (Figure 13.4). There is no predilection for involvement of just the medial or just the lateral regions of the substantia nigra. Lewy bodies are absent.

The white matter of the cerebral cortex may be uninvolved or may show evidence of gliosis. Leukodystrophy is not part of the spectrum of DLDH.

Mann and colleagues (Mann et al., 1993; Cooper et al., 1995) have applied immunohistochemical methods to classify FTD cases. Use of antibodies to tau identified a subset of patients with AD, Pick body-positive PiD, and corticobasal degeneration/dementia with swollen chromatolytic neurons. The fact that not all patients showed tau immunostaining suggests that not all cases involve tau pathology. If that is true, this is further evidence that Pick body- and ballooned cell-positive cases are biochemically distinct from DLDH cases with no tau staining. On the other hand, if tau immunostaining is somehow a variable marker of neuronal dysfunction, then it may not be positive in all cases.

Ballooned neurons were further detected with alphaB-crystallin. Cases with MND had positive staining with ubiquitin. Patients who showed staining with none of these constituted instances of DLDH, that is, they lacked ballooned neurons or other inclusions. These immunohistological findings tell us that DLDH is heterogeneous pathologically, and that there is a subset of patients who lack a unique positive immunohistochemical signature.

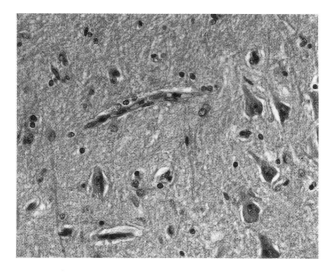

FIGURE 13.3. Hippocampus showing cell loss in the CA1 region. Transition zone between the CA1 and CA2 regions of hippocampal formation in a patient with DLDH. The field was chosen to illustrate the presence of pyramidal neurons in the CA2 region and the virtual absence of neurons in the adjacent CA1 region. Gliosis was modest (Original magnification 624×).

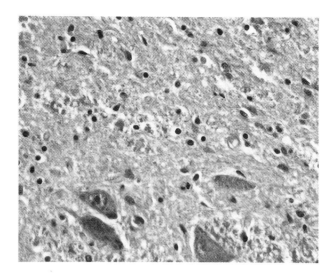

FIGURE 13.4 Histological changes in the substantia nigra. Loss of pigmented neurons is particularly prominent. In this section, a few remaining pigmented neurons were captured in the photographic field for orientation. In the remainder of the substantia nigra, marked dropout of pigmented neurons was obvious, with many microscopic fields totally devoid of neurons (Original magnification 480×).

There is no cholinergic deficit in most of the DLDH-like cases in which the assay has been reported (Houropian et al., 1984; Mehler et al., 1987; Gilbert et al., 1988; Knopman et al., 1990). Ultimately, this finding indicates only that the basal forebrain nuclei are not lesioned by the DLDH processes. Three groups have reported dopaminergic deficits in DLDH-like patients, however (Houropian et al., 1984; Gilbert et al., 1988; Yamada et al., 1992). This finding is consistent with the neuropathological involvement of the substantia nigra. Dopaminergic neurons that project to the neocortex and hippocampus are located contiguous to the nigra in the ventral tegmental area.

The heterogeneity of the described cases with DLDH will make more sense once the molecular genetics of these disorders has been clarified. Phenotypic variations that form the basis for clinical and pathological classification may or may not turn out to be predictive of the genotype.

GENETICS OF DLDH

It has been recognized that a number of DLDH patients had strong family histories of similar illnesses. This has been a major impetus to the study of the disorders that have the DLDH pathological phenotype. In our initial series, we ascertained a positive family history of dementia or (in one case) amyotrophic lateral sclerosis (Knopman et al., 1990). Over the next several years, siblings of our patients came to autopsy and pathological confirmation of a second family member was obtained in two additional instances.

It is likely that the DLDH-like disorders will be genetically heterogeneous (Ashworth et al., 1995). Among the families with DLDH-like pathology, there are now some whose molecular basis is being established. For thalamic pathology, at least one group of patients with nonspecific histology has been linked to the prion gene, the fatal familial insomnia cases (Manetto et al., 1992; Petersen et al., 1992). For most other instances of DLDH-like pathology, there have been no abnormalities in the prion gene (Collinge and Palmer, 1993; Diedrich et al., 1992; Petersen et al., 1992; Clinton et al., 1993).

Prominent cortical, amygdala, striatal, and mesencephalic pathology that lacked typical distinctive histological features was seen in one family originally described by Lynch et al. (1994) who showed linkage to the q21–22 region of chromosome 17. In the originally described family, the neuropathology closely resembled the DLDH profile in that there was widespread neuronal loss and gliosis in cortical and subcortical regions but prominent argyrophilic inclusions in neurons (Sima et al., 1996). Evidence for linkage has been expanded to a dozen other families, including some with pure cortical pathology. Several also have had prominent neurofibrillary tangles or some other form of tau pathology (Sumi et al., 1992). However, tau pathology is absent in others (Foster et al., 1997). The families linked to chromosome 17 who had DLDH-like pathology were originally described under a variety of labels, including *disinhibition-dementia-parkinsonism-amyotrophy complex* (Lendon et al., 1994), *progressive subcortical gliosis* (Lanska et al., 1993), and *PiD* (Schenk, 1958). These labels demonstrate the phenotypic variation that may arise and give pause to those who wish to classify patients based solely on pathology. It seems almost heretical to conjecture that the presence or absence of neurofibrillary tangles may represent a phenotypic variation that is not predictive of the genotype, but the genetic evidence is pointing in that direction (Foster et al., 1997). Further investigations of the chromosome 17-linked families may help clarify this issue.

A very interesting finding to emerge from investigations with chromosome 17 families is that a family known widely in the literature as the Schenk family has shown linkage to the q21–22 region of chromosome 17 (Schenk, 1958; Groen and Endtz, 1982). The Schenk family has been regarded as an example of autosomal dominant PiD, but a careful reexamination of the neuropathology reveals that the findings are of DLDH in that there are neither Pick bodies nor ballooned neurons (Heutink et al., 1997).

Another gene may also turn out to have important links to DLDH cases. Brown et al. (1995) have reported linkage to a 12-centimorgan region of chromosome 3 in a family (originally reported by Gydesen et al., 1987) with a dementing disorder plus a gait abnormality. This family had clinical presentations that included a frontal lobe syndrome as well as a parietal lobe (AD-like) syndrome. The pathology has been reported to be primarily cortical.

Some familial MNDs have been linked to mutations of the Cu-Zn superoxide dismutase (Rosen et al., 1993), but to my knowledge, there has been no linkage to cases with dementia plus MND.

CONCLUSIONS

DLDH is a pathologically defined entity that may represent one etiological molecular mechanism but more likely represents several. Over the next decade, we can expect that more and more familial dementing disorders with DLDH pathology will be linked to specific genes. The relationship of DLDH to disorders with distinctive histopathological features, in particular PiD with Pick bodies and ballooned neurons, remains to be clarified. While it is obvious that they share a clinical phenotype and some aspects of the pathological phenotype (mainly the topographic distribution of cell loss), Pick body-positive PiD and DLDH have an uncertain relationship.

ACKNOWLEDGMENTS

The author would like to thank Dr. Angeline Mastri for originally identifying this entity in our dementia brain bank and enlisting my assistance in developing the clinical pathological correlations. I would also like to thank Dr. Joo Ho Sung for many helpful discussions concerning the neuropathological findings of this disorder.

REFERENCES

Adams RD, Van Bogaert L, Vander Eecken H (1964): Striato-nigral degeneration. J Neuropathol Exp Neurol 23:584–608.

Ashworth A, Brown J, Gydesen S, Sorensen SA, Rossor MN, Hardy J, Collinge J (1995): Frontal lobe or "nonspecific" dementias are genetically heterogeneous. Neurology 45:1781.

Boller F, Lopez OL, Moossy J (1989): Diagnosis of dementia: Clinicopathologic correlations. Neurology 39:76–79.

Braak H, Braak E (1989): Cortical and subcortical argyrophilic grains characterize a disease associated with adult onset dementia. Neuropathol Appl Neurobiol 15:13–26.

Brandt J, Bylsma FW, Gross R, Stine OC, Ranen N, Ross CA (1996): Trinucleotide repeat length and clinical progression in Huntington's disease. Neurology 46:527–531.

Brown J, Ashworth A, Gydesen S, Sorenson A, Rossor M, Hardy J, Collinge J (1995): Familial nonspecific dementia maps to chromosome 3. Hum Mol Genet 4:1625–1628.

Brun A (1987): Frontal lobe degeneration of non-Alzheimer type. I. Neuropathology. Arch Gerontol Geriatr 6:193–208.

Brun A (1993): Frontal lobe degeneration of the non-Alzheimer type revisited. Dementia 4:126–131.

Caselli RJ, Windebank AJ, Petersen RC, Komori T, Parisi JE, Okazaki H, Kokmen E, Iverson R, Dinapoli RP, Graff-Radford NR (1993): Rapidly progressive aphasic dementia and motor neuron disease. Ann Neurol 33:200–207.

Clinton J, Mann DMA, Roberts GW (1993): Frontal lobe dementia is not a variant of prion disease. Neurosci Lett 164:1–4.

Collinge J, Palmer MS (1993): Prion disease in humans and their relevance to other neurodegenerative diseases. Dementia 4:178–185.

Constantinidis J, Richard J, Tissot R (1974): Pick's disease: Histological and clinical correlation. Eur Neurol 11:208–217.

Cooper PN, Jackson M, Lennox G, Lowe J, Mann DMA (1995): Tau, ubiquitin and alphaB-crystallin immunohistochemistry define the principal causes of degenerative frontotemporal dementia. Arch Neurol 52:1011–1015.

Deymeer F, Smith TW, DeGirolami U, Drachman DA (1989): Thalamic dementia and motor neuron disease. Neurology 39:58–61.

Dickson DW, Davies P, Bevona C, Van Hoeven KH, Factor SM, Grober E, Aronson MK, Crystal HA (1994): Hippocampal sclerosis: A common pathological feature of dementia in very old (≥ 80 years of age) humans. Acta Neuropathol 88:212–221.

Diedrich JF, Knopman DS, List JF, Olson K, Frey WH II, Emory CR, Sung JH, Haase AT (1992): Deletion in the prion protein gene in a demented patient. Hum Mol Genet 1:443–444.

Foster NL, Wilhelmsen K, Sima AAF, Jones MZ, D'Amato C, Gilman S, et al (1997): Frontotemporal dementia and Parkinsonism linked to chromosome 17: A consensus. Ann Neurol 41:706–715.

Furtado S, Suchowersky O, Rewcastle B, Graham L, Klimek L, Garber A (1996): Relationship between trinucleotide repeats and neuropathological changes in Huntingtons's disease. Ann Neurol 39:132–136.

Galasko D, Hansen LA, Katzman RA (1994): Clinical-neuropathological correlations in Alzheimer's disease and related dementias. Arch Neurol 51:888–895.

Gearing M, Mirra SS, Hedreen JC, Sumi SM, Hansen LA, Heyman A (1995): The consortium to establish a registry for Alzheimer's Disease (CERAD). Neurology 45:461–466.

Giannakopoulos P, Hof PR, Bouras C (1995): Dementia lacking distinctive histopathology: Clinicopathological evaluation of 32 cases. Acta Neuropathol 89:346–355.

Gilbert JJ, Kish SJ, Chang LJ, Morito C, Shannak K, Hornykiewicz O (1988): Dementia, parkinsonism, and motor neuron disease: Neurochemical and neuropathological correlates. Ann Neurol 24:688–691.

Groen JJ, Endtz LJ (1982): Hereditary Pick's disease. Second reexamination of a large family and discussion of other hereditary cases, with particular reference to electroencephalography and computed tomography. Brain 105:443–459.

Gustafson L (1987): Frontal lobe degeneration of non-Alzheimer type. II. Clinical picture and differential diagnosis. Arch Gerontol Geriatr 6:209–223.

Gustafson L (1993): Clinical picture of frontal lobe degeneration of non-Alzheimer type. Dementia 4:143–148.

Gydensen S, Hagen S, Klinken L, Abelskov J, Sorensen SA (1987): Neuropsychiatric studies in a family with presenile dementia different from Alzheimer and Pick disease. Acta Psychiatr Scand 76:276–284.

Heutink P, Stevens M, Rizzu P, Bakker E, Kros JM, Tibben A, Niermeijer MF, van Duijn CM, Oostra BA, van Swieten JC (1997): Hereditary frontotemporal dementia is linked to chromosome 17q21–q22: A genetic and clinico pathological study of three Dutch families. Ann Neurol 41:150–159.

Horoupian DS, Thal L, Katzman R, Terry RD, Davies P, Hirano A, DeTeresa R, Fuld PA, Petito C, Blass J, Ellis JM (1984): Dementia and motor neuron disease: Morphometric, biochemical, and Golgi studies. Ann Neurol 16:305–313.

Hyman BT (1996): Alzheimer's disease or Alzheimer's disease? Clues from molecular epidemiology. Ann Neurol 40:135–136.

Itagaki S, McGeer PL, Akiyama H, Beattie BL, Walker DG, Moore GRW, McGeer EG (1989): A case of adult onset dementia with argyrophilic grains. Ann Neurol 26:685–689.

Joachim CL, Morris JH, Selkoe DJ (1988): Clinically diagnosed Alzheimer's disease: Autopsy results in 150 cases. Ann Neurol 24:50–56.

Kertesz A, Hudson L, Mackenzie IRA, Munoz DG (1994): The pathology and nosology of primary progressive aphasia. Neurology 44:2065–2072.

Kim RC, Collins GH, Parisi JE, Wright AW, Chu YB (1981): Familial dementia of adult onset with pathological findings of a nonspecific nature. Brain 104:61–78.

Kirshner HS, Tanridag O, Thurman L, Whetsell WO Jr (1987): Progressive aphasia without dementia: Two cases with focal spongiform degeneration. Ann Neurol 22:527–532.

Knopman DS (1993): Overview of dementia lacking distinctive histology: Pathological designation of a progressive dementia. Dementia 4:132–136.

Knopman DS, Mastri AR, Frey WH II, Sung JH, Rustan T (1990): Dementia lacking distinctive histologic features: A common non-Alzheimer degenerative dementia. Neurology 40:251–256.

Lendon CL, Shears S, Busfield F, Talbot CJ, Renner J, Morris JC, Goate AM (1994): Molecular genetics of hereditary dysphasic dementia. Neurobiol Aging 15(Suppl 1):S128.

Lynch T, Sano M, Marder KS, Bell KL, Foster NL, Defendini RF, Sima AA, Keohane C, Nygaard TG, Fahn S (1994): Clinical characteristics of a family with chromosome 17-linked disinhibition-dementia-parkinsonism-amyotrophy complex. Neurology 44:1878–1884.

Manetto V, Medori R, Cortelli P, Montagna P, Baruzzi A, Hauw J, Vanderhaegen JJ, Mailleux P (1992): Fatal familial insomnia: Clinical and pathological study of five new cases. Neurology 42:312–319.

Mann DMA, South PW (1993): The topographic distribution of brain atrophy in frontal lobe dementia. Acta Neuropathol 85:334–340.

Mann DMA, South PW, Snowden JS, Neary D (1993): Dementia of frontal lobe type: Neuropathology and immunochemistry. J Neurol Neurosurg Psychiatry 56:605–614.

Masse G, Mikol J, Brion S (1981): Atypical presenile dementia: Report of an anatomo-clinical case and review of the literature. J Neurol Sci 52:245–267.

Mehler MF, Horoupian DS, Davies P, Dickson D (1987): Reduced somatostatin-like immunoreactivity in cerebral cortex in nonfamilial dysphasic dementia. Neurology 37:1448–1453.

Moossy J, Martinez AJ, Hanin I, Rao G, Yonas H, Boller F (1987): Thalamic and subcortical gliosis with dementia. Arch Neurol 44:510–513.

Morita K, Kaiya H, Ikeda T, Namba M (1987): Presenile dementia combined with amyotrophy: A review of 34 Japanese cases. Arch Gerontol Geriatr 6:263–277.

Neary D, Snowden JS (1991): Dementia of the frontal lobe type. In Levin HS, Eisenberg H, Benton AL (eds): Frontal Lobe Function and Dysfunction. New York: Oxford University Press, pp 304–317.

Neary D, Snowden JS, Mann DMA (1993): Familial progressive aphasia: Its relationship to other forms of lobar atrophy. J Neurol Neurosurg Psychiatry 56:1122–1125.

Neary D, Snowden JS, Mann DMA, Northen B, Goulding PJ, Macdermott N (1990): Frontal lobe dementia and motor neuron disease. J Neurol Neurosurg Psychiatry 53:23–32.

Neary D, Snowden JS, Northen B, Goulding P (1988): Dementia of frontal lobe type. J Neurol Neurosurg Psychiatry 51:353–361.

Neumann MA, Cohn R (1967): Progressive subcortical gliosis, a rare form of presenile dementia. Brain 90:405–418.

Peavy GM, Hertzog AG, Rubin NP, Mesulam M-M (1992): Neuropsychological aspects of dementia of motor neuron disease: Report of two cases. Neurology 42:1004–1008.

Petersen RB, Tabaton M, Berg L, Schrank B, Torack RM, Leal S, Julien J, Vital C, Deleplanque B, Pendelburg WW (1992): Analysis of the prion protein gene in thalamic dementia. Neurology 42:1859–1863.

Prusiner SB, Hsiao KK (1994): Human prion diseases. Ann Neurol 35:385–395.

Risse SC, Raskind MA, Nochlin D, Sumi SM, Lampe TH, Bird TD, Cubberley L, Peskind ER (1990): Neuropathological findings in patients with clinical diagnoses of probable Alzheimer's disease. Am J Psychiatry 147:168–172.

Rosen DR, Siddique T, Patterson D, Figlewicz DA, Sapp P, Hentati A, Donaldson D, Goto J, O'Reagan JP, Deng HX (1993): Mutations in Cu/Zn superoxide dismutase gene are associated with familial amyotrophic lateral sclerosis. Nature 362:59–62.

Rosenberg RN (1995): Autosomal dominant cerebellar phenotypes: The genotype has settled the issue. Neurology 45:1–5.

Schenk VWD (1959): Re-examination of a family with Pick's disease. An Hum Genet 23:325–333.

Sima AAF, Defendini R, Keohane C, D'Amato C, Foster NL, Parchi P, Gambetti P, Lynch T, Wilhelmsen KC (1996): The neuropathology of chromosome 17-linked dementia. Ann Neurol 39:734–743.

Snowden JS, Neary D, Mann DMA, Goulding PJ, Testa HJ (1992): Progressive language disorder due to lobar atrophy. Ann Neurol 31:174–183.

Torack RM, Morris JC (1986): Mesolimbic dementia. A clinicopathological case study of a putative disorder. Arch Neurol 43:1074–1078.

Turner RS, Kenyon LC, Trojanowski JQ, Gonatas N, Grossman M (1996): Clinical, neuroimaging and pathologic features of progressive nonfluent aphasia. Ann Neurol 39:166–173.

Verity MA, Roitberg B, Kepes JJ (1990): Mesolimbocortical dementia. Clinicopathological studies on two cases. J Neurol Neurosurg Psychiatry 53:492–495.

Verity MA, Wechsler AF (1987): Progressive subcortical gliosis of Neumann: A clinicopathologic study of two cases with review. Arch Gerontol Geriatr 6:245–261.

Wade JPH, Mirsen TR, Hachinski VC, Fisman M, Lau C, Merskey H (1987): The clinical diagnosis of Alzheimer's disease. Arch Neurol 44:24–29.

Wechsler AF, Verity MA, Rosenschein S, Fried I, Scheibel AB (1982): Pick's disease. A clinical, computed tomographic, and histologic study with Golgi impregnation observations. Arch Neurol 39:287–190.

Wikstrom J, Paetau A, Palo J, Sulkava R, Haltia M (1982): Classic amyotrophic lateral sclerosis with dementia. Arch Neurol 39:681–683.

Yamada T, McGeer PL, McGeer EG (1992): Some immunohistochemical features of argyrophilic grain dementia with normal cortical choline acetyltransferase levels but extensive subcortical pathology and markedly reduced dopamine. J Geriatr Psychiatry Neurol 5:3–13.

Disinhibition-Dementia-Parkinsonism-Amyotrophy Complex in New York and Ireland and Its Relationship to Pick Complex

TIMOTHY LYNCH

Department of Neurology, Columbia University, College of Physicians and Surgeons, New York, NY, 10032

INTRODUCTION

Dementia is defined as a decline in memory and other cognitive functions (such as judgment or abstract thought) (McKhann et al., 1984), associated with impairment in occupational or social functioning (American Psychiatric Association, 1987). Dementia may be caused by more than 60 disorders (Cummings and Benson, 1992), most of which are progressive and have no specific treatment. It is difficult to ascertain the relative frequency of the different dementing disorders, as specific biological markers are lacking and clinical syndromes have been inadequately defined (Schoenberg, 1986; Kokmen et al., 1988; Cummings and Benson, 1992). The three most common causes of dementia are Alzheimer's disease (AD), accounting for 55–60% of dementia (Evans et al., 1989), vascular dementia, accounting for 15–20% (Tatemichi et al., 1992), and frontotemporal dementia (FTD), which may account for 10–15% (Knopman et al., 1990; Brun et al., 1994). Other, less common causes include diffuse Lewy body disease, Parkinson's disease, brain tumors, acquired immunodeficiency syndrome, neurosyphilis, Huntington's disease, and prion disorders (Schoenberg, 1986; Cummings and Benson, 1992).

Recognition of the role of genetics and its contribution to our understanding of dementia has increased significantly in the past decade. A person with AD is 40 times more likely to have two or more first-degree relatives with dementia than is an age-matched, nondemented control (Hofman et al., 1989). A primary research focus in dementia has been familial AD, resulting in the identification of several disease-associated mutations in different chromosomal regions (Goate et al., 1991; St George-Hyslop et al., 1992; Rogaev et al., 1995; Sherrington et al.,

Pick's Disease and Pick Complex, Edited by Andrew Kertesz and David G. Munoz
ISBN 0-471-17792-X ©1998 Wiley-Liss, Inc.

TABLE 14.1   Frontotemporal Dementias (Pick Complex)

Frontotemporal Dementias	Authors
Pick's Disease	Constantinidis et al. (1974), Pick (1892)
Disinhibition-dementia-parkinsonism-amyotrophy (DDPAC)	Lynch et al. (1994a)
Frontal lobe degeneration of non-AD type	Gustafson (1987)
Dementia lacking distinctive histological features	Knopman et al. (1990)
Dementia of frontal lobe type	Neary et al. (1988)
Nonspecific familial presenile dementia	Kim et al. (1981), Brown et al. (1995)
Primary progressive aphasia	Mesulam (1982), Kertesz et al. (1994)
Hereditary dysphasic (disinhibition) dementia	Morris et al. (1984), Lynch et al. (1996)
Focal cortical atrophies (e.g., CBD)	Rebeiz et al. (1968)
Thalamic dementia	Deymeer et al. (1989)
Presenile dementia with MND	Morita et al. (1987), Lynch et al. (1994b)
Progressive subcortical gliosis	Petersen et al. (1995)
Long-duration Creutzfeldt-Jakob disease	Neumann and Cohn (1987)
Rapidly progressive pallido-ponto-nigral degeneration	Wszolek et al. (1992)

Abbreviations: CBD = corticobasal degeneration.

1995). This work has contributed to the understanding of AD. FTD, both less frequent and seemingly more clinically diverse (Table 14.1), has received less attention.

CLASSIFICATION OF FTD

Frontal dementia syndromes have been ascribed many different names, making the classification of FTD confusing (Table 14.1). A consensus statement proposed the following clinico-pathological classification (Brun et al., 1994):

Clinical: Frontotemporal dementia (FTD)
Pathological: Frontotemporal atrophy
Microscopic: Frontal lobe degeneration characterized by spongiform change
             Pick-type characterized by gliosis and Pick bodies
             Motor neuron disease (MND) type characterized by spongiform change

FTD (PICK COMPLEX)

The clinical significance of selective frontal and frontotemporal cortical degeneration was pointed out by Arnold Pick more than one hundred years ago (Pick, 1892). Much confusion has persisted regarding the differences between Pick's lobar atrophy (nonspecific, circumscribed atrophy) and Pick's disease (PiD) (with specific histological features). In the past, dementia of frontal lobe type has been synonymous with PiD and its characteristic pathology. Recently, frontotemporal degenerations have been redefined and separated from PiD (Brun et al., 1994). It has been suggested that many of these frontotemporal dementing disorders comprise the same clinicopathological complex, namely, the Pick complex (Kertesz et al., 1994, 1996). PiD (circumscribed atrophy, neuronal loss, gliosis, and Pick bodies) is a rare dementia; however, the Pick complex, including PiD, appears to be a common cause of dementia. The clinical phenotypes of the disease are summarized in Table 14.1.

In the initial clinical stages, FTD differs from AD due to more marked personality changes, loss of social awareness and judgment, hyperorality, progressive diminution of speech, and relative preservation of spatial orientation and the ability to calculate (Constantinidis et al., 1974; Neary et al., 1988; Brun et al., 1994; Royall et al., 1994; Barber et al., 1995; Levy et al., 1996). Cranial imaging of FTD shows lobar atrophy, single photon emission computed tomography (SPECT) studies reveal decreased frontotemporal cortical glucose perfusion (Neary et al., 1987), and positron emission tomography (PET) studies reveal decreased frontotemporal cortical glucose metabolism (Figure 14.1) (Brun et al., 1994; Lynch et al., 1994b). In contrast, functional imaging in AD reveals posterior cerebral hypoperfusion or hypometabolism. However, in advanced stages, FTD becomes difficult to distinguish from AD due to the severity of the cognitive deficits present in both. In addition, the neuropathological definition of FTD is less clear than that of AD due to the absence of distinctive intracellular or extracellular markers in FTD.

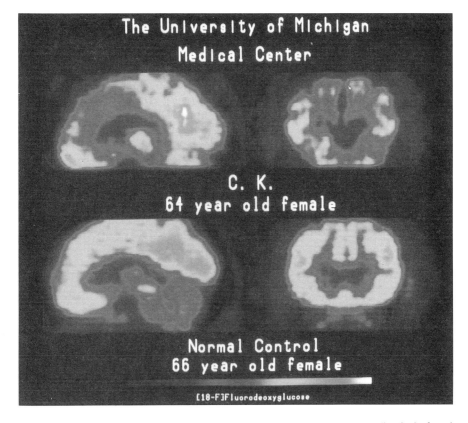

FIGURE 14.1. Positron emission tomography demonstrating decreased glucose metabolism in the frontal lobes and cingulate gyrus (III-35). (Permission to publish this image was kindly given by Norman Foster MD, Department of Neurology, University of Michigan Medical Center.) Figure also appears in color section.

TABLE 14.2 Frequency of FTD in Autopsy Series of Dementia

Authors	No. of Autopsies	No. (%) of FTD	FHx Dementia
Malamud and Waggoner (1943)	NA	16 pedigrees	yes
Tomlinson et al. (1970)	50	5 (10%)	NA
Heston (1978)	85	11 (13%)	63%
Sulkava et al. (1983)	27	2 (7.5%)	NA
Clark et al. (1986)	92	16 (17%)	NA
Gustafson (1987)	158	16 (10%)	50%
Neary et al. (1987)	136	26 (19%)	46%
Joachim et al. (1988)	150	2 (1.5%)	NA
Knopman et al. (1990)	460	28 (6%)	57%
Hulette et al. (1992)	186	9 (4.8%)	NA
Gustafson (1993)	400	36 (9%)	NA

Abbreviations: FTD = frontotemporal dementia; FHx = family history; NA = information not available.

EPIDEMIOLOGY OF FTD

The epidemiology of FTD is incompletely characterized, partially due to past difficulty distinguishing this syndrome from AD. The frequency of FTD ranges from 1.5% to 19% in dementia autopsy series (Table 14.2). Both "dementia lacking distinctive histologic features" and PiD contributed 3% each to all cases of dementia in one series (Table 14.2) (Knopman et al., 1990). However, these two syndromes comprised 17% of the postmortem diagnoses of those patients who died before age 70. PiD has represented as little as 2% to as much as 25% of dementias in other series (Table 14.2), differences that may reflect methodological or geographical factors. The morbidity risk for PiD is estimated as 500 per million for the Swedish population (Sjogren, 1952; Gustafson, 1987). PiD accounts for an estimated 24 per 100,000 deaths in Minnesota compared to 70 per 100,000 for AD in the same area (Heston, 1978). These data suggest that the prevalence of FTD (or Pick complex) may be underestimated.

FAMILIAL INCIDENCE OF FTD

Hereditary disease may occur more frequently in FTD compared to AD (Table 14.2). Dementia was noted among family members in more than 30% of families of index cases with pathologically confirmed PiD (Sjogren, 1952; Heston, 1978). Among 14 families with a member dying with dementia lacking distinctive histological features, 8 had additional family members affected with dementia or MND (Knopman et al., 1990). Reviews of PiD have identified more than 40 families with multiply affected members (Zerbin-Rudin, 1971). One family with "Pick's disease" had more than 25 affected members; however, no Pick bodies were present at autopsy (Sanders et al., 1939; Schenk, 1959; Groen and Endtz, 1982). The trait in this family has since been mapped to chromosome 17q21–22 (Heutink et al., 1997). The likeliest mode of inheritance in these families is autosomal dominant with high penetrance (Table 14.2).

CLINICAL FEATURES OF FAMILIAL FRONTOTEMPORAL DEMENTIA (DISINHIBITION-DEMENTIA-PARKINSONISM-AMYOTROPHY COMPLEX)

We identified an Irish-American family (family Mo) with disinhibition, frontal lobe dementia, parkinsonism, and amyotrophy and named the condition *disinhibition-dementia-parkinsonism-amyotrophy complex (DDPAC)* (Lynch et al., 1994b). DDPAC can be included among the frontotemporal dementias (or Pick complex). It provides an excellent example of a familial frontotemporal dementia and demonstrates the features found in the Pick complex (Wilhelmsen et al., 1991; 1994a, 1994b, 1995, 1996; Lynch et al., 1994a, 1994b; Sima et al., 1994, 1995). We sought to determine (1) whether all affected family members had a common clinical-pathological phenotype and (2) whether the condition was due to a common environmental exposure, the co-occurrence of common neurodegenerative diseases, or inheritance of an autosomal dominant gene mutation. Our hypotheses were that (1) affected family members, dispersed geographically, would have the same clinicopathological characteristics, confirming an autosomal dominant mode of inheritance and (2) genetic linkage analysis in family Mo would identify the chromosomal location of the disease gene (Wilhelmsen et al., 1994a). We also sought to assess whether other familial neurodegenerative conditions with similar clinical-pathological phenotypes may share the same gene locus (allelic) with DDPAC. I will refer to these latter points briefly as they are dealt with in Chapter 18.

We studied the clinical and pathological features of family Mo (Figure 14.2), with 13 members affected by a seemingly diverse set of progressive neurological and psychiatric disorders (Lynch et al., 1994b). Patient III-57 was the subject of a separate case report; he was described as having familial PiD at autopsy (Gaughran et al., 1994). The following case histories illustrate the clinical condition and highlight the intrafamilial diversity found in DDPAC.

DDPAC Case Histories

Proband III-39.   A 41-year-old Irishman presented in 1975 with difficulty walking and an insidious personality change. He had completed 2 years of college education prior to becoming a successful businessman. He neither smoked nor drank alcohol. At age 25, his behavior became erratic; he was noted to be increasingly compulsive and aggressive. His wife complained that "he was sexually inappropriate . . . he acted weird and would stay outside the house for hours sitting in the car." He separated from his wife at age 29 and lived alone thereafter.

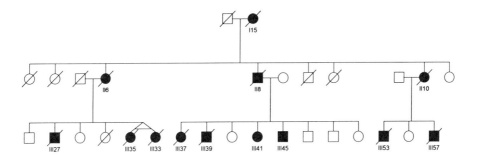

FIGURE 14.2. First three generations of the family Mo (DDPAC) pedigree; all affected individuals are indicated by a blackened symbol.

His family noted that he dressed inappropriately and became shy with strangers, whereas he had always been gregarious. He developed a huge appetite for sweet food and, although an athlete, tended toward obesity.

By age 41 he had developed a festinating gait and fell occasionally. Subsequently, he developed bradykinesia. At age 42, a diagnosis of Parkinson's disease was made and carbidopa/levodopa was commenced, without effect. His speech became soft and slurred. He complained of drooling and had difficulty coughing, clearing his throat, swallowing, and turning in bed. Orthostatic symptoms developed, and he became incontinent. Examination revealed involuntary moaning, slurred speech, and palilalia with tachyphemia. Kayser-Fleischer rings were absent. Eye movements were normal, and glabellar tap, snout, and jaw jerk reflexes were present. Marked facial hypomimia, bradykinesia with moderate rigidity, and difficulty rising from a chair were noted. Gait was shuffling and short-stepped, and the pull test was positive. Reflexes were brisk and plantars flexor. Amantadine was commenced, with minimal effect.

Normal investigations included visual field examination, complete blood count, coagulation screen, electrolytes, serum calcium, liver function tests, thyroid function tests, venereal disease research laboratory (VDRL), serum ceruloplasmin, urinalysis, urine copper, chest and skull x-rays, isotope brain scan, computed tomography (CT) brain scan, cerebrospinal fluid, electrocardiogram, and electroencephalogram.

At age 43 he was mildly demented and had increasing difficulty managing his business. According to his family, he behaved "childishly." He complained of difficulty "catching his breath" and remained awake at night because he believed he needed to take voluntary breaths. Carbon dioxide retention with an altered level of consciousness was documented, and central neurogenic hypoventilation was diagnosed. The nocturnal hypoventilation and hypercapnia were unresponsive to carbidopa/levodopa. A phrenic nerve pacemaker was inserted.

At age 44 he developed acute cholecystitis requiring a cholecystectomy. A deltoid muscle biopsy revealed minor nonspecific abnormalities. At 45, 8 months prior to death, fasciculations developed and an electromyogram confirmed the presence of diffuse denervation and fasciculations. Brisk tendon jerks, ankle clonus, glabellar tap, snout reflex, and bilateral Hoffman's signs were noted. His central respiratory failure progressed, and a tracheotomy was performed. Following prolonged nocturnal cardiorespiratory arrest, he remained in a vegetative state and was ventilated for 7 months, dying at age 43. An autopsy was performed.

Patient III-35. A 54-year-old Irish-American woman, monozygotic twin sister to III-33, with no significant past medical or psychiatric history, developed an insidious personality change and progressive intellectual decline. Her husband noticed that she sometimes became confused about what food to buy in a food store. She received a high school education but, like her twin sister, always performed poorly academically, and both were described as "simple-minded." She worked as a cashier in a department store and retired at age 61. Always quiet-spoken, she became passive and withdrawn, with a marked lack of initiative, by age 59. Memory difficulties ensued, and she lost the ability or interest in cooking or maintaining her personal hygiene.

Examination at age 64 revealed a hypokinetic, quiet woman unable to follow commands. She had no delusions, hallucinations, or illusions. She had little spontaneous speech but responded when questioned. Her speech was slurred and monotonous, and she was unable to name body parts, tell the time, or orient herself in time and place. She did not know her own address or telephone number. She scored 7 on the modified mini-mental state (mMMS) score, 21 on the short blessed test, and 55 on the Wechsler Memory Scale score. The Wechsler Adult Intelligence Scale-Revised (WAIS-R) scored 54 full scale, with a 54 verbal IQ and a 59 performance IQ. Boston naming scored 2 out of 60, 0 on verbal fluency, 2 out 10 words in selective reminding, 8 on the self-rating Hamilton score, and 4 on the Hachinski score. Proverb interpretation and similarities were impaired (e.g., the orange-apple comparison elicited "both are good"). The patient's tone was increased symmetrically, but no tremor was seen. Carbidopa/ levodopa was commenced, with little effect. Higher doses induced vomiting. Reflexes were brisk, including the jaw jerk. Normal investigations included VDRL, fluorescent treponema antibody (FTA), serum protein electrophoresis (SPEP), an erythrocyte sediment rate of 15, and an electroencephalogram.

Six months later, the patient required supervision while eating, dressing, bathing, grooming, and toileting. Her Schwab and England activities of daily living scale was 40%. Examination revealed poor pursuit eye movements with overshoot dysmetria on saccades, intact vertical gaze, a "vacant look," a masked facies, a blink rate of four per minute, mild bradykinesia, poor arm swing when walking, and a slightly flexed posture. Her balance was intact. No tremor was noted. Her weight increased, and she became incontinent. Insidious progression of the dementia resulted in admission to a nursing home facility.

At age 65 the patient was lethargic but rousable and oriented to name only. Speech was slurred and nonfluent and naming was poor, with marked perseveration. She was unable to obey commands or repeat sentences. She was oriented to person and named 1 object out of 10; her digit span was 4 forward and 0 reverse. She was unable to perform serial sevens, spell "world" backward, make change, recall any objects at 5 minutes, name any past presidents, repeat and obey commands, read, write, or copy designs. Extraocular eye movements were full. Marked bradykinesia, cogwheel rigidity, hypometria, and retrocollis were evident. Gait was unsteady, with decreased arm swing and stooped posture. Reflexes were brisk and symmetrical, with prominent snout, glabellar, palmomental, jaw jerk, and flexor plantar responses. At age 64 a deoxyglucose positron emission tomography (PET) scan showed hypometabolism bilaterally in the frontotemporal lobes and cingulate gyrus, with relative sparing of the posterior lobes (Figure 14.1). She died at the age of 65. An autopsy was performed.

Demographic Features and Symptoms of DDPAC

We examined and performed neuropsychological testing on 33 family members. We identified 13 affected family members by history and examined 7 affected family members. We obtained clinical information from available medical records, and from unaffected family members, to determine a diagnosis in the six historically affected members who died prior to the onset of our study (Lynch et al., 1994b). We were unable to obtain sufficient clinical information regarding individual I-15; therefore our data are based on 12 of the 13 affected cases (Tables 14.3 and 14.4; Figure 14.2). The family believe that I-15 died from a dementing-parkinsonian disease. I-15 had six siblings, all of whom migrated to the United States; we traced descendants of one of the siblings, including a nephew of I-15 who was alive at age 103, with late-onset dementia consistent with the diagnosis of AD. All of his children were over 70 years of age and have no personality change, dementia, parkinsonism, or MND.

We estimated the average age at onset of DDPAC to be 45. The full clinical picture developed over 5–10 years, and the average duration of disease was 13 years. Affected family members presented with prodromal psychiatric symptoms including alcoholism in five, depressive symptoms in five, hypersexuality in four, hyperreligiosity in three, shoplifting in two, and restlessness, wandering, and compulsive behaviors in others (Table 14.3). Frank psychosis with auditory hallucinations and paranoid ideation, reminiscent of the positive symptoms of schizophrenia, was seen in others (Lynch et al., 1994b). We noted poor school performance in some, but not all, of the affected members. Divergent initial diagnoses included "catatonic schizophrenia" (III-27), depression, alcoholism, and Korsakoff's psychosis (III-57). In-patient psychiatric care was required in three.

Table 14.3 Symptoms Found in DDPAC

Pedigree ID	Onset (yr)	Disease Duration	Autopsy	First Symptom	Early Wt Gain (Sweets)	Alcohol Abuse	Depression	Other Symptoms	Late Mutism
I-15	N/A	N/A	No	N/A	N/A	N/A	N/A	N/A	N/A
II-6	48	16	No	PC	Yes	No	N/A	N/A	N/A
II-8	53	10	No	PC	Yes	No	N/A	Shy, apathy, repetitive, roaming	Yes
II-10	56	13	No	PC	Yes	No	No	Poor planning & organization, crude, apathy	Yes
III-27	27	8	Yes[1]	PC	N/A	No	Yes	"Catatonic schizophrenia"	Yes
III-33	52	13	Yes	PC	Yes	Yes	Yes	S/lifter, somnolent	Yes
III-35	54	12	Yes	PC	Yes	No	No	Apathy, slovenly, h/religious, somnolent	Yes
III-37	52	8	Yes	PC	Yes	No	No	Mouthing objects, roaming, "childish"	Yes
III-39	25	18	Yes	PC/PD	Yes	No	No	Sexually aggressive, "childish"	Yes
III-41	46	>15	Alive	PC	Yes	Yes	Yes	Anxious, compulsive, h/religious	Yes
III-45	45	>11	Alive	PC	Yes	Yes	Yes	Initially hypersexual, "childish"	Yes
III-53	30	23	Yes	PC	Yes	Yes	Yes	Restless, agitated, aggressive, "childish," s/lifter	Yes
III-57	35	20	Yes	PC	Yes	Yes	Yes	Aggressive, "childish," "Korsakoff's"	Yes

N/A = not available; S/lifter = shoplifter: H/religious = hyperreligious.
[1]Autopsy material not available.

TABLE 14.4 Neurological Signs Found in DDPAC

Pedigree ID	Frontal Signs	Postural Instability	Brady	Rigidity	L-dopa Response	Eye Move	Late Dysphagia	Pyram signs	Fascicul	Other	CT/MRI Atrophy	rCBF/PET Hypoactivity
I-15	N/A	N/A	N/A	N/A	N/A	N/A	N/A	N/A	N/A	N/A	N/A	N/A
II-6	N/A	Yes	Yes	Yes	N/A	N/A	Yes	N/A	N/A	"Beri-beri"	N/A	N/A
II-8	N/A	Yes	Yes	Yes	N/A	N/A	Yes	N/A	N/A	N/A	N/A	N/A
II-10	N/A	Yes	Yes	Yes	N/A	N/A	Yes	N/A	N/A	N/A	N/A	N/A
III-27	N/A	N/A	N/A	N/A	N/A	N/A	N/A	N/A	N/A	Neuroleptic hypo	N/A	N/A
III-33	Yes	Yes	Yes	Yes	No	Slow sacc	Yes	No	No	Anosmia	Yes	N/A
III-35	Yes	Yes	Yes	Yes	No	Slow sacc	Yes	Yes	No	Retrocollis	Yes	Frontotemp/limbic
III-37	Yes	Yes	Yes	Yes	Halluc	Norm	Yes	No	No	N/A	Yes	Frontotemp
III-39	Yes	Yes	Yes	Yes	No	Norm	Yes	Yes	Yes	Ondine's curse	Yes	N/A
III-41	Yes	Yes	Yes	Yes	No	Sq wave	Yes	Yes	No	Syndactyl, echolalia	Yes	Frontotemp
III-45	Yes	Yes	Yes	Yes	No	Eye apraxia	Yes	Yes	No	Myoclonus, echolalia	N/A	N/A
III-53	Yes	Yes	Yes	Yes	No	Slow sacc	Yes	Yes	No	Tongue rolling, seiz	Yes	N/A
III-57	N/A	Yes	Yes	Yes	No	Norm	Yes	No	No	Neuroleptic hypo	N/A	N/A

N/A = not available; Norm = normal; Sq wave = square wave jerks present with eye fixation; Sacc = saccades; Seiz = seizure; Halluc = hallucinations; Frontotemp = frontotemporal; limbic = limbic lobe; Hypo = neuroleptic-induced hypotension; Eye apraxia = eyelid-opening apraxia.

An insidious personality change developed in all affected family members following the prodromal symptoms; this was often dismissed by family members for several years. A variety of early clinical features were noted, including disinhibition in 13; hyperphagia in 11; wandering or persistent pacing and a stereotyped, ritualized, compulsive daily routine in 3; and aggressive behavior in 2. All affected family members had two or more symptoms associated with the human Kluver-Bucy syndrome (Kluver and Bucy, 1939; Cummings and Duchen, 1981). Eleven had increased appetite and weight gain, with a particular craving for sweets. One (III-33) regularly ate food from the garbage can, while others tended to "cram food into [their mouths] in such a manner as to be at risk from choking." There was a progression from childish, disinhibited behavior to a withdrawn, abulic state with emotional blunting in all. Patient III-53 was arrested for shoplifting, and III-39 and II-52 both developed severe hypotension following administration of a neuroleptic.

Neuropsychologic assessment revealed early memory loss, poor general knowledge, and poor constructions (perseverative), with preservation of orientation, praxis, language, and calculation until late in the disease course. Early difficulty with retrieval naming (e.g., "name as many animals as you can in one minute") was noted. Inappropriate behavior, lack of regard for normal social interactions, and unconcern about poor test performance were noted during testing. Adynamic speech, echolalia, and perseverations progressing to mutism were noted in serial testing of some affected members (III-37, III-41, III-45). The neurobehavioral pattern was consistent with a frontal lobe dementia (Lynch et al., 1994b).

Physical Signs in DDPAC

We found axial, truncal, and limb rigidity, bradykinesia, postural instability, dementia, and, terminally, an akinetic mute state in all affected family members examined (Table 14.4). All seven affecteds examined had postural instability and frontal lobe release signs (palmomental, grasp reflex), and one had retrocollis (Table 14.4). Clinical amyotrophy with weakness, wasting, fasciculations, ankle clonus, and bilateral Hoffman's signs developed in the late stages of the disease in III-39. Hyperreflexia was observed in III-35, III-41, and III-53, and Hoffman and Babinski signs were present in III-53 and III-41, without wasting or fasciculations. Poor saccadic eye movements were observed in three, but ocular movements were full in all. We noted square wave jerks late in the disease course in III-41. Patient III-45 developed apraxia of eyelid opening and stimulus-sensitive cortical myoclonus (Table 14.4). Eleven affecteds became mute, incontinent, and cachectic in the terminal stages; III-45 has yet to reach this stage in the disease (Table 14.4). Seizures occurred rarely (III-41, III-53), and none had a significant response to levodopa (Table 14.4). One (III-39) had a short-lived, inadequate response to dopa agonists. In summary, all affected family members developed disinhibition, dementia, and parkinsonism, and one (III-39) developed central hypoventilation and amyotrophy (Lynch et al., 1994b).

INVESTIGATIONS IN DDPAC

Routine laboratory tests including complete blood count, serum electrolytes, serum calcium, phosphate, and magnesium, serum and urine copper, ceruloplasmin, vitamin B_{12}, folate, VDRL, and lysosomal enzyme assay were normal in all.

Electrophysiology

Electromyography demonstrated diffuse denervation in one affected member (III-39) corresponding to the diffuse clinical fasciculations and wasting; two others (III-35 and III-41) had normal studies. Nerve conduction studies were normal in all three. Electroencephalography revealed normal recordings in six and a nonspecific, dysrhythmic pattern in one.

Radiology

Computed tomography or magnetic resonance imaging in five affected family members revealed ventricular dilation with prominent cortical sulci and moderate to severe atrophy, involving primarily the frontal lobes in III-37. Isotope brain scans were normal in III-39 and III-53. Regional cerebral blood flow revealed hypoactivity in the frontal lobes bilaterally in two, with the later development of frontoparietal lobe hypoactivity in one (Table 14.4). Fluorodeoxyglucose positron emission tomography in one (III-35) revealed hypometabolism in the frontotemporal lobes and cingulate gyrus bilaterally (Figure 14.1).

PATHOLOGY IN DDPAC

The mean duration to death was 13 years, and the range was 5 to 23 years (Table 14.3). Neuropathology was available on six affected patients who had been studied and examined in life (III-33, III-35, III-37, III-39, III-53, III-57). We studied postmortem brain and brainstem tissue from these six individuals; only three spinal cords were available for examination (III-33, III-37, III-39). Varying pathological diagnoses were made for the six patients who came to autopsy, reflecting the worldwide dispersion of family Mo and resulting in some delay in the identification of the syndrome as familial. A consensus meeting among the three neuropathologists involved determined that there was a common pathologic phenotype (Sima et al., 1996).

Gross Brain Specimens

All six affected family members showed moderate to severe basal ganglia, as well as frontal and temporal lobe atrophy; asymmetrical atrophy was not noted. The severity of gyral atrophy varied among family members and was evident in anterior and inferior regions of the temporal lobes, the prefrontal regions, and the anterior cingulate (Figure 14.3). Brain weights varied from 970 to 1350 g. The substantia nigra was depigmented in all. The cerebral white matter and cerebellum were normal.

Microscopic Pathological Changes

Microscopic changes were uniform in their distribution, but their severity varied. Changes consisted of circumscribed neuronal loss, gliosis and laminar spongiosis of the limbic neocortical areas, and frontal, temporal, and occipital association areas. The most severely affected areas were, in descending order, the prepiriform, anterior temporal, entorhinal, visual association (area 18), anterior cingulate, prefrontal, and insular regions. The superficial neocortical laminae showed modest neuronal attrition and patchy astrocytosis. Generally, the astrogliosis appeared to exceed the severity of neuronal loss. In the most severely affected cortical areas, neuronal loss and gliosis were seen throughout the thickness of the cortex, and the underlying white matter showed axonal loss, myelin pallor, and mild astrogliosis, with sparing of the U fibers. There was a sharp demarcation between severely affected cortices and seemingly normal cortex. In five family members, there was a striking spongy rarefaction of the neuropil confined to the inner border of the plexiform layer and the second cortical layer, with reduction in the small pyramidal cells. In III-53 the spongiform change was more extensive in the temporal and frontal cortex. Ballooned neurons were infrequently seen in two (III-35 and III-53) (Figure

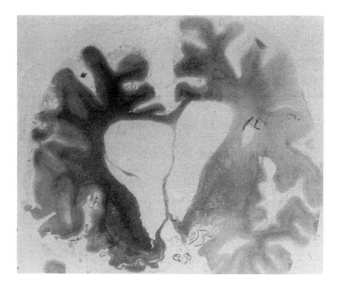

FIGURE 14.3. Neuropathological coronal section (III-53) demonstrating severe temporal and frontal atrophy. (Permission to publish this image was kindly given by K. Keohane FRCPath, Department of Neuropathology, Cork University Hospital, Cork, Ireland.) Figure also appears in color section.

14.4), and very rare Pick bodies were seen in one (III-53) but were not confirmed by ultrastructural studies. Spheroids were also present. Virtually no large multipolar nerve cells remained in the second layer of the entorhinal cortex. Pyramidal cell loss was substantial in the broad third layer, especially in its outer half. No abnormalities were detected in the pre- or parasubicular sectors of the parahippocampal periallocortex. The nerve cells of the hippocampal formation (CA1 to CA3) appeared normal, but a marked cortical deafferentiation of the formation was evident along a shrunken, rarefied, and gliotic perforant pathway, most striking in the molecular layer of the dentate gyrus (Figure 14.5). The endfolium showed a proliferation of astrocytes, with frequent hypertrophy of the cell bodies (Sima et al., 1996). The changes in the prefrontal cortex and the deafferentiation of the hippocampus formation probably account for the frontal lobe release signs and profound dementia seen in DDPAC.

Subcortical Structures

The subcortical structures affected included the amygdala, substantia nigra, ventral globus pallidus, periaqueductal gray, ventral hypothalamus, and caudate nucleus. The rostral and ventral parts of the caudate nucleus, nucleus accumbens, putamen, medial pallidum, and claustrum were most severely affected, whereas the caudal and dorsal parts of the basal ganglia appeared virtually normal. The pigmented and nonpigmented cell populations of the substantia nigra were decimated in all (Figure 14.6), correlating with the severe parkinsonism found in DDPAC. Nerve cell loss and astrocytosis in the amygdala were severe. The severe involvement of the anterior temporal cortices and both amygdala may correlate with the hyperorality and altered sexual behavior found in DDPAC, which is reminiscent of that found in the Kluver-Bucy syndrome (Kluver and Bucy, 1939; Cummings and Duchen, 1981). The locus ceruleus, by contrast, was only slightly affected. Other subcortical structures including the red nucleus, pontine

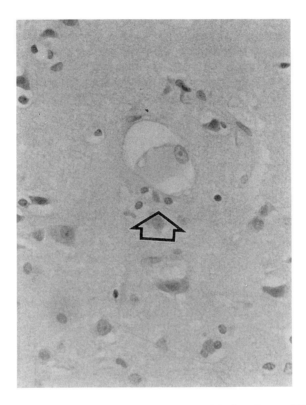

FIGURE 14.4. Ballooned neuron (arrow) seen in the third layer of the frontal cortex (H&E stain). (Permission by R. DeFendini M.D., Department of Neuropathology, Columbia-Presbyterian Medical Center, New York). Figure also appears in color section.

nuclei, thalamic nuclei, and substantia innominata were only minimally involved (Sima et al., 1996). Mild neuronal loss was found in the inferior olivary nucleus and dorsal vague nucleus. The cerebellar nuclei and cortex were normal. Two individuals (III-33 and III-39), including one with muscle fasciculations, had spinal anterior horn cell loss and fibrillary astrocytosis; these findings varied with regard to level and side in the cord (Figure 14.7).

Neuronal and Glial Cytoplasmic Inclusions

Argyrophilic neuronal cytoplasmic inclusions, with abnormal filaments, were noted in brainstem nuclei (third nerve nucleus, dorsal raphe nucleus), ventral hypothalamus, subthalamic nucleus, periaqueductal gray, pars compacta of the substantia nigra, red nucleus, and globus pallidus. The inclusions stained with Bielschowsky's silver impregnation and were composed of haphazardly arranged spicules. Oligodendroglial argyrophilic tangle-like inclusions were widespread in white matter structures. These stained positive for ubiquitin and tau but negative for beta-amyloid, phosphorylated neurofilament, and glial fibrillary acidic protein. These inclusions were similar to those found in multiple system atrophy (MSA) (Papp et al., 1989),

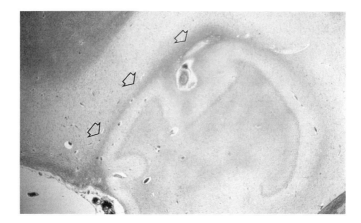

FIGURE 14.5. Deafferentiation of the hippocampus from the entorhinal cortex, as judged by a severely gliotic perforant pathway (arrows) (PTH stain). (Permission by A.A.F. Sima M.D., PR.D., Department of Pathology and Neurology, Wayne State University and Detroit Medical Center). Figure also appears in color section.

confirming that glial cytoplasmic inclusions are neither specific nor pathognomonic for MSA (Lynch and Sima, 1996). The subcortical neuronal inclusions stained positive for phosphorylated neurofilament and ubiquitin and negative for beta-amyloid and tau, consistent with non-AD tangles. Ballooned neurons stained positive for phosphorylated neurofilaments and variably positive for ubiquitin and tau. In areas of neuronal loss and gliosis, numerous ubiquitin-positive granules and spheroids were seen. Lewy bodies, neurofibrillary tangles (NFTs), or neuritic plaques of the AD type were present in insignificant numbers (Sima et al.,

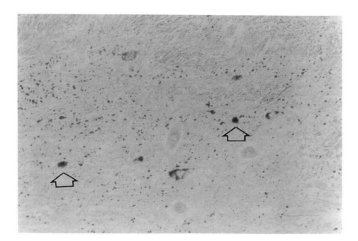

FIGURE 14.6. Neuronal loss with extracellular pigment (arrows) in the substantia nigra (Bielschowsky stain). (Permission by A.A.F. Sima M.D., PR.D., Department of Pathology and Neurology, Wayne State University and Detroit Medical Center). Figure also appears in color section.

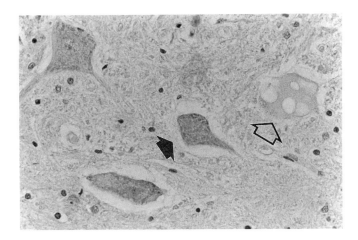

FIGURE 14.7. Abnormal shrunken cervical anterior horn cells (closed arrow) with vacuolation in another anterior horn cell (open arrow) (H&E stain). (Permission by R. DeFendini M.D., Department of Neuropathology, Columbia-Presbyterian Medical Center, New York). Figure also appears in color section.

1996). Western blot analysis of brain extracts from the cerebellum of member III-35 was negative for protease-resistant PrP. No immunoreactive deposits of PrP were detected in any of the sections. Intraneuronal inclusions were identified by ultrastructural study in three brains and consisted of 10- to 14-nm filaments showing a three-dimensional lattice-like arrangement with variable periodicity. The distribution of these neuronal intracytoplasmic inclusions was similar to the tangle distribution found in progressive supranuclear palsy (PSP), although they differed from the straight tubular structures found in PSP.

GENETIC STUDIES IN DDPAC

Chapter 18 describes the genetic studies in family Mo; therefore, I will only comment briefly on the significance of the genetics in DDPAC. The benefits of molecular genetics include the ability (1) to identify genes not detected by biochemical analysis; (2) to characterize etiological relationships between clinical diseases; (3) to provide presymptomatic testing; and (4) to develop a foundation for genetic therapy. We identified 13 affected individuals from the pedigree (Figure 14.2, Tables 14.3 and 14.4). There were seven affected women and six affected men, with a female:male ratio of 2:1 in the second generation, and 4:5 in the third generation. Female-to-female transmission and female-to-male transmission were seen four times. Male-to-male transmission occurred twice. By age 50, 10 of 21 children of affected parents had symptoms, a pattern consistent with a highly penetrant autosomal dominant condition. We mapped DDPAC to chromosome 17q21–22 within a 12-cM (sex-averaged) region between D17S800 and D17S787 (Lynch et al., 1994b; Wilhelmsen et al., 1994a). Two-point lod scores were calculated for all markers using Ilink (form LINKAGE programs, version 5.05) (Lathrop et al., 1985). Lod scores consistent with linkage were obtained for microsatellite polymorphisms associated with the HOX2B (Lod_{max} 3.03 with $Lod_{max} = 0$) and GP3A (Lod_{max} 3.28 with $Lod_{Max} = 0$) loci on chromosome 17q21–23 (Wilhelmsen et al., 1994a). A lod score greater than 3 is considered proof that a marker and a trait are linked (Morton, 1955). The maximum multipoint lod score was 4.2, and the support interval was 10.9 cM (sex-averaged) (Wilhelmsen et al., 1994a). All affected individuals have inherited the same haplotype for markers across the interval.

SIMILAR NEURODEGENERATIVE CONDITIONS

Idiopathic Parkinson's Disease, PSP, and Familial AD

These diseases differ from DDPAC (clinical presentation, the absence of Lewy bodies, amyloid plaques or NFTs). However, NFTs similar to those found in AD were shown in a chromosome 17-linked family with presenile dementia and psychosis (Sumi et al., 1992; Bird et al., 1997). DDPAC differs clinically and pathologically from PSP (Steele et al., 1964; de Yebenes et al., 1995). However, familial multiple-system tauopathy with presenile dementia, another chromosome 17-linked disorder, shares many clinical and pathological features with PSP (Spillantini et al., 1997). It remains unclear how helpful NFTs are in making clear diagnoses in the realm of neurodegenerative disease. Indeed, the existing clinicopathological classification of many neurodegenerative disorders may need to be revised following the identification of the DDPAC disease gene.

Frontal Lobe Dementia, Parkinsonism, and Amyotrophy

Some forms of these disorders share many clinical features with DDPAC (Sanders et al., 1939; Schenk, 1959, Haberlandt, 1964; Neumann and Cohn, 1967; Schaumburg and Suzuki, 1968; Staal and Went, 1968; Hughes et al., 1973; Pinsky et al., 1975; Bonduelle, 1976; Ball, 1980; Burnstein, 1981; Hudson, 1981; Kim et al., 1981; Groen and Endtz, 1982; Mata et al., 1983; Horoupian et al., 1984; Morris et al., 1984; Schmitt et al., 1984; Clark et al., 1986; Dickson et al., 1986; Brun, 1987; Constantinidis, 1987; Gustafson, 1987, 1993; Morita et al., 1987; Gilbert et al., 1988; Mann et al., 1988; Neary et al., 1988; Deymeer et al., 1989; Rosenberg et al., 1989; Hsiao and Prusiner, 1990; Knopman et al., 1990; Neary et al., 1990; Gunnarsson et al., 1991; Miller et al., 1991; Caselli et al., 1992, 1993; Hulette and Crain, 1992; Sumi et al., 1992; Woods and McKee, 1992; Miller et al., 1995; Mitsuyama, 1993; Brun et al., 1994; Kertesz et al., 1994; Brown et al., 1995; Denson and Wszolek, 1995). The personality change and dementia are similar to those in PiD and other forms of frontal lobe dementia (Brun et al., 1994). Although many of the clinical characteristics of PiD are found in all affected DDPAC family members, the strict pathological criteria (presence of Pick bodies) are not met (Mendez et al., 1993). DDPAC shares many similarities and overlap with lobar atrophies (Mann et al., 1988; Caselli et al., 1992; Neary et al., 1993; Kertesz et al., 1994), hereditary dysphasic dementia (Morris et al., 1984), pallido-ponto-nigral degeneration (Wszolek et al., 1992), progressive subcortical gliosis (Neumann and Cohn, 1967; Lanska et al., 1994; Petersen et al., 1995), and corticobasal degeneration (CBD) (Rebeiz et al., 1968; Mori et al., 1994). CBD differs with its sporadic occurrence, later age at onset, rapid course, and asymmetrical involvement of the parietal lobe.

Rare descriptions of sporadic (Froment, 1925; Decourt et al., 1934; Roger and Cain, 1947; Cordier, 1951; Greenfield and Mattews, 1954; Legrand et al., 1959; Brait et al., 1973; Gilbert et al., 1988) and familial parkinsonism-amyotrophic lateral sclerosis (ALS) (Van Bogaert and Radermecker, 1954; Brait et al., 1973; Alter and Schaumann, 1976) do not match the pathology in this kindred. Of note, Roy et al. (1988) described an Irish family with autosomal dominant parkinsonism, depression, weight loss, and central hypoventilation similar to those found in III-39. However, the neuropathology in that and other similar kindreds (Perry et al., 1975; Purdy et al., 1979) differed from DDPAC, and linkage studies have not been performed on these pedigrees. The dementia-parkinsonism-ALS complex of Guam is clinically similar to DDPAC but differs pathologically (Table 14.5) (Hirano et al., 1961a, 1961b). However, the DDPAC locus remains a strong candidate locus for the Guamanian disease, and a study addressing the inheritance pattern of the disease with an accompanying linkage study remains to be done.

There are other sporadic (Myrianthopoulos and Smith, 1962; Boudouresques et al., 1967; Hudson, 1981; Delisle et al., 1987; Morita et al., 1987; Gilbert et al., 1988) and familial forms (Haberlandt, 1964; Caidas et al., 1966; Bonduelle, 1976; Burnstein, 1981; Horoupian et al., 1984; Schmitt et al., 1984; Delisle et al., 1987; Gilbert et al., 1988; Neary et al., 1990) of dementia-parkinsonism-ALS with varying pathology; some closely match the clinical and pathological findings in DDPAC; some may be the same disease. No consistent name has been assigned to these familial conditions, probably reflecting the confusion associated with intrafamilial phenotypic heterogeneity and the limitations of clinicopathological analysis in syndromes with overlapping features of common neurodegenerative diseases. The identification of a disease gene responsible for DDPAC may allow these conditions, and other similar familial neurodegenerative diseases, to be tested to determine whether they are the same or distinct disorders. This may help resolve the taxonomic difficulties in classifying neurodegenerative diseases.

Linkage Studies in other FTD Families

Validation of the importance of this chromosomal region in FTD has come from subsequent studies in which additional families with autosomal dominant, highly penetrant FTD and parkinsonism have been linked to the same chromosomal region (Tables 14.5 and 14.6) (Foster et al., 1997). These familial disorders have been named under different guises, including *pallido-ponto-nigral degeneration* (Wilker et al., 1996), *progressive subcortical gliosis* (Petersen et al., 1995), *hereditary-dysphasic-disinhibition-dementia* (Lendon et al., 1996; and Lendon et al., in press; Lynch et al., 1996), *hereditary frontotemporal dementia* (Heutink et al., 1997), *FTD family from Duke* (Yamaoka et al., 1996), *familial presenile dementia with psychosis associated with cortical neurofibrillary tangles and degeneration of the amygdala* (Sumi et al., 1992; Bird et al., 1997), *familial multiple system tauopathy with presenile dementia* (Spillantini et al., 1996, 1997; Murrell et al., 1997), *chromosome 17-linked rapidly progressive familial FTD* (Basun et al., 1997) and *FTD family from Australia* (Tables 14.5 and 14.6) (Dark et al., 1997; Baker et al., 1997).

Rapidly progressive autosomal dominant parkinsonism-dementia with pallido-ponto-nigral degeneration began in the fifth decade; 32 affected individuals had a neurodegenerative disease similar, but not identical, to that of the DDPAC family (Tables 14.5 and 14.6). DDPAC differed with regard to the later development of parkinsonism, the amyotrophy, the absence of abnormal ocular motility, and the presence of motor neuron pathology (Table 14.6). The PPND trait showed linkage to the same locus on chromosome 17q21 (Wilker et al., 1996); the gene was localized to the 10-cM region between D17S250 and D17S943 (Tables 14.5 and 14.6) (Wilker et al., 1996).

Progressive subcortical gliosis (PSG) described in two families. It was very similar to DDPAC except that the degree of white matter astrocytosis in PSG far outweighed that seen in DDPAC and there was no sharp demarcation between affected and unaffected cortices (Tables 14.5 and 14.6) (Lanska et al., 1994). In collaboration with Petersen, Gambetti, and Lanska, we studied one of the PSG families for the segregation pattern of markers from chromosome 17q21–22. Data were consistent with linkage of this trait to chromosome 17q21–22 (Petersen et al., 1995).

Hereditary dysphasic disinhibition dementia (HDDD) presented with insidious personali-

TABLE 14.5 Neuropathology of Kindreds with FTD Linked to Chromosome 17

			Definite Linkage								Probable Linkage			
	DDPAC	PPND	HDDD	HFTD Family 1	Aust Family	Duke 1684 Family	FMST	Seattle Family A	PSG Family A	Karolinska Family	HFTD Family 2	HFTD Family 3	Seattle Family B
Macroscopic													
Number of patients	6	10	4	5	4	3	9	5	5	3	5	1	4
Brain weight (grams)	870–1350	N/A	740–1340	855–1230	N/A	990	N/A	870–1210	850–1040	935–1440	730–1250	1170	N/A
Asymmetric atrophy	0	0	0	+	N/A	0	0	0	0	+	2/5	0	+
Distribution of atrophy	F-T	F-T	F-T-P	F-T	F-T	F-T-P-O	F-T	F-T-P	F-T	F-T-P	F-T	F-T	F-T
Basal ganglia atrophy	+	+	+	+	N/A	+	+	0	+	+	+	+	+
SN depigmentation	+++	+	+	4/14	1/4	+	+	0	+++	+/–	++	+	+
Microscopic													
Neuronal loss	+++	+++	+++	+++	+++	+++	+++	+++	++	+++	+++	+++	+++
Gray matter gliosis	++	++	+	+	+	+	++	+	+++	++	++	++	++
Neuronal cyto inclusions	++	+	N/A	0	0	0	+++	+++	+	0	0	0	0
Glial cyto inclusions	++	+	N/A	0	0	0	+++	0	+	0	+	0	0
Ballooned cells	+	+	+	+	+	0	+	0	+	0	+	0	0
Neuropil vacuolation	++	0	+	+	+	+	+	0	++	+	+	+	++
White matter gliosis	++	+	+	++	N/A	+	++	+/–	+++	++	++	0	+
Lewy bodies, AD-like plaques	0	0	0	0	0	0	0	0	0	0	0	0	0

DDPAC = disinhibition-dementia-parkinsonism-amyotrophy complex; PPND = pallido-ponto-nigral-degeneration; HDDD = hereditary dysphasic disinhibition dementia; HFTD = hereditary frontotemporal dementia; Aust = Australian family with autosomal dominant non-Alzheimer's dementia; Duke = Duke family 1684 with FTD; FMST = familial multiple system tauopathy with presenile dementia; Seattle = Seattle family with presenile dementia, psychosis, cortical neurofibrillary tangles, and degeneration of the amygdala; PSG = progressive subcortical gliosis; Cyto = cytoplasmic tau-positive inclusions (neuronal and glial inclusions stained tau and argyrophilic positive); 0 = absent; + = mild; ++ = moderate; +++ = severe; +/– = sometimes present; N/A = not available ; F = frontal lobe; T = temporal lobe; P = parietal lobe; O = occipital lobe; C = cingulate gyrus.

TABLE 14.6 Kindreds with FTD Linked to Chromosome 17

	Definite Linkage								Probable Linkage				
	DDPAC	PPND	HDDD	HFTD Family 1	Aust Family	Duke 1684 Family	Seattle Family A	FMST	PSG Family A	Karolin Family	HFTD Family 2	HFTD Family 3	Seattle Family B
Number of patients	13	35	21	49	26	16	18	41	17	6	34	30	7
Mean age at onset (yr)	45	43	63	51	N/A	55	51.4	49	47	51	46.5	63.4	54.7
(range, yr)	(25–56)	(32–58)	(48–75)	N/A	(39–64)	(45–63)	(+/−7.4)	(39–55)	(41–58)	(42–55)	(+/−3.5)	(57–75)	(+/−7.5)
Duration (yr)	13	9	7	8	N/A	9.2	13.8	10.6	11	3	8.3	N/A	10
(Range, yr)	(5–23)	(2–17)	(4–17)	(4–16)	(4–14)	(6–13)	(+/−7.8)	(1–22)	(7–17)	(2–4)	(+/−2.7)	N/A	(+/−5.2)
Presenting SX													
Personality change	12	10	0	49	+	++	+++	++	++	++	++	+++	+++
Psychosis	+	0	0	++	0	0	+++	0	+	0	+	+	+
Dementia	0	5	6 of 9	++	+	++	+	+	+	0	++	+	+
Parkinsonism	1	14	+	+	+	+	0	0	+	+	0	0	+
Aphasia	0	0	3 of 9	0	0	0	0	0	+	++	0	0	++
Later Features													
Dementia	13	26	18	49	++	+++	+++	+++	+++	+++	+++	+++	+++
S/nuclear gaze	0	15	0	0	0	0	0	0	0	0	0	0	0
Parkinsonism	11	25	++	10	++	++	+	++	+++	++	++	++	++
Pyramidal signs	3	16	+	7	+	+	+	++	++	+	+	+	+
ALS	1	0	0	0	0	0	0	0	0	0	0	0	0
Aphasia/mutism	+++	+++	19 of 21	+++	++	++	++	+++	+++	+++	+++	+++	+++
Lod score (affecteds only)	>3	6.8	3.7	>3	>3	>5	>3	>3	1.6	2.7	1.6	2.6	1.1

DDPAC = disinhibition-dementia-parkinsonism-amyotrophy complex; PPND = rapidly progressive autosomal dominant parkinsonism and dementia with pallido-ponto-nigral-degeneration; HDDD = hereditary dysphasic disinhibition dementia; HFTD = hereditary FTD in Dutch families; Aust = Australian family with autosomal dominant non-AD dementia; Duke = Duke family 1684 with FTD; FMST = familial multiple system tauopathy with presenile dementia; Seattle = Seattle family with presenile dementia, psychosis, cortical neurofibrillary tangles, and degeneration of the amygdala; PSG = progressive subcortical gliosis; Karolin = Karolinska FTD family; yr = years; Sx = symptoms; 0 = absent; + = mild; ++ = moderate; +++ = severe; N/A = not available. S/nuclear = supranuclear gaze palsy; parkinsonism = rigidity, bradykinesia, postural instability, *no* tremor, levodopa unresponsive.

ty change, alcohol abuse, hyperphagia, dysphasia, dementia and parkinsonism with focal cerebral atrophy, cortical spongiform change and degeneration of substantia nigra, but lacking definitive AD pathology, Pick inclusions, or prion protein on immunostaining (Tables 14.5 and 14.6). HDDD differed from DDPAC in that it occurred at an older age, presented with aphasia, and was notable for argyrophilic senile plaques and hippocampal involvement (Table 14.5). HDDD showed linkage (lod score 3.68) to 17q21–22 (Lendon et al., 1996; Lynch et al., 1996; and Lendon et al., in press).

Other hereditary FTD families showing linkage to 17q21–22 include three Dutch hereditary FTD families (HFTD) (Heutink et al., 1997). One of these families had previously been described as having hereditary PiD without Pick bodies (Sanders et al., 1939; Schenk, 1959; Groen and Endtz, 1982). The clinical and pathological features were similar to those in DDPAC (Tables 14.5 and 14.6). An Australian non-AD dementia family with features similar to those of DDPAC showed linkage to 17q21–22 (Baker et al., 1997; Dark et al., 1997). An FTD family (Duke family 1684), very similar to the DDPAC family, showed linkage to 17q21–22 (Yamaoka et al., 1996). A family with presenile dementia with psychosis associated with cortical NFTs (Seattle family A) showed linkage to 17q21–22 (Sumi et al., 1992; Bird et al., 1997); it has some similarities with DDPAC, with marked psychosis (schizophrenia-like), auditory hallucinations, paranoia, and bizarre behavior, but differed due to the presence of AD-like NFTs and the absence of ballooned neurons or substantia nigra involvement (Tables 14.5 and 14.6). Familial multiple system tauopathy with presenile dementia (FMST) showed linkage to 17q21–22 (Spillantini et al., 1996, 1997; Murrell et al., 1997). FMST differed from DDPAC by disequilibrium at onset, supranuclear gaze palsy, and widespread tau-positive glial and neuronal inclusions and twisted NFTs, but was similar with amyotrophy in two. A Swedish FTD family (Karolinska family) showed linkage to 17q21–22; it was very similar to DDPAC but differed due to later age at onset and shorter duration (Tables 14.5 and 14.6) (Basun et al., 1997; Foster et al., 1997; Froelich et al., in press).

In summary, the chromosome 17-linked dementias are highly penetrant, autosomal dominant, progressive neurodegenerative disorders presenting between the ages of 25 and 75 and resulting in an insidious personality change, apathy, stereotypic compulsive behavior, psychosis, hyperphagia, mutism, dementia, and parkinsonism in surprisingly varying combinations and severity (Table 14.6) (Foster et al., 1997). The duration of the illness varies from approximately 1 year to 25 years. Most patients show focal cerebral atrophy, cortical spongiform change, gliosis, and degeneration of the substantia nigra, but all lack definitive AD pathology, Lewy bodies, or Pick bodies (Table 14.5). Distinctive pathological features are absent in most cases, although some families show profound tau pathology, as evidenced by argentophilic- and tau-staining neuronal and glial inclusions. The significant differences in clinical and pathological phenotypes between families have resulted in delayed recognition of their biological relationship; this intrafamilial phenotypic variation (phenotypic heterogeneity) confirms that a common genotype can lead to variable phenotype, possibly via the interaction of other genes, environmental influences, and epigenetic phenomena. Indeed, the monozygotic twins III-33 and III-35 (Figure 14.2) developed the disease at different ages and died 3 years apart (Table 14.3). An NIH-funded consensus meeting was convened to determine the common features among these frontotemporal dementia parkinsonism-linked to chromosome 17 families (Tables 14.5 and 14.6) (Foster et al., 1997). Although showing linkage to a common locus does not necessarily indicate that these families suffer from the same genetic disease, it does point to an important role for this chromosomal region in dementia. The disorders may result from a common mutation at the same gene, from different mutations at the same gene, or from mutations at different genes at the same locus. It is likely that different mutations in a single gene are responsible for these varied clinical phenotypes, and it is also likely that the gene mutations are gain-of-function mutations resulting in a novel function for the gene product.

GENETIC HETEROGENEITY IN FAMILIAL FTD

Genetic heterogeneity, present in familial AD, is also present in familial FTD; a Danish family with autosomal dominant presenile dementia lacking specific pathological features showed linkage to chromosome 3 and, surprisingly, not to chromosome 17 (Brown et al., 1995). Twenty individuals over three generations developed personality change, memory loss, hyperorality, nonfluent aphasia, dementia, and later parkinsonism and corticospinal tract signs (Gydesen et al., 1987). The age at onset was between 50 and 67, and the duration of disease varied from 7 to 20 years. Generalized atrophy, neuronal loss, and gliosis were found at autopsy (Gydesen et al., 1987). This family can be classified under the Pick complex; it is similar to DDPAC in many features but differs in its older age at onset, lack of substantia nigra and spinal cord involvement, and absence of tau-positive neuronal and glial inclusions. The identification of this second locus for FTD confirms that more than one disease gene (genetic heterogeneity) is responsible for familial FTD. The establishment of biological and genetic markers for these chromosome 3-linked and 17-linked dementias will help to clarify any clinical, pathological, molecular, and biochemical interrelationships.

CONCLUSION

DDPAC is similar to many familial neurodegenerative diseases (Table 14.1). These conditions can all be incorporated under the term the *Pick complex*. All are highly penetrant, autosomal dominant, clinically heterogeneous, fatal neurodegenerative disorders. The DDPAC disease locus on chromosome 17 was the first frontal lobe dementia locus identified. Other FTD pedigrees have shown linkage to same locus on chromosome 17 (Sumi et al., 1992; Petersen et al., 1995; Lendon et al., 1996; Lendon et al., in press; Lynch et al., 1996; Spillantini et al., 1996, 1997; Murrell et al., 1997; Wilker et al., 1996; Yamaoka et al., 1996; Basun et al., 1997; Bird et al., 1997; Foster et al., 1997; Heutink et al., 1997; Baker et al., 1997), thus confirming its importance and proving that these FTDs are not due to environmental influence or epigenetic phenomena. Knowledge of the function of the DDPAC locus may contribute to our understanding of the pathogenesis and pathophysiology of neurodegenerative diseases.

REFERENCES

Alter M, Schaumann B (1976): A family with amyotrophic lateral sclerosis and Parkinsonism. J Neurol 212:281–284.

Alzheimer A (1910): Uber eigenartige Krankheitsfalle des spateren Alters. Z Gesamte Neurol Psychiatr 4:356–385.

American Psychiatric Association (1987): Diagnostic and Statistical Manual of Mental Disorders, Rev. (DSM-III-R). Washington, DC: APA.

Baker M, Kwok JBJ, Kucera S, Crook R, Farrer M, Houlden H, Isaacs A, Lincoln S, Onstead L, Hardy J, Wittenberg L, Dodd P, Webb S, Hayward N, Tannenberg T, Andreadis A, Hallupp M, Schofield P, Dark F, Hutton M (1997): Localization of fronto-temporal dementia with parkinsonism in an Australian kindred to chromosome 17q21–22. Ann Neurol 42:794–798.

Ball MJ (1980): Features of Creutzfelt-Jakob disease in brains of patients with familial dementia of Alzheimer type. Can J Neurol Sci 7:51–57.

Barber R, Snowden JS, Craufurd D (1995): Frontotemporal dementia and Alzheimer's disease: Retrospective using information from informants. J Neurol Neurosurg Psych 59:61–70.

Basun H, Almkvist O, Axelman K, Brun A, Campbell TA, Collinge J, Forsell C, Froelich S, Wattlund L, Wetterberg L, Lannfelt L (1997): Clinical characteristics of a chromosome 17-linked rapidly progressive familial frontotemporal dementia. Arch Neurol 54:539–544.

Bird TD, Wijsman EM, Nochlin D, Leehey M, Sumi SM, Payami H, Poorkaj P, Memens RN, Rafkind M, Schellenberg GD (1997): Chromosome 17 and hereditary dementia: Linkage studies in three non-Alzheimer families and kindreds with late-onset FAD. Neurology 48:949–954.

Bonduelle M (1976): Amyotrophic lateral sclerosis. In Vinken PJ, Bruyn GW (eds): Handbook of Clinical Neurology. New York: Elsevier, pp 281–338.

Boudouresques J, Toga M, Roger J, Khalil R, Vigouroux RA, Pellet W, Hassoun JJ (1967): [Dementia, amyotrophic lateral sclerosis, extrapyramidal syndrome. Anatomical study. Nosological discussion]. Rev Neurol (Paris) 116:693–704.

Brait K, Fahn S, Schwarz GA (1973): Sporadic and familial parkinsonism and motor neuron disease. Neurology 23:990–1002.

Brown J, Ashworth A, Gydesen S, Sorensen A, Rossor M, Hardy J, Collinge J (1995): Familial non-specific dementia maps to chromosome 3. Hum Mol Genet 4:1625–1628.

Brun A (1987): Frontal lobe degeneration of non-Alzheimer type. I. Neuropathology. Arch Gerontol Geriatr 6:193–208.

Brun A, Englund B, Gustafson L, Passant U, Mann DMA, Neary D, Snowden JS (1994): Clinical and neuropathological criteria for frontotemporal dementia. The Lund and Manchester Groups. J Neurol Neurosurg Psychol 57:416–418.

Burnstein MH (1981): Familial amyotrophic lateral sclerosis, dementia, and psychosis. Psychosomatics 22:151, 155–151, 157.

Caidas M, Marcutu V, Vuia O (1966): Sclerose laterale amyotrophique associee a la demence et au parkinsonisme. Acta Neurol Psychiatr Belg 66:719–731.

Caselli RJ, Jack CR Jr, Petersen RC, Wahner HW, Yanagihara T (1992): Asymmetric cortical degenerative syndromes: Clinical and radiologic correlations. Neurology 42:1462–1468.

Caselli RJ, Windebank AJ, Petersen RC, Komori T, Parisi JE, Okazaki H, Kolemen E, Iverson R, Di Napoli, RP, Gruff Radford NR, Stein SD (1993): Rapidly progressive aphasic dementia and motor neuron disease. Ann Neurol 33:200–207.

Clark AW, White CL, Manz HJ, Parhad IM, Curry B, Whitehouse PJ, Lehmann J, Coyle JT (1986): Primary degenerative dementia without Alzheimer pathology. Can J Neurol Sci 13:462–470.

Constantinidis J (1987): A familial syndrome: A combination of Pick's disease and amyotrophic lateral sclerosis. Encephale 13:285–293.

Constantinidis J, Richard J, Tissot R (1974): Pick's disease: Histological and clinical correlation. Eur Neurol 11:208–217.

Cordier J (1951): Syndrome parkinsonien avec des amyotrophies rappelant la sclerose amyotrophique et d'orgine post traumatique. Acta Neurol Belg 51:194–205.

Cummings JL, Benson DF (1992): Dementia: A Clinical Approach. Butterworths.

Cummings JL, Duchen LW (1981): Kluver-Bucy syndrome in Pick disease: Clinical and pathologic correlations. Neurology 31:1415–1422.

Dark, F (1997): A family with autosomal dominant non-Alzheimer's presenile dementia. Austral N Zeal J Psychiatry 31:139–144.

Decourt J, Mathieu PS, Mayer P (1934): Syndrome de sclerose laterale amyotrophique consecutif a une encephalite lethargique. Signes extrapyramidaux associes. Rev Neurol 2:596–600.

Delisle MB, Gorce P, Hirsch E, Hauw JJ, Rascol A, Bouissou H (1987): Motor neuron disease, parkinsonism and dementia. Report of a case with diffuse Lewy body-like intracytoplasmic inclusions. Acta Neuropathol (Berl) 75:104–108.

Denson MA, Wszolek ZK (1995): Familial Parkinsonism: Our experience and review. Parkinsonism Related Dis 1:35–46.

De Yebenes JG, Sarasa JL, Daniel SE, Lees AJ (1995): Familial progressive supranuclear palsy. Description of a pedigree and review of the literature. Brain 118:1095–1103.

Deymeer F, Smith TW, Degirolami U, Drachman DA (1989): Thalamic dementia and motor neuron disease. Neurology 39:58–61.

Dickson DW, Horoupian DS, Thal LJ, Davies P, Walkley S, Terry RD (1986): Kluver-Bucy syndrome and amyotrophic lateral sclerosis: A case report with biochemistry, morphometrics, and Golgi study. Neurology 36:1323–1329.

Evans DA, Funkenstein H, Albert MS (1989): Prevalence of Alzheimer's disease in a community population of older persons: Higher than previously reported. JAMA 262:2551–2556.

Foster NL, Wilhelmsen KC, Sima AAF, Jones MZ, D'Amato C, Gilman S, and the participants of the Chromosome 17-Related Dementia Conference (1997): Frontotemporal dementia and parkinsonism linked to chromosome 17: A consensus. Ann Neurol 41:706–716.

Froelich S, Basun H, Forsell C, Lannfelt L: Mapping of a disease locus for familial rapidly progressive frontotemporal dementia to chromosome 17q21–22. Am J Med Genet (in press).

Froment J (1925): Sclerose laterale amyotrophique et encephalite epidique. Rev Neurol 32:842–843.

Gaughran F, Keohane C, Buckley M (1994): Familial dementia with Pick's cells. A case report of probable familial Pick's disease. Ir J Psychol Med 11:34–38.

Gilbert JJ, Kish SJ, Chang LJ, Morito C, Shannak K, Hornykiewicz O (1988): Dementia, parkinsonism, and motor neuron disease: Neurochemical and neuropathological correlates. Ann Neurol 24:688–691.

Goate A, Chartier Harlin MC, Mullan M, Brown J, Crawford F, Fidani L, Giuff RA, Haymes A, Irving N, James L (1991): Segregation of a missense mutation in the amyloid precursor protein gene with familial Alzheimer's disease. Nature 349:704–706.

Greenfield JG, Mattews WB (1954): Post-encephalitic parkinsonism with amyotrophy. J Neurol Neurosurg Psychiat 17:50–56.

Groen JJ, Endtz LJ (1982): Hereditary Pick's disease: Second re-examination of the large family and discussion of other hereditary cases, with particular reference to electroencephalography, a computerized tomography. Brain 105:443–459.

Gunnarsson LG, Dahlbom K, Stranfman E (1991): Motor neuron disease and dementia reported among 13 members of a single family. Acta Neurol Scand 84:429–433.

Gustafson L (1987): Frontal lobe degeneration of non-Alzheimer type. II. Clinical picture and differential diagnosis. Arch Gerontol Geriatr 6:209–223.

Gustafson L (1993): Clinical picture of frontal lobe degeneration of non-Alzheimer type. Dementia 4:143–148.

Gydesen S, Hagen S, Klinken L, Abeiskov J, Sorensen SA (1987): Neuropsychiatric studies in a family with presenile dementia different from Alzheimer and Pick disease. Acta Psychiatr Scand 76:276–284.

Haberlandt WF (1964): Amyotrophische lateralsklerose. Klinisch—pathologische und genetisch—demographische Studie. Stuttgart: Gustav Fischer Verlag, pp 1–185.

Heston LL (1978): The clinical genetics of Pick's disease. Acta Psychiatr Scand 57:202–206.

Heutink P, Stevens M, Rizzu P, Bakker E, Kros JM, Tibben A, Niermeijer MF, Van Duijn CM, Oostra BA, Van Swieten JC (1997): Hereditary frontotemporal dementia is linked to chromosome 17q21–22: A genetic and clinicopathological study of three Dutch families. Ann Neurol 41:150–159.

Hirano A, Kurland LT, Krooth RS, Lessell S (1961a): Parkinsonism-dementia complex, an endemic disease on the island of Guam. I. Clinical features. Brain 84:642–661.

Hirano A, Malamud N, Kurland LT (1961b): Parkinsonism-dementia complex, an endemic disease on the island of Guam. II. Pathologic features. Brain 84:662–679.

Hofman A, Schulte W, Tanja TA, Van Duijn CM, Haaxma R, Lameris AJ, Otten VM, Saan RJ (1989): History of dementia and Parkinson's disease in 1st-degree relatives of patients with Alzheimer's disease. Neurology 39:1589–1592.

Horoupian DS, Thal L, Katzman R, Terry RD, Davies P, Hirano A, Deteresa R, Fuld PA, Petito C, Blass J (1984): Dementia and motor neuron disease: Morphometric, biochemical, and Golgi studies. Ann Neurol 16:305–313.

Hsiao K, Prusiner SB (1990): Inherited human prion diseases. Neurology 40:1820–1827.

Hudson AJ (1981): Amyotrophic lateral sclerosis and its association with dementia, parkinsonism and other neurological disorders: A review. Brain 104:217–247.

Hughes CP, Myers FK, Smith K, Torack RM (1973): Nosologic problems in dementia. A clinical and pathologic study of 11 cases. Neurology 23:344–351.

Hulette CM, Crain BJ (1992): Lobar atrophy without Pick bodies. Clin Neuropathol 11:151–156.

Joachim CL, Morris JH, Selkoe DJ (1988): Clinically diagnosed Alzheimer's disease: Autopsy results in 150 cases. Ann Neurol 24:50–56.

Kertesz A, Hudson L, Mackenzie IR, Munoz DG (1994): The pathology and nosology of primary progressive aphasia. Neurology 44:2065–2072.

Kertesz A, Kalvach P (1996): Arnold Pick and German neuropsychiatry in Prague. Arch Neurol 53:935–938.

Kertesz A, Lynch T, Morris JC, Munoz DG, Wilhelmsen KC (1996): The Pick complex. A recently hypothesized link between focal atrophies, dementia, parkinsonism, and ALS (abstract). Winter Conf Brain Res.

Kim RC, Collins GH, Parisi JE, Wright AW, Chu YB (1981): Familial dementia of adult onset with pathological findings of a "non-specific" nature. Brain 104:61–78.

Kluver H, Bucy PC (1939): Preliminary analysis of the function of the temporal lobe in monkey. Arch Neurol Psychiatry 42:979–1000.

Knopman DS, Mastri AR, Frey WH, Sung JH, Rustan T (1990): Dementia lacking distinctive histologic features: A common non-Alzheimer degenerative dementia. Neurology 40:251–256.

Kokmen E, Chandra V, Schoenberg BS (1988): Trends in incidence of dementing illness in Rochester, Minnesota, in three quinquennial periods, 1960–1974. Neurology 38:975–980.

Lanska DJ, Currier RD, Cohen M, Gambetti P, Smith EE, Bebin J, Jackson JF, Whitehouse PJ, Marksbury WR (1994): Familial progressive subcortical gliosis. Neurology 44:1633–1643.

Lathrop GM, Lalouel JM, Julier C, Ott J (1985): Multilocus linkage analysis in humans: Detection of linkage and estimation of recombination. Am J Hum Genet 37:482–498.

Legrand R, Linquette M, Delahousse J, Gerard A (1959): A propos d'un nouveau cas d'association d'une maladie de Parkinson et d'une sclerose laterale amyotrophique. Rev Neurol 101:191–193.

Lendon CL, Shears S, Busfield F, Talbot CJ, Renner J, Morris JC, Goate AM (1994): Molecular genetics of hereditary dysphasic dementia (abstract). Neurobiol Aging 15(Suppl 1):S128.

Lendon CL, Lynch T, Norton J, Busfield F, Craddock N, Chakraverty S, Gopalakrishnan G, Shears SD, Grimmett W, Wilhelmsen KC, Hanson L, McKeel DW, Morris JC, Goate AM: Hereditary Dysphasic Disinhibition Dementia: A frontal lobe dementia linked to 17q21–22. Neurology (in press).

Levy ML, Miller BL, Cummings JL, Fairbanks LA, Craig A (1996): Alzheimer disease and frontotemporal dementia. Arch Neurol 53:687–690.

Lynch T, Bell K, Sano M, Marder K, Nygaard T, Keohane C, Defendini R, Fahn S, Mayeux R, Wilhelmsen KC (1994a): The clinical and pathologic presentation of Moynihan's disease: Familial dementia-parkinsonism-amyotrophy complex (abstract). Neurology 44, A260.

Lynch T, Sano M, Marder KS, Bell KL, Foster NL, Defendini RF, Sima AAF, Keohane C, Nygaard TG, Fahn S, Mayeux R, Rowland LP, Wilhelmsen KC (1994b): Clinical characteristics of a family with chromosome 17-linked disinhibition-dementia-parkinsonism-amyotrophy complex. Neurology 44:1878–1884.

Lynch T, Sima AAF (1996): Glial cytoplasmic inclusions in multiple system atrophy. Ann Neurol 39:123.

Lynch T, Lendon CL, Busfield F, Morris JC, Craddock N, Fahn S, Wilhelmsen KC, Goate A (1996): Hereditary dysphasic dementia (HDD) and disinhibition-dementia-parkinsonism-amyotrophy complex (DDPAC) are linked to the *wld* locus on chromosome 17q21–22 (abstract). Mov Disord 11(Suppl 1):86.

Lynch T, Vu T, Pech RS, Goldman JE, Hays AP, Rowland LP (1994c): Amyotrophic lateral sclerosis and dementia: A retrospective review of autopsy cases (abstract). Ann Neurol 36:321.

Malamud N, Waggoner W (1943): Genealogic and clinicopathologic study of Pick's disease. Arch Neurol Psychol 50:288–303.

Mann DM, Marcyniuk B, Yates PO, Neary D, Snowden JS (1988): The progression of the pathological changes of Alzheimer's disease in frontal and temporal neocortex examined both at biopsy and at autopsy. Neuropathol Appl Neurobiol 14:177–195.

Mata M, Dorovini Zis K, Wilson M, Young AB (1983): New form of familial Parkinson-dementia syndrome: Clinical and pathologic findings. Neurology 33:1439–1443.

McKhann G, Drachman D, Folstein M, Katzman R, Price D, Stadlan EM (1984): Clinical diagnosis of Alzheimer's disease: Report of the NINCDS-ADRDA Work Group under the auspices of Department of Health and Human Services Task Force on Alzheimer's Disease. Neurology 34:939–944.

Mendez MF, Selwood A, Mastri AR, Frey WH (1993): Pick's disease versus Alzheimer's disease: A comparison of clinical characteristics. Neurology 43:289–292.

Mesulam MM (1982): Slowly progressive aphasia without generalized dementia. Ann Neurol 11:592–598.

Miller BL, Chang L, Mena I, Boone K, Lesser IM (1993): Progressive right frontotemporal degeneration: Clinical, neuropsychological and SPECT characteristics. Dementia 4:204–213.

Miller BL, Cummings JL, Villanueva Meyer J, Boone K, Mehringer CM, Lesser IM, Mena I (1991): Frontal lobe degeneration: Clinical, neuropsychological, and SPECT characteristics. Neurology 41:1374–1382.

Mitsuyama Y (1993): Presenile dementia with motor neuron disease. Dementia 4(3–4):137–142.

Mori H, Nishimura M, Namba Y, Oda M (1994): Corticobasal degeneration: A disease with widespread appearance of abnormal tau and neurofibrillary tangles, and its relation to progressive supranuclear palsy. Acta Neuropathol (Berl) 88:113–121.

Morita K, Kaiya H, Ikeda T, Namba M (1987): Presenile dementia combined with amyotrophy: A review of 34 Japanese cases. Arch Gerontol Geriatr 6:263–277.

Morris JC, Cole M, Banker BQ, Wright D (1984): Hereditary dysphasic dementia and the Pick-Alzheimer spectrum. Ann Neurol 16:455–466.

Morton NE (1955): Sequential tests for detection of linkage. Am J Hum Genet 7:277–318.

Murrell JR, Koller D, Faroud T, Goedert M, Spillantine MG, Edenberg HJ, Farlow MR, Ghetti B (1997): Familial multiple system tauopathy with presenile dementia is localized to chromosome 17. Am J Hum Genet 61:1131–1138.

Myrianthopoulos NC, Smith JK (1962): Amyotrophic lateral sclerosis with progressive dementia and with pathologic changes of the Creutzfeldt-Jakob syndrome. Neurology 12:603–610.

Neary D, Snowden JS, Mann DM (1993): The clinical pathological correlates of lobar atrophy. Dementia 4:154–159.

Neary D, Snowden JS, Mann DM, Northen B, Goulding PJ, MacDermott N (1990): Frontal lobe dementia and motor neuron disease. J Neurol Neurosurg Psychiatry 53:23–32.

Neary D, Snowden JS, Northen B, Goulding P (1988): Dementia of frontal lobe type. J Neurol Neurosurg Psychiatry 51:353–361.

Neary D, Snowden JS, Shields RA, Burjan AW, Northen B, MacDermott N, Prescott ME, Testa HJ (1987): Single photon emission tomography using 99mTc-HM-PAO in the investigation of dementia. J Neurol Neurosurg Psychiatry 50:1101–1109.

Neumann MA, Cohn R (1967): Progressive subcortical gliosis, a rare form of presenile dementia. Brain 90:405–418.

Neumann MA, Cohn R (1987): Long-duration Jacob-Creutzfeldt disease. Arch Gerontol Geriatr 6:279–287.

Papp MI, Kahn JE, Lantos PL (1989): Glial cytoplasmic inclusions in the CNS of patients with multiple system atrophy (striatonigral degeneration, olivopontocerebellar atrophy and Shy-Drager syndrome). J Neurol Sci 94:79–100.

Perry TL, Bratty PJ, Hansen S, Kennedy J, Urquhart N, Dolman CL (1975): Hereditary mental depression and Parkinsonism with taurine deficiency. Arch Neurol 32:108–113.

Petersen RB, Tabaton M, Chen SG, Monari L, Richardson SL, Lynch T, Manetto V, Lanska DJ, Markesbury WR, Currier RD, Autilio-Gambetti L, Wilhelmsen KC, Gambetti P (1995): Familial progressive subcortical gliosis: Presence of prions and linkage to chromosome 17. Neurology 45:1062–1067.

Pick A (1892): Uber die Beziehungen der senilen Hirnatrophie zur Aphasie. Prag Med Wochenschr 17:165–167.

Pinsky L, Finlayson MH, Libman I, Scott BH (1975): Familial amyotrophic lateral sclerosis with dementia: A second Canadian family. Clin Genet 7:186–191.

Purdy A, Hahn A, Barnett HJ, Bratty P, Ahmad D, Lloyd KG, McGeer EG, Perry TL (1979): Familial fatal Parkinsonism with alveolar hypoventilation and mental depression. Ann Neurol 6:523–531.

Rebeiz JJ, Kolodny EH, Richardson EPJ (1968): Corticodentatonigral degeneration with neuronal achromasia. Arch Neurol 18:20–33.

Rogaev EI, Sherrington R, Rogaeva EA (1995): Familial Alzheimer's disease in kindreds with missense mutations in a gene on chromosome 1 related to the Alzheimer's disease type 3 gene. Nature 376:775–778.

Roger H, Cain J (1947): De l'association d'un syndrome parkinsonien et d'un syndrome d'atrophie musculaire avec contractions fibrillaires d'origine encephalique probable, rappelant le sclerose laterale amyotrophique. Bull Acad Nat Med 131:461–465.

Rosenberg RN, Green JB, White CL, Sparkman DR, Dearmond SJ, Kepes JJ (1989): Dominantly inherited dementia and parkinsonism, with non-Alzheimer amyloid plaques: A new neurogenetic disorder. Ann Neurol 25:152–158.

Roy EP, Riggs JE, Martin JD, Ringel RA, Gutmann L (1988): Familial parkinsonism, apathy, weight loss, and central hypoventilation: Successful long-term management. Neurology 38:637–639.

Royall DR, Mahurin RK, Cornell J (1994): Bedside assessment of frontal degeneration: Distinguishing Alzheimer's disease from non-Alzheimer's cortical dementia. Expt Aging Res 20:95–103.

Sanders J, Schenk VWD, Van Veen P (1939): A family with Pick's disease. In Anonymous (ed): Verhandelingen der Koninklijke Nederlandsche Akademie van Wetenschappen, Part 38, No 3. Amsterdam: Noord-Hollandsche Vitgeversmij.

Schaumburg HM, Suzuki K (1968): Non-specific familial presenile dementia. J Neurol Neurosurg Psychiatry 31:479–486.

Schenk VWD (1959): Re-examination of a family with Pick's disease. Ann Hum Genet 23:325–333.

Schmitt HP, Emser W, Heimes C (1984): Familial occurrence of amyotrophic lateral sclerosis, parkinsonism, and dementia. Ann Neurol 16:642–648.

Schoenberg BS (1986): Epidemiology of Alzheimer's disease and other dementing illnesses. J Chronic Dis 39:1095–1104.

Sherrington R, Rogaev E, Liang Y (1995): Cloning of a gene bearing missense mutations in early-onset familial Alzheimer's disease. Nature 375:754–760.

Sima AAF, D'Amato C, Defendini RF, Jones MZ, Foster NL, Lynch T, Wilhelmsen KC (1994): Primary limbic lobe gliosis; familial and sporadic cases (abstract). Brain Pathol 4:538.

Sima AAF, D'Amato C, Foster NL, Lynch T, Defendini RF, Wilhelmsen KC (1995): Neuronal and glial inclusions in familial progressive limbic lobe sclerosis (abstract). J Neuropathol Exp Neurol 54:459.

Sima AAF, Defendini R, Keohane C, D'Amato C, Foster NL, Parchi P, Gambetti P, Lynch T, Wilhelmsen KC (1996): The neuropathology of Chromosome 17-linked dementia. Ann Neurol 39:734–744.

Sjogren T (1952): A genetic study of morbus Alzheimer and morbus Pick. Acta Psychiatr Neurologica Scand Suppl 82:1–66.

Spillantini MG, Crowther RA, Goedert M (1996): Comparison of the neurofibrillary pathology in Alzheimer's disease and familial dementia with tangles. Acta Neuropathol 92:42–48.

Spillantini MG, Goedert M, Crowther RA, Murrell Jr, Farlow MR, Ghetti B (1997): Familial multiple system tauopathy with presenile dementia: A disease with abundant neuronal and glial tau filaments. Proc Natl Acad Sci USA 94:4113–4118.

St George-Hyslop PH, Haines J, Rogaev E, Mortilla M, Vaula G, Pericak-Vance MA, Foncin J-F, Montesi M, Bruni A, Sorbi S, Rainero I, Pinessi L, Pollen D, Polinsky R, Nee L, Kennedy J, Macciardi F, Rogeava E, Liang Y, Alexandrova N, Lukiw W, Schlumpf K, Tanzi R, Tsuda T, Farrer L, Cantu J-M, Duara R, Amaducci L, Bergamini L, Gusella J, Roses AD, Crapper McLachlan D (1992): Genetic evidence for a novel familial Alzheimer's disease locus on chromosome 14. Nat Genet 2:330–334.

Staal A, Went LN (1968): Juvenile amyotrophic lateral sclerosis-dementia complex in a Dutch family. Neurology 18:800–806.

Steele PS, Richardson JC, Olszewski J (1964): Progressive supranuclear palsy: A heterogeneous degeneration involving the brainstem, basal ganglia and cerebellum with vertical gaze and pseudobulbar palsy, nuchal dystonia and dementia. Arch Neurol 10:333–359.

Sulkava R, Haltia M, Paetau A, Wikstrom J, Palo J (1983): Accuracy of clinical diagnosis in primary degenerative dementia: Correlation with neuropathological findings. J Neurol Neurosurg Psychiatry 46:9–13.

Sumi SM, Bird TD, Nochlin D, Raskind MA (1992): Familial presenile dementia with psychosis associated with cortical neurofibrillary tangles and degeneration of the amygdala. Neurology 42:120–127.

Tatemichi TK, Desmond DW, Mayeux R (1992): Dementia after stroke: Baseline frequency, risks, and clinical features in a hospitalized cohort. Neurology 42:1185–1193.

Tomlinson BE, Blessed G, Roth M (1970): Observations on the brains of demented old people. J Neurol Sci 11:205–242.

Van Bogaert L, Radermecker MA (1954): Scleroses laterales amyotrophiques typiques et paralysies agitantes hereditaires, dans une meme famille, avec une forme de passage possible entre les deux affections. M sch Psychiatry Neurol 127:185–203.

Wilhelmsen KC, Defendini R, Dooneief G, Bell K, Marder K, Sano M, Fohn S, Mayeux R (1991): Identification of a kindred with autosomal dominant thalamic dementia (abstract). Neurology 41:214s.

Wilhelmsen KC, Lynch T, Arwert F, Wszolek Z (1995): Two large parkinsonian kindreds linked to *wld* on chromosome 17q21–22 (abstract). Ann Neurol 38:301.

Wilhelmsen KC, Lynch T, Pavlou E, Higgins M, Nygaard TG (1994a): Localization of disinhibition-dementia-parkinsonism-amyotrophy complex to 17q21–22. Am J Hum Genet 55:1159–1165.

Wilhelmsen KC, Nygaard T, Pavlou E, Lynch T (1994b): A genetic localization of Moynihan's disease: Familial dementia-parkinsonism-amyotrophy complex. Neurology 44(Suppl 2):A361–A362.

Wilhelmsen KC, Wszolek ZK, Currier RC, Lanska DJ (1996): The clinical spectrum of chromosome 17q21–22-linked degenerative syndromes (abstract). Neurology 46(Suppl):A188.

Wilker M, Wszolek ZK, Wolters ECH, Rooimans MA, Pals G, Pfeiffer RF, Lynch T, Rodnitzky RL, Wilhelmsen KC, Arwert F (1996): Localization of the gene for rapidly progressive autosomal dominant parkinsonism and dementia with pallido-ponto-nigral degeneration to chromosome 17 q21. Hum Mol Genet 5:151–154.

Woods BT, McKee AC (1992): Case records of the Massachusetts general Hospital. Case 6-1992. N Engl J Med 326:397–405.

Wszolek ZK, Pfeiffer RF, Bhatt MH, Schelper RL, Cordes M, Snow BJ, Rodnitzky RL, Wolters EC, Arwert F, Calne DB (1992): Rapidly progressive autosomal dominant parkinsonism and dementia with pallido-ponto-nigral degeneration. Ann Neurol 32:312–320.

Yamaoka LH, Welsh-Bohmer KA, Hulette CM, Gaskell PC, Murray M, Rimmler JL, Helms BR, Guerra M, Roses AD, Schmechel DE, Paricak-Vance MA (1996): Linkage of frontotemporal dementia to chromosome 17: Clinical and neuropathological characterization of phenotype. Am J Hum Genet 59:1306–1312.

Zerbin-Rüdin E (1967): Hirnatropische Progresse. In Beker PE (ed): Ein Kurzes Handbuch. Stuttgart: Thieme.

CHAPTER 15

The Pathology of Pick Complex

DAVID G. MUNOZ

Departments of Pathology and Clinical Neurological Sciences, University of Western Ontario, London, Ontario, N6A 5C1, Canada

INTRODUCTION

There can be no argument that among the degenerative diseases of the nervous system, a cluster of conditions stands out by their clinical and pathological similarities. Selective atrophy of specific cortical areas in a symmetric or asymmetric fashion is a common gross finding, and the term *lobar atrophies* has been applied to this group. The first example of these conditions was reported by Arnold Pick, who in 1892 described circumscribed atrophy of the anterior forebrain in an aphasic and demented patient. A long line of historical tradition has associated the term *Pick's disease* with all brains showing this pattern of atrophy, although others have required the additional presence of the specific histological abnormalities—rounded argyrophilic neuronal cytoplasmic inclusions and ballooned cells—described by Alois Alzheimer (1911). Over the last few years, several distinct conditions have been delineated within this cluster, but all too often patients demonstrate overlap between the rigidly defined diseases. We have attempted to integrate both diversity and group coherence of manifestations and lesions by proposing the term *Pick complex,* which has the additional advantage of respecting tradition while shaking off rigid usage constraints (Kertesz et al., 1994). The concept is compatible with consideration of the diverse disease entities as separate diseases or, alternatively, as polar types within a spectrum of disease sharing some common mechanisms. At present, our knowledge of the genetic and/or environmental factors responsible for the development of these diseases does not allow a definite choice between these two views. Furthermore, more complex alternatives are suggested by recent developments in other dementing illnesses. Mutations in diverse genes can give rise to clinically and pathologically indistinguishable Alzheimer's disease (Sandbrink et al., 1996), while mutations in the prion protein gene can be manifested as Jakob-Creutzfeldt disease or several other syndromes, including Gerstmann-Straussler-Scheinker disease (Prusiner & Hsiao, 1994). Even the same mutation can produce such widely divergent syndromes as Jakob-Creutzfeldt disease and fatal familial insomnia, depending on the associ-

Pick's Disease and Pick Complex, Edited by Andrew Kertesz and David G. Munoz
ISBN 0-471-17792-X   ©1998 Wiley-Liss, Inc.

ated genetic polymorphism at another site (Gambetti et al., 1995). It would not be surprising if similar patterns become evident as the Pick complex is dissected out.

The first attempt to introduce order into the diversity of cases with a frontotemporal pattern of cortical atrophy was presented by Constantinidis, who in a series of papers proposed a simple histology-based classification: Type A showed Pick bodies and ballooned neurons, type B ballooned neurons only, and type C neither lesion (Constantinidis et al., 1974). Subsequently, several entities, including a generalized form of Pick's disease, corticobasal degeneration, frontal lobe degeneration, and dementia of the motor-neuron disease type were introduced in a somewhat hesitant manner, characterized by major modifications in the pathological criteria in successive publications. A contemporary working classification (Cooper et al., 1995; Jackson and Lowe, 1996) is based on the immunoreactivity for tau and ubiquitin of neuronal inclusions. It considers ballooned neurons a nonspecific element potentially present in all subtypes and thus establishes the overlap between Constantinidis' subtypes. Constantinidis' Pick's disease type B could correspond to corticobasal degeneration, dementia of motor neuron disease type, or frontal lobe degeneration. This scheme has been modified by Feany et al. (1996), who emphasized the importance of glial alterations. This chapter expands these frameworks by proposing diagnostic criteria and incorporating glial pathology while attempting to explore in greater detail the shared and unique features of each entity and adding two more varieties to the group. It is based on the examination of 29 brains with a final diagnosis of one of the variants of Pick complex, as well as a critical review of the literature.

Pick complex thus encompasses Pick body dementia, corticobasal degeneration, dementia with ubiquitinated tau-negative noneosinophilic inclusions (UTNNEI), basophilic inclusion body disease, dementia lacking distinctive histopathology, and the several variants linked to chromosome 17. *Dementia with UTNNEI,* a term introduced here, is equivalent to dementia of the motor-neuron disease type (Okamoto et al., 1992), and *basophilic inclusion body disease* is considered synonymous with the generalized form of Pick's disease as reported by Munoz-Garcia and Ludwin (1984).

Clinical presentations observed in patients with Pick complex include frontal lobe-type dementia, primary progressive aphasia, and syndromes of apraxia and movement disorders, as reviewed in other chapters. Since the proposed classification in this chapter is based entirely on histology, and since the clinical syndromes are largely dependent on the distribution of the atrophy, it follows that each of the entities making up the Pick complex can have diverse clinical manifestations, and conversely, the clinical syndromes have a variable structural basis. Although such lack of direct correlation can be frustrating to the clinician until diagnostic methods other than autopsy become practical, it is the author's belief that histopathology is the best currently available clue to the pathogenesis. Thus this approach is more likely to be able to accommodate the expected advances obtained by application of biochemistry and genetics to these diseases. The different entities comprising the Pick complex often share histological features, and thus it was deemed appropriate to introduce the characteristic lesions seen under the microscope prior to discussing their combination in separate but overlapping diseases. We will consider in turn lesions in neuronal perikarya, abnormalities in glia, and disorders of neuropil.

A DICTIONARY OF LESIONS IN PICK COMPLEX

Neuronal Perikarya

Inclusions in neuronal perikarya can be rounded, Pick body-like, or fibrillary, adapting one of the diverse shapes of neurofibrillary tangles. Alterations in the cytoplasm without a defined condensation are here considered diffuse inclusions. Based on the composition, as revealed by histochemistry and immunohistochemistry, rounded inclusions can be classified as Pick bodies, UTNNEI, and basophilic bodies. Neurofibrillary tangles can be classified into Alzheimer type, progressive supranuclear palsy type, and chromosome 17-linked dementia type. Corticobasal degeneration-type inclusions can adopt rounded or fibrillary configurations. Diffuse inclusions comprise ballooned neurons and dispersed tau immunoreactivity. All these lesions are summarized in Table 15.1.

Rounded inclusion type R-I: Pick body.   Pick bodies are distinctive by their large size, roughly similar to that of the cell nucleus, their often perfectly round shape, and the intense argyrophilia on the Bielchowsky or Bodian stain (Figure 15.1a), which contrast with their weakly basophilic and relatively inconspicuous appearance on hematoxylin and eosin (Color Plate 1a). Although a single inclusion in each affected neuron is typical, neurons with two or three bodies are often encountered (Feany et al., 1996). Not all Pick bodies are round, and particularly at sites other than the hippocampus, irregularly shaped bodies may predominate. In the locus ceruleus lobulated, cloverleaf-like Pick bodies are described as the characteristic finding (Takauchi et al., 1995) (Color Plate 1b). The general absence of staining of Pick bodies with the Gallyas silver stain (Braak and Braak, 1989) comes as a surprise, since this method prominently demonstrates all other forms of neurofibrillary pathology. Pick bodies do not take the stains for amyloid (i.e., Congo red and thioflavin S).

The antigenic expression of Pick bodies is far less consistent than that of neurofibrillary tangles, and significant variation from case to case, and even between regions in a given case, is to be expected. Probably corresponding to the unusual failure to stain by the Gallyas method, only some antibodies against tau, such as PHF1 and Tau-1, recognize Pick bodies consistently. Others, including ALZ-50 (Love et al., 1988; Cochran et al., 1994) and tau-2, label only a subset (Color Plate 1c). Pick bodies in the dentate fascia, hippocampus, and adjacent temporal cortex tend to show wider tau immunoreactivity than those in the frontal cortex. Additionally, Delacourte et al. (Chapter 16, this volume) have shown that Pick bodies do not contain the region of tau encoded by exon 10, and that their constituent tau proteins are not phosphorylated at specific sites where neurofibrillary tangle-derived tau proteins are. These results explain the differences from neurofibrillary tangles discussed above but not the interregional variation within a case. No cytoskeletal proteins other than tau are consistently associated with Pick bodies. Staining for microtubule-associated protein 2 (MAP-2) demonstrates a few bodies (Murayama et al., 1990), but most commonly the inclusion does not stand out from the surrounding perikaryon (Color Plate 1d). Tubulin has been reported as a component of Pick bodies, but this seems to be due to cross-reactivity of antitubulin antibodies with MAPs (Munoz-Garcia and Ludwin, 1984). Similarly, immunoreactivity for neurofilament proteins is usually observed for tau cross-reactive antibodies only (Murayama et al., 1990). However cases have been reported with argyrophilic inclusions that are tau negative and consistently (Yokoo et al., 1994) or variably (Horoupian and Dickson, 1991) decorated with neurofilament antibodies. Although immunoreactivity for ubiquitin was recognized early (Lowe et al., 1988) and has been used as a histological criterion for the identification of Pick bodies (Cooper et al., 1995; Jackson and Lowe, 1996), only a minority are intensely labeled (Love et al., 1988; Murayama et al., 1990) (Color Plate 1e). In the author's experience, the vast majority of bodies barely stand above the background level, but even this contrasts with the total absence of labeling of the lesions of corticobasal degeneration (type R/F). Others have found that ubiquitin immunoreactivity of neuronal inclusions did not discriminate among Pick body dementia, corticobasal degeneration, and progressive supranuclear palsy (Feany et al., 1996). There is a large region of overlap in the immunoreactive profile of Pick bodies and Alzheimer-type neurofibrillary tangles (NT-I). Both are recognized by antibodies directed against the N-terminal but not the C-termi-

TABLE 15.1 Neuronal Inclusions

Name	Type	Bielchowsky	Gallyas	Congo Red	Tau	Ubiquitin	Neurofilament	Chromogranin A	Seen in:
Rounded Inclusions									
Pick body	R-I	+	–	–	+	+	–	+	PiD
UTNNEI	R-II	–	–	–	–	+	–	–	UTNNEI Dementia,
ALS									
Basophilic	R-III	–	–	–	–	–	–	–	BIBD
Neurofibrillary Tangles									
Alzheimer-type	NT-I	+	+	+	+	+	–	–	AD, PiD, others
PSP-type	NT-II	+	+	–	+	+	–	–	PSP, PiD, CBD
Ch-17-type	NT-III	+	?	?	–	?	+	?	Ch-17
Rounded/Fibrillary Inclusions									
CBD-type	R/F	+	+	–	+	–	–	–	CBD
Diffuse Perikaryal Inclusions									
Pick cells	DP-I	–	–	–	–		+	–	Pick complex
Dispersed tau	DP-II	–	–	–	+		–	–	PiD, CBD, DLDH

Abbreviations: AD = Alzheimer's disease; ALS = amyotrophic lateral sclerosis; BIBD = basophilic inclusion body disease; CBD = corticobasal degeneration; Ch-17 = chromosome 17-linked dementia;

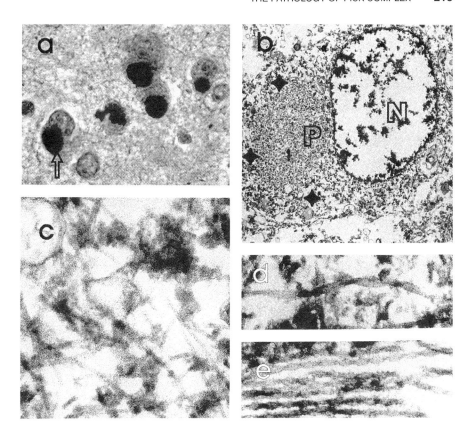

FIGURE 15.1. Pick bodies (R-I). (a) The Bielchowsky stain demonstrates several Pick bodies (one labeled by an arrow) in neocortical neurons. (b) At the ultrastructural level, a Pick body (outline P, delineated by black diamonds) appears as a non-membrane-bound distinct area in the neuronal cytoplasm. Outline N designates the nucleus. (c) High-power electron microscopy demonstrates the straight fibrils and dense osmophilic granules that make up the Pick body. (d) Long-period twisted fibrils are occasionally intermingled with the more common straight filaments in Pick bodies, as seen under high-power electron microscopy. (e) Paired helical filaments from a neurofibrillary tangle of type NT-I at the same magnification as (d) demonstrate a shorter period.

nal segment of β-amyloid precursor protein (Yasuhara et al., 1994a), as well as phosphoinositide-specific phospholipase C isozyme (Shimohama et al., 1993). Proteoglycans, present in several types of neuronal fibrillary inclusions, are thought to play an active role in their formation, perhaps by conferring resistance to proteases (DeWitt et al., 1994). Pick bodies contain both heparan sulfate, and condroitin sulfate proteoglycans. Although they lack the physical structure of amyloid, the P component, a common element of all amyloids, is also expressed in Pick bodies (Kalaria et al., 1991). In contrast to the above similarities, the proliferation-associated antigen Ki-67 is found in neurofibrillary tangles in a variety of disorders, including Pick's disease, but is not detectable in Pick bodies (Smith and Lippa, 1995). A particularly useful marker in the differential diagnosis of Pick bodies is chromogranin A, the major protein of large dense core synaptic vesicles (Yasuhara et al., 1994c). Most Pick bodies are intensely labeled (Color Plate 1f), whereas other round inclusions, including rounded/fibrillary inclusions of corticobasal type (R/F), are not. However, Pick bodies are weakly labeled in neurons, such as hippocampal CA1 pyramidal cells, that normally express chromogranin A at low levels. Dentate granule cells provide an interesting insight into the formation of Pick bodies. Normally, these neurons do not demonstrate chromogranin A immunoreactivity in the perikaryon, but only in their terminals in the mossy fibers. However, all Pick bodies in this layer are labeled, indicating that the formation of the Pick body disrupts the anterograde axonal transport of vesicles. In addition, Pick bodies express the other two proteins associated with large dense core synaptic vesicles, chromogranin B and secretoneurin (Bergmann et al., 1996). Synaptophysin, a membrane protein selectively associated with small clear synaptic vesicles, is also present in a subset of Pick bodies, although far less prominently than chromogranin A.

The ultrastructure of Pick bodies has been the subject of confusion because the original reports, erroneously describing normal neurofilaments as their major component (Wisniewski et al., 1972), have been repeatedly cited (Lowe et al., 1988). In fact, Pick bodies consist of non-membrane-bound, randomly arranged aggregates of fibrils with an average diameter of 15 nm (Figure 15.1b). Their larger diameter, absence of side arms, and straight rather than wandering course facilitate their distinction from neurofilaments (Brion and Mikol, 1971; Munoz-Garcia and Ludwin, 1984) (Figure 15.1c). Some bodies contain, in addition, twisted fibrils with maximum and minimum diameters of 26 and 13 nm, respectively, and a period of 140 to 200 nm (Figure 15.1d), longer than that of paired helical filaments of Alzheimer's neurofibrillary tangles (Figure 15.1e). These long-period, twisted tubules initially reported by Munoz-Garcia and Ludwin (1984) have now been confirmed in numerous reports, with minor differences in the measurements (Yoshimura, 1989; Kato and Nakamura, 1990; Murayama et al., 1990; Takauchi et al., 1995). Scattered among the fibers are dense osmophilic granules, probably derived from the rough endoplasmic reticulum. The regular presence of vesicles is the likely correlate of the chromogranin A immunoreactivity described earlier.

The heterogeneity encountered in immunohistochemistry has its ultrastructural correlate in single case reports of unusual patterns. The fibrils constituting Pick bodies appeared indistinguishable from paired helical filaments of Alzheimer's neurofibrillary tangles in one case (Schochet et al., 1968). In another case, true neurofilaments were encountered in Pick bodies, thus confirming the neurofilament immunoreactivity observed by light microscopy (Yokoo et al., 1994). This case provides an interesting example of the overlap between rounded inclusions, since 25-nm tubular profiles coated with granular material, characteristic of the basophilic body inclusion (type R-III (vide infra), were also present. Wisniewski et al.'s (1972) original hypothesis that the composition of the Pick body is determined by the cytoskeletal components present in the cell body at the onset of the pathological process is consistent with the observed variability in ultrastructure. The differences in argyrophilia (Color Plate 3g) and antigenic expression (Color Plate 3h) among adjacent bodies in a single case are remarkable, without parallel in other neurodegenerative diseases, and not yet addressed at the biochemical level.

Rounded inclusion type R-II: UTNNEI.   The proposed name *ubiquinated tau-negative noneosinophilic inclusions* (*UTNNEI*) refers to a previously unnamed, but well-described inclusion encountered in the perikarya of dentate granular cells and neocortical neurons in a subset of patients with Pick complex, some of whom also suffer from motor neuron disease. The shape varies from round to arciform, as if molded by the nucleus, and the size is equivalent to that of a Pick body (Color Plate 2a). The inclusions are not visible in routine or silver stains and are not stained by either Congo red or aniline dyes. Although intensely immunoreactive for ubiquitin, UTNNEI are not labeled by tau, neurofilament, tubulin, actin, desmin, or β-amyloid antibodies. At the ultrastructural level, the inclusions consist of loosely arranged 10- to 15-nm-wide fibrils associated with granular material (Okamoto et al., 1991). Similar inclusions can be seen in small neurons in the superficial layers of the temporal cortex, including the lateral part of the entorhinal cortex and the frontal cortex body (Color Plate 2b), but not the hippocampus proper, parietal or occipital cortices, basal ganglia, cerebellum, or brain stem (Okamoto et al., 1992). The shape but not the immunohistochemical profile of UTNNEI sets them apart from the skein-like inclusions found in motor neurons in patients with amyotrophic lateral sclerosis. The lack of eosinophilia distinguishes UTNNEI from cortical Lewy bodies.

Rounded inclusion type R-III: Basophilic.   The inclusions that give basophilic inclusion body disease its name have been described in a handful of cases, presenting either as motor neuron disease or as dementia of frontal type. The shape and size of the basophilic inclusions in cortical and most subcortical neurons are comparable to those of Pick bodies (Color Plate 2c), but in motor neurons their irregular outline suggests a derivation form aggregated Nissl substance (Munoz-Garcia and Ludwin, 1984). The inclusions are stained by methyl-green pyronin but show inconsistent, generally poor argyrophilia on Bodian stain, often limited to a dark, thin rim outlining the body (Figure 15.2a). They are not stained by the Gallyas method and are not generally recognized by antibodies to tau or neurofilaments, but they are immunoreactive for chromogranin A. Ultrastructurally, they consist of randomly arranged aggregates of 13- to 25- (average, 15) nm-wide fibrils covered almost entirely by granular and fuzzy material (Figure 15.2b,c). In addition, wider structures, up to 55 nm in diameter, recognizable as altered rough endoplasmic reticulum, are present in the inclusion. Munoz-Garcia and Ludwin (1984) proposed that coating of granular material prevented antibodies against cytoskeletal components from gaining access to the underlying fibrils.

Neurofibrillary tangle type NT-I: Alzheimer type.   Classical flame-shaped neurofibrillary tangles of the Alzheimer type can be stained with Congo red or thioflavin T, as well as with all the silver stains, including Bielchowsky and Gallyas (Figure 15.2d). They are recognized by all antibodies against tau (Color Plate 1c) and ubiquitin, but not by antibodies against neurofilament epitopes that do not cross-react with tau. These tangles are common findings in the brains of patients with most varieties of Pick complex, sometimes in numbers that fall within the expected range for the individual's age, but not rarely at much greater densities. Questions of double diagnosis (Pick complex plus Alzheimer's disease) or overlap, which may be raised in these cases, are discussed below. NT-I tangles can also be found in subcortical sites, especially the nucleus basalis of Meynert, the locus ceruleus, and the raphe nuclei. Although in these locations the tangles adopt a globose morphology, they retain their affinity for Congo red and thioflavin.

Neurofibrillary tangle type NT-II: Progressive supranuclear palsy type.   These are globose tangles with the appearance of balls of yarn, typically located in subcortical neurons. Although their reactivity with silver stains and cytoskeletal antibodies is similar to that of NT-I tangles, NT-II tangles fail to stain with Congo red and thioflavin, and thus can be distinguished from Alzheimer-type tangles of similar morphology. They are stained by Gallyas and thus are easily separated from subcortical Pick bodies, which are not (Figure 15.2e). NT-II tangles are integral components of progressive supranuclear palsy, as well as several varieties of Pick complex, including Pick body dementia.

Neurofibrillary tangle type NT-III: Chromosome 17-linked dementia type.   This type of tangle, so far described only in subcortical neurons in patients with chromosome 17-

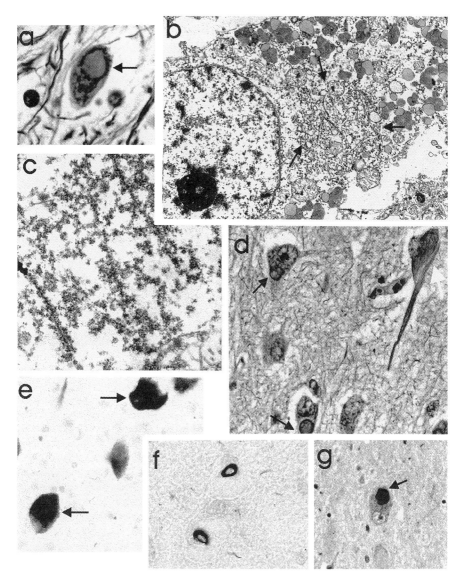

FIGURE 15.2. Other neuronal inclusions. (a) A type R-III (basophilic) inclusion demonstrates a narrow rim of argyrophilia (arrow), as demonstrated by the Bodian method. The core of the inclusion is unstained. (b) Under low power at the ultrastructural level, type R-III inclusions (arrows) appear very similar to Pick bodies, consisting of non-membrane-bound aggregates of randomly oriented linear structures. (c) Under high-power electron microscopy, the fibrils constituting R-III inclusions are densely coated by granular material resembling ribosomes. (d) Neurofibrillary tangles of Alzheimer type, type NT-I (upper left), can be found in neurons adjacent to others bearing Pick bodies (arrows). Bodian stain, CA1 sector of the hippocampus. (e) Neurofibrillary tangles of type NT-II (arrows) demonstrated by the Gallyas method in the substantia nigra in a patient suffering from Pick body dementia. (f) The ring shape is the most characteristic form of rounded/fibrillary inclusions of corticobasal degeneration type, as revealed by the Gallyas method in the neocortex of a patient with this disease. (g) Some rounded/fibrillary inclusions of corticobasal degeneration type adopt a spherical shape (arrow) and are thus indistinguishable from Pick bodies using any stain that labels both. Tau immunohistochemistry, periaqueductal neuron, in a patient with corticobasal degeneration.

linked dementia, appears as an argyrophilic spicular mass on Bielchowsky's silver stain. It is immunoreactive for phosphorylated neurofilament and ubiquitin, but not for tau or β-amyloid. At the electron microscopic level, it is made up of a lattice-like arrangement of 10- to 14-nm-diameter filamentous structures. The lattice demonstrates variable periodicity (Sima et al., 1996).

Rounded/Fibrillary inclusions (R/F): Corticobasal degeneration type. This type of inclusion is remarkable for the variety of shapes it adopts, even within a small area. The distinctive ring shape (Figure 15.2f) is found intermingled with arciform, ball (Figure 15.2g), and flame-shaped configurations, but the pattern is recognizable even in a reduced sample. These inclusions are best seen with the Gallyas stain and somewhat less so with the Bielchowsky stain. They do not stain with Congo red or thioflavin. Their immunoreactivity for tau contrasts with the lack of staining by ubiquitin antibodies. Unlike type NT-I tangles, R/F inclusions favor the small neurons in layers II and III. The ball-shaped inclusions are indistinguishable from Pick bodies on Bielchowsky stain, but unlike the latter, they are stained by Gallyas and lack chromogranin A and ubiquitin immunoreactivity. At the ultrastructural level, they are made up of 15-nm-wide straight tubules (Wakabayashi et al., 1994) identical to those described in progressive supranuclear palsy and the common form of Pick body.

Diffuse perikaryal lesion type DP-I: Ballooned neuron. This distinctive lesion is known by a variety of names: *ballooned, swollen,* or *achromatic neurons* and *Pick cells.* On hematoxylin and eosin stain, the rounded outline of the large perikaryon is filled with pinkish homogeneous cytoplasm devoid of Nissl substance but sometimes containing vacuoles, which may be associated with a granule, as in the granulovacuolar degeneration seen in hippocampal pyramidal neurons in Alzheimer's disease. The nucleus is displaced to the periphery. Pick cells are variable, usually weakly stained on Bodian and Bielchowsky silver stains, and are not recognized on Gallyas stain. Antibodies directed against phosphorylated neurofilaments (normally restricted to axons) such as SMI-31 or NF2F11 selectively label many of these neurons and thus allow their recognition at low power. αB-Crystallin is an alternative marker, favored in Cooper et al.'s (1995) classification of lobar atrophies. A weak ubiquitin immunoreactivity is consistently present, whereas chromogranin A, although occasionally detectable (Yasuhara et al., 1994c), is not always encountered. Some Pick cells show diffuse or focal cytoplasmic immunoreactivity for tau (Murayama et al., 1990) (Color Plate 2d), which together with the occasional presence of a central condensation reminiscent of a Pick body has raised the question of whether ballooned neurons could be the precursors of Pick bodies. This seems unlikely, since ballooned neurons are located in the deep layers of the cortex, contrasting with the preferential distribution of Pick bodies in the superficial layers. Electron microscopic examination of Pick cells does not provide additional insights: the cytoplasm shows a paucity of organelles and absence of rough endoplasmic reticulum. Neurofilaments constitute the main fibrillary elements, but occasional 15-nm straight tubules and even twisted profiles can be detected (Munoz-Garcia and Ludwin, 1984; Murayama et al.,1990).

Ballooned neurons are consistently present in Pick body dementia and corticobasal degeneration, and in some cases of dementia of motor neuron disease type, basophilic inclusion body disease, and dementia lacking distinctive histology. Similar neurons are seen in a variety of unrelated diseases. The pattern of expression of heat shock proteins of ballooned neurons in Pick complex—positive protein 27 and negative 72—is different from that in swollen neurons seen in amyotrophic lateral sclerosis, axonal reaction, and pellagra but identical to that of the swollen neurons of Creutzfeldt-Jakob disease (Kato et al., 1992).

Diffuse perikaryal lesion type DP-II: Dispersed tau immunoreactivity.   Labeling by tau antibodies in a dense granular pattern of perikarya and proximal dendrites of neurons demonstrating normal shape and no obvious inclusions is a common finding in Pick body dementia, corticobasal degeneration, and some cases of dementia lacking distinctive histopathology (Scheltens et al., 1994) (Color Plate 3a).

Glial Lesions

All glial lesions reported in the Pick complex are detected by their tau immunoreactivity, and so far can be separated on the basis of shape only. Unfortunately, a plethora of names has developed, so that the reader is often left wondering whether different names refer to the same or different lesions. The proposed classification, summarized in Table 15.2, attempts to smooth over minor details to emphasize distinctive entities.

Astroglial inclusion type A-I: Thorny astrocyte.   This type of astrocytic tau inclusion is characterized by dense punctate tau immunoreactivity filling the perikaryon and extending into the proximal processes. The latter are stubby, with sharp angles, and thus are reminiscent of thorns (Figure 15.3a). The appearance of A-1 inclusions is somewhat different on Gallyas-stained sections, where A-1 inclusion bearing astrocytes are crisscrossed by strands of fibrillary material. Type A-1 inclusions are abundant in affected gray and white matter in Pick body dementia, and can be present in corticobasal degeneration along with the more characteristic A-II inclusion.

Astroglial inclusion type A-II: Glial plaque.   Tau accumulates in the terminal, curled branches of star-shaped astrocytes, which may thus resemble a senile plaque minus the amyloid. Unlike the solid pattern in elongated neuritic processes observed in senile plaque, tau immunoreactivity in terminal astrocytic branches is arranged as rings surrounding small empty spaces (Figure 15.3b). Occasionally the astrocytic perikaryon is also labeled, and the underlying structure of the false plaque is revealed (Color Plate 2e). Glial plaques often coalesce, and by losing their individuality become part of the extensive cortical network of tau-immunoreactive processes. Glial plaques are the hallmark of corticobasal degeneration, although less well developed structures of similar appearance can be found in Pick body dementia.

Astroglial inclusion type A-III: Rounded.   This type of inclusion, resembling a miniature Pick body, has been described by Feany et al. (1996) in astrocytes in some cases of Pick

TABLE 15.2   Glial Inclusions

Name	Type	Bielchowsky	Gallyas	Tau	Seen in:
Astroglial					
Thorny	A-I	−	+	+	PiD, others
Glial plaque	A-II	+	+	+	CBD
Rounded	A-III	+	+	+	PiD, DLDH
Oligodendroglial					
Coiled body	O-I	+	+	+	CBD, PiD, UTNNEI

Abbreviations: CBD = corticobasal degeneration; DLDH = dementia lacking distinctive histopathology; UTNNEI = ubiquitinated tau-negative noneosinophilic inclusions; PiD = Pick body dementia.

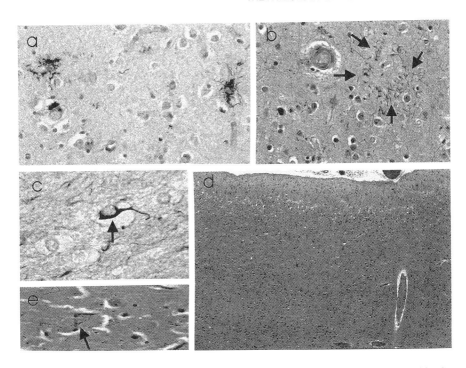

FIGURE 15.3. Glial and neuropil lesions. (a) Thorny astrocytes (A-I inclusions) demonstrated by the Gallyas method in the neocortex of a patient with Pick body dementia. (b) A glial plaque (A-II inclusion) in the neocortex of a patient with corticobasal degeneration is outlined by small arrows. Bielchowsky stain. (c) A coiled body (O-I inclusion, arrow) in a white matter oligodendrocyte (Gallyas stain). (d) Superficial linear spongiosis (N-I) is present in the upper layer II in a patient with corticobasal degeneration. H&E stain. (e) Braak's argyrophilic grains appear as small, spindle-shaped argyrophilic structures (arrow). CA1 sector of the hippocampus. Bielchowsky stain.

body dementia. The present author has found them in a small fraction of patients with this condition, as well as in some patients with dementia lacking distinctive histopathology (Color Plate 2f). The inclusions are made up of 15-nm straight tubules, identical to those found in Pick bodies, and thus are different from the glial cytoplasmic inclusions of multiple system atrophy (Caselli et al., 1993). However, A-III inclusions are stained by the Gallyas silver method and cannot be considered the glial counterpart of Pick bodies. The astrocytic nature of the containing cells has not been proven beyond doubt, and A-III lesions may be contained in oligodendrocytes.

Oligodendroglial inclusion type O-I: Coiled body.   Oligodendroglial O-I inclusions, also referred to as *oligodendroglial microtubular masses* (Yamada and McGeer, 1990), are best appreciated on Gallyas silver stains. The classical appearance, referred to as *coiled bodies,* consists of bundles of argyrophilic fibrils tightly embracing the nucleus and extending into one or several processes (Figure 15.3c). Tau immunostains show a wider spectrum of morphological appearances: some cells demonstrate an oblong cytoplasm, whereas other appear distended, with sparse short processes issuing from the perikaryon (Color Plate 2g). Several papers indicate that these inclusions are not recognized by ubiquitin antibodies (Horoupian and Chu, 1994; Wakabayashi et al., 1994); however, in this author's experience, they often are. In contrast to the cytoplasmic oligodendroglial inclusion of multiple-system atrophy, they are not visible on hematoxylin and eosin-stained sections and are not well demonstrated by the Bielchowsky method (Horoupian and Chu, 1994). The electron microscope reveals 15-nm-wide straight tubules similar to those seen in neuronal inclusions type R-I, NT-II, and R/F (Wakabayashi et al., 1994). The same straight tubules can be demonstrated in the inner and outer loops of myelin sheaths, where they constitute the substrate of the argyrophilic threads in white matter (Ikeda et al., 1994).

The oligodendroglial inclusions, which can be located in both gray and white matter, show identical morphology in all variants of lobar atrophy. However, they vary greatly in their areal density, being much more numerous in corticobasal degeneration, particularly in the white matter.

Neuropil Lesions

Neuropil abnormalities include the gliosis associated with atrophy in the affected areas and the impressive superficial linear spongiosis. As viewed with either silver stains or immunohistochemical procedures, the myriad processes encountered in the neuropil often represent a complex mixture of neuronal, astrocytic, and oligodendroglial abnormalities in which it may be impossible to ascertain the nature of individual elements. We can, however, separate abnormalities detected on tau and ubiquitin immunostains.

Neuropil lesion N-I: Superficial linear spongiosis. In its most distinctive form, this lesion consists of a narrow band of closely packed small empty spaces, or vacuoles, located at the junction of cortical layers I and II. The vacuoles do not appear to compress or indent adjacent neuronal cell bodies (Figure 15.3d). In severely affected areas, spongiosis may extend toward the white matter to include the entire layer III. However, unlike the transcortical spongiosis seen in prion diseases, the spongiosis of the Pick complex never spreads uniformly throughout the thickness of the cortex. Superficial linear spongiosis is seen in all varieties of the Pick complex, although not in every region in all cases. For example, it is often not detectable in severely atrophic areas in Pick body dementia, but it will be found at the transition to normal cortex.

Neuropil lesion N-II: Tau abnormalities. Neuropil threads appear as slender processes of uniform thickness with an irregular, randomly oriented course. They are seen in Pick body dementia but are even more abundant in corticobasal degeneration. The processes of thorny and glial plaque astrocytes and the occasional oligodendrocyte also contribute to the cortical and subcortical networks observed with silver stains and tau immunostains. Tau abnormalities in the white matter are almost exclusively of glial origin, predominantly astrocytic in Pick body dementia and oligodendrocytic in corticobasal degeneration (see Figure 14.5e).

Braak's argyrophilic grains are distinctive spindle-shaped small structures scattered in the neuropil, visible with silver stains only. Their oval outline is often sharpened to a pointed edge, from which a thin thread extends to other grains (Figure 15.3e). They are found in the CA1 sector of the hippocampus, the subiculum, and layer pre-β of the entorhinal cortex, as well as in the amygdala and the hypothalamus. Braak and Braak described these structures in demented patients lacking other lesions and construed them as the marker of a separate form of dementia (Braak and Braak, 1987, 1989). However, others have reported the association with progressive supranuclear palsy (Masliah et al., 1991). Martinez-Lage and Munoz (1996) have confirmed this association, and have shown that the grains can be found in over 10% of autopsied patients over the age of 65, as well as in patients with Pick body dementia, corticobasal degeneration, and dementia with motor neuron disease. The distribution of the grains, and their consistent association with superficial linear spongiosis and ballooned neurons, suggest that they belong to the Pick complex family of lesions.

Neuropil lesion N-III: Ubiquitin-immunoreactive neurites.   Elongated, thick neurites with an irregular course, immunoreactive for ubiquitin but not for tau, can be found scattered in all layers and in random orientation in patients with dementia of motor neuron disease type (Munoz, unpublished observation). In addition, vertically oriented neurites have been described in the upper cortical layers in association with superficial linear spongiosis in five patients with frontal lobe degeneration without associated motor neuron disease (Tolnay & Probst, 1995).

Patterns of Atrophy

There is no direct association between any of the varieties of the Pick complex and involvement of specific areas. On the contrary, it would appear that each entity can selectively involve any combination of areas from among those favored by the complex as a group. Thus, frontal predominance is common, but other patients show preferential involvement of temporal lobes, parietal lobes, or the motor strip. It would be extremely unusual, on the other hand, to find atrophy of the occipital lobes, if this ever occurs. A distinctive pattern of severe atrophy of the subiculum (Color Plate 3c) is very common in all varieties but is not present in every case. Subcortical structures that may be involved include the amygdala, neostriatum, nucleus basalis of Meynert, thalamus, hypothalamus, subthalamic nucleus, red nucleus, periaqueductal gray, substantia nigra, locus ceruleus, motor nuclei of the brainstem, and anterior horn of the spinal cord. Structures consistently spared include the optic nerves and tracts, the geniculate bodies, the pontine nuclei and brainstem nuclei other than the ones mentioned above, and the cerebellar cortex. The clinical manifestations depend on the areas involved rather than the underlying histology.

THE HISTOLOGICAL VARIETIES OF PICK COMPLEX

Pick Body Dementia

Pick body dementia can be operationally defined by the presence of Pick bodies in the granular cell layer of the dentate fascia. Although Pick bodies in the neocortex can be recognized by the use of the markers discussed above (Bielchowsky positive, Gallyas and Congo red negative, tau and chromogranin A positive, ubiquitin weakly positive), a simple silver stain or tau immunostain does not allow distinction from round corticobasal-type neurofibrillary tangles (NT-III). However, no other disease shows abundant round argyrophilic inclusions in the dentate, and this author has never encountered or seen a description of a case with Pick bodies elsewhere that failed to show Pick bodies in the dentate. Additional Pick bodies, as well as ballooned neurons, may be present in the hippocampal pyramidal cell layer, the neocortex, and subcortical sites.

The cortical atrophy is often severe, deserving the epithet *walnut-like* but not quite the hyperbolic *knife edge*. The brain weight is often reduced to less than 1000 g, although brain weights within the normal range can be encountered. The distinctive feature of the atrophy is its sharp margin on abutting normal-appearing cortex (Figure 15.4a). The atrophy is usually symmetrical, but striking asymmetry has been reported. The distribution of the atrophy is by no means constant. The frontal lobes are most commonly affected. Preferential involvement of

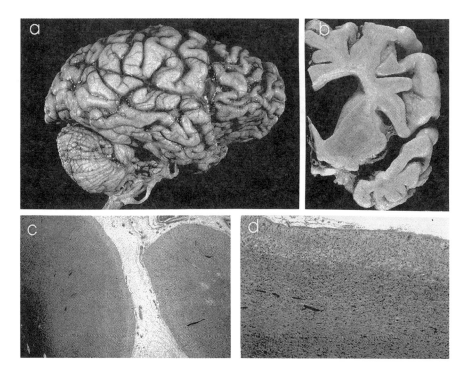

FIGURE 15.4. Pick body dementia. (a) Severe atrophy of the frontal lobes, sparing the precentral gyrus, and the inferior and anterior portions of the temporal lobes. (b) The atrophy of the frontal and temporal cortices and white matter contrasts with the preservation of the shape of the caudate. (c) Abrupt transition from the normal superior temporal gyrus (left) to the middle temporal (right) is illustrated in this low-power photograph of an H&E-stained section. (d) Superficial linear spongiosis is best demonstrated in areas with an intermediate degree of atrophy. H&E stain.

the convexities or the medial and basal surfaces can be encountered, but in most cases there is a sharp transition to normal-appearing cortex at the precentral sulcus. When the temporal lobes are affected, the atrophy typically spares the posterior third of the superior temporal gyrus. Frontal and temporal atrophy are often but not always combined. Less common patterns include atrophy restricted to the parietal lobes (Cambier et al., 1981) or to the hippocampal formation and basal temporal cortex. At the opposite extreme, pancortical atrophy sparing the striate cortex alone has been reported (Cochran et al., 1994). It is tempting to assume that the location of the atrophy determines the clinical syndrome, which may take the form of a frontal lobe syndrome or, as in Arnold Pick's first case, progressive aphasia. However, proof of this is difficult to obtain, in part because the clinical syndrome evolves as the disease progresses. For example, previously talkative frontal patients become mute. One of the best pieces of evidence supporting the contention above is provided by patients presenting with the clinical picture of amyotrophic lateral sclerosis, but with histological features of Pick body dementia, including argyrophilic Pick bodies in the dentate fascia. The motor deficits can be ascribed to posterior extension of the frontal atrophy to include the precentral gyrus (Sam et al., 1991). The external appearance of the brain does not allow differentiation from other lobar atrophies. In contrast to the consistent demonstration of atrophy in the hippocampus and amygdala, coronal sections may show no gross abnormalities in the basal ganglia (Figure 15.4b) or else reveal atrophy of the neostriatum or the thalamus. The substantia nigra may appear normal or depigmented. The white matter underlying the affected areas show grayish discoloration.

The abrupt transition from well-preserved to severely atrophic cortex is maintained at the microscopic level (Figure 15.4c). The affected cortex is devastated, as over 90% of the neuronal population is lost. Large neurons in layers III and V appear to be preferentially spared. The prominent cell bodies of reactive astrocytes render the gliosis much more conspicuous than in Alzheimer's disease. Superficial linear spongiosis may be obscured by the severe cortical atrophy and has to be sought at the transition between affected and unaffected cortex (Figure 15.4d). This author firmly rejects the use of the absence of superficial spongiosis as a diagnostic criterion for Pick body dementia (Mann et al., 1993).

In addition to their presence in numerous perikarya in the granular cell layer of the dentate fascia (Color Plate 1e,f)—necessary for diagnosis of Pick body dementia—Pick bodies are usually found in the pyramidal cell layer of the CA2 and CA1 sectors of the hippocampus and in the subiculum (Color Plate 1c,d). Granulovacuolar degeneration and Hirano bodies are commonly located in the same neuronal populations. Pick bodies are often but not always found in the neocortex (Figure 15.1a), where they are arranged in a bilaminar distribution, with a prominent band in layer II and upper layer III and a lesser one in layer VI, although occasional bodies are scattered in all layers (Hof et al., 1994). The small pyramidal neurons of layer II and upper layer III, where most Pick bodies reside, are the source of projections to neighboring cortical areas. This is in contrast to the large neurons in layers III and V preferentially affected by neurofibrillary tangles in Alzheimer's disease, which are the origin of long cortico-cortical projections. Pick bodies in layer VI could be expected to interfere with cortical projections to the thalamus. The functional implications of these anatomical observations remain obscure. Occasional Pick bodies can also be found beyond the areas of atrophy, in regions that are not even microscopically gliotic, such as the parietal lobes. They are, however, entirely absent from the striate cortex (Yoshimura, 1989). Unlike neurofibrillary tangles, little remains of most Pick bodies following the death of the containing neuron; thus Pick bodies are difficult to find in severely atrophic cortical areas. However, a few extracellular Pick bodies can be demonstrated in the dentate fascia. These structures, stained by Bodian stain but not by tau antibodies, demonstrate intermingling of straight fibrils with glial bundles (Izumiyama et al., 1994). We have also observed that they induce the formation of clusters of dystrophic neurites loaded with chromogranin A (Munoz, unpublished observation).

Extracortical Pick bodies can be found in the amygdala, anterior olfactory nucleus, and claustrum, as well as in the large neurons of the neostriatum, the anterior and dorsomedial nuclei of the thalamus, the subthalamic nucleus, the hypothalamus (particularly the mamiloinfundibular nucleus), the periaqueductal gray, superior colliculus, red nucleus, substantia nigra, locus ceruleus, and dorsal vagal nuclei. They have even been reported in the basis pontis and anterior horn motor neurons. They are absent from the cerebellum, including the dentate nucleus, and the lateral geniculate (Arima, 1989). Quantitative studies have failed to demonstrate any correlation between the number of Pick bodies and age of onset, disease duration, or degree of cortical atrophy (Hansen et al., 1988).

Ballooned neurons (DP-I) or Pick cells are always present in the deep layers of the cortex in Pick body dementia, although in highly variable numbers. Neuropil threads are well demonstrated on tau immunostains, as well as on the Bielchowsky—but not Gallyas—stain (Murayama et al., 1990). In addition, Braak's argyrophilic grains (Braak and Braak, 1987, 1989) are often seen in the hippocampus and the entorhinal cortex. Golgi impregnations have not been helpful, in spite of the excitement generated by the unusually long, unbranched basilar dendrites without spines reported in one case. The authors concluded that the pattern was unique and probably congenital (Wechsler et al., 1982). However, this finding has not been confirmed in other Golgi studies, which simply report nonspecific dendritic swellings similar to those seen in Alzheimer's and Jakob-Creutzfeldt diseases (Ferrer et al., 1990). The Di-I fluorescent stain, which is able to trace processes after postmortem injection, reveals peculiar neuritic aggregates not associated with amyloid deposits, astrocytes, or capillaries. These neuritic clusters have been interpreted as a peculiar neuritic response to the loss of specific populations of neurons (Sinha et al., 1993).

Tau immunoreactivity in glia is expressed predominantly in astroglia, which take the form of thorny astrocytes. These cells are relatively rare in the cortex and underlying white matter but much more abundant in subcortical structures. The neostriatum, thalamus, globus pallidus, and internal capsule may be peppered with them, contrasting with their absence in the optic tracts. The presence of thorny astrocytes appears unrelated to the distribution of neuronal lesions. For example, thorny astrocytes can be the only tau lesion in the dorsolateral nucleus of the thalamus or the dentate nucleus of the cerebellum. Only a fraction of thorny astrocytes are demonstrated on Gallyas stains. Oligodendroglial inclusions—coiled bodies—are present but rare in Pick body dementia.

Microglial activation is easily demonstrated in the affected cortex and underlying white matter but not in the spared regions. Unexpectedly, the CA1 sector of the hippocampus, and particularly the granular layer of the dentate gyrus, show a reduced density of microglial cells in comparison to controls (Paulus et al., 1993). Antibodies to components of the complement's classical pathway label Pick bodies and astrocytes in the brains of patients with Pick body dementia. Some groups have also found complement membrane attack complex (Yasuhara et al., 1994b), while others deny the presence of the terminal components C9 and membrane attack complex, possibly because of the additional presence of inhibitory proteins (Singhrao et al., 1996). It is at present unclear whether neurons synthesize complement proteins—as they are known to do *in vitro*—or internalize them following binding to their membrane. Removal from the neuronal surface of C3 fragments, potent activators of microglia, would explain the lack of microglia activation in regions where Pick bodies are abundant, such as the dentate fascia (Paulus et al., 1993).

The mechanisms of neuronal death in Pick body dementia are not known. There are numerous discrepancies between the distribution of Pick bodies and achromatic neurons and neuronal loss. The dentate granular layer is the region most densely endowed with Pick bodies, but neuronal loss is minimal. Cell counts demonstrate marked losses in cortical layers III and V even if these neurons do not tend to develop Pick bodies (Hof et al., 1994). Although Pick bodies appear in the large neurons in the neostriatum, the preferential loss of small perikarya results in an increased density of large neurons. There is a substantial loss of pigmented neurons in the substantia nigra, which affect exclusively the pigmented neurons, but Pick bodies are rare in this area (Uchihara et al., 1990). We can conclude that the development of Pick bodies is not necessarily part of the process leading to cell death in Pick body dementia. Loss of white matter volume and normal color can be detected grossly, and corresponds microscopically to loss of axons and myelin accompanied by prominent gliosis. Whether this simply reflects cortical neuronal loss or, as one may suspect, additional damage to axons or myelin we do not know.

A limited number of studies have addressed neurotransmitter alterations in Pick body dementia. Normal cortical levels of choline acetyltransferase and acetylcholinesterase are consistently found, contrasting with the marked loss observed in Alzheimer's disease. However, the hypothalamus and nucleus basalis of Meynert show decreased levels of these cholinergic enzymes compared to controls. Contrasting with the reduced levels in Alzheimer's disease, cortical somatostatin remains unaltered in Pick body dementia (Wood et al., 1983). The functional significance of these observations remains obscure. An interesting correlation has been suggested with the reverse pattern of serotonin and imipramine binding found in the hypothalamus of patients with dementia with Pick bodies in contrast to Alzheimer's disease, which may be related to the characteristic gluttony and reduced feeding, respectively, observed in these diseases (Sparks and Markesbery, 1991).

Pathologists often encounter brains in which pathology pointing to other degenerative diseases is superimposed on the typical findings of Pick body dementia. Most commonly, the question arises in regard to Alzheimer's disease. Neurofibrillary tangles of the Alzheimer type (NT-I) in the hippocampus and entorhinal cortex are very common (Color Plate 1c, Figure 15.2d), and neocortical β-amyloid plaques are present in approximately half of the cases. NT-I tangles can also be seen in the cortex, occupying their usual location in Alzheimer's disease in layers III and V, and thus in a distribution complementary to that of Pick bodies (Hof et al., 1994). In some cases, the density of lesions reaches the diagnostic criteria for Alzheimer's disease (Berlin, 1949), which has led some authors to raise the hypothesis that Alzheimer's disease and Pick body dementia constitute two polar types of a continuous spectrum (Cole et al., 1979; Morris et al., 1984). However, there are multiple contrasting features between the two entities. Differences in the distribution of the lesions are highlighted by positron emission tomography, which demonstrates parietal hypometabolism in Alzheimer's disease in contrast to the frontal hypoactivity of Pick body dementia. At the microscopic level, there is a contrasting pattern of involvement of regions of the hippocampal formation and layers in the neocortex. The differences in abnormal tau proteins demonstrated by Delacourte and his colleagues (Chapter 16, this volume) are reflected in the contrasting staining pattern in Gallyas and thioflavin S stains and in several antibodies. When amyloid deposits are present in Pick body dementia, their rather homogeneous cortical distribution, including the calcarine cortex, contrasts with the lobar restriction of Pick-related pathology. In parallel with current views regarding the relationship of Alzheimer's and Parkinson's diseases (Saitoh et al., 1995), it is reasonable to hypothesize that although Alzheimer's disease and Pick body dementia are distinct entities, the risk of developing one is increased by having the other. The sharing of mechanisms of progression, such as, for example, aberrant phosphorylation of cytoskeletal elements, or impaired axonal transport may be relevant in this respect. A possible model of this interaction is provided by aged transgenic mice expressing the human medium-weight neurofilament protein, which develops accumulation of neurofilaments in the shape of both neurofibrillary tangles (in layers III and V) and of Pick bodies (in layer II) (Vickers et al., 1994).

The area of overlap with progressive supranuclear palsy relates to the presence in some cases of Pick body dementia of globose neurofibrillary tangles of type NT-2. The distribution is similar in both diseases, including the thalamus, neostriatum, substantia nigra, locus ceruleus, and nucleus basalis of Meynert Case reports of patients who fulfill strict pathological diagnostic criteria for both diseases are on record (Arima et al., 1992). However, the abnormal tau proteins are different, and it seems reasonable to apply to progressive supranuclear palsy the hypothesis outlined above regarding overlap with Alzheimer's disease.

Most cases of Pick body dementia are sporadic. Although the literature contains reports of several large families carrying the diagnosis of Pick's disease, careful reading reveals that the diagnosis is based on the presence of lobar atrophy, or at most of ballooned neurons, and therefore is not acceptable by current criteria (Lowenberg et al., 1936; Malamud and Waggoner, 1943; Schenk, 1959; Groen and Endtz, 1982). This author is not aware of any reports of families with Pick body dementia as defined above.

Corticobasal Degeneration

The nosology of corticobasal degeneration—also named *corticobasal ganglionic degeneration*—has been clouded by the confusion derived from using the same name to refer to a pathological entity with several possible clinical manifestations, and the first recognized form of the latter, a peculiar movement disorder. In addition, accurate descriptions of the characteristic histopathology have emerged slowly, on multiple attempts over several years. In what is now considered the first account of the disease, Rebeiz et al. (1967) reported, under the name *corticodentatonigral degeneration with neuronal achromasia,* a degenerative disease of late adult life in which neuronal loss in the regions indicated was associated with the presence of ballooned neurons in the cortex. Gibbs et al. (1989) added the presence in the substantia nigra of inclusions construed as unique but now recognized as globose neurofibrillary tangles. A contemporary operational definition of corticobasal degeneration would include the following:

1. Lobar atrophy
2. Cortical ballooned neurons (DP-I)
3. Cortical rounded/fibrillary corticobasal degeneration-type inclusions
4. Subcortical rounded/fibrillary corticobasal degeneration-type inclusions and/or NT-II tangles
5. Cortical glial plaques (A-II astrocytic inclusions)
6. Massive white matter oligodendroglial tau inclusions (O-I)

The cortical atrophy is usually milder than in Pick body dementia, and the brain weight almost always exceeds 1000 g and not infrequently 1200 g (Figure 15.5a). The distribution of the atrophy can be correlated with one of the three clinical presentations: frontal lobe type dementia, movement disorder, or primary progressive aphasia (Lippa et al., 1991). Thus atrophy of the frontal lobes would give rise to dementia, atrophy of the superior parietal regions and the precentral gyri to the peculiar movement disorder, and involvement of the frontal operculum and anterior superior temporal gyrus to primary progressive aphasia. The temporal and occipital lobes are spared. As In Pick body dementia, evolution of the disease often adds further manifestations to the presenting syndrome and thus blurs clean clinicopathological correlations. The margins of the atrophy are not sharp, and the degree of asymmetry, if any, is well below that expected from the clinical manifestations. Depigmentation of the substantia nigra and locus ceruleus is a consistent finding. It may represent the only gross subcortical pathology or may be accompanied by discoloration of the globus pallidus and dorsomedial thalamic atrophy.

On microscopic examination of the atrophic cortex, the prominent superficial linear spongiosis (N-I) is more impressive than the moderate degree of neuronal loss (Figure 15.3d). Swollen, achromatic neurons—Pick cells (DP-I)—are easily found in the infragranular layers. Their immunohistochemical profile—αB-crystallin and phosphorylated neurofilaments in many and tau in a minority—is no different from that in Pick body dementia. Ultrastructurally, 20-nm-wide fibrils coated with granular material have been reported in addition to the expected neurofilaments (Wakabayashi et al., 1994). Ballooned neurons are most abundant in regions where the atrophic cortex abuts spared areas (Horoupian and Chu, 1994). The initial reports, based on the use of conventional silver stains, denied or minimized argyrophilic pathology (Gibb et al., 1989; Riley et al., 1990). It is only with the application of the Gallyas silver stain that a pervasive network of threads in both gray and white matter (N-II) becomes manifest (Figure 15.5e). Recognition of this pattern allows the pathologist to reach a tentative spot diagnosis. Rounded/fibrillary inclusions are preferentially located in neurons in layer II and upper layer III, as in Pick body dementia. They are pleomorphic, their appearance ranging from diffuse argyrophilia, to flame-shaped tangles, to the more common ring or arciform shapes. In their rounded configuration, they resemble Pick bodies, particularly on Bielchosky's stain (Fig-

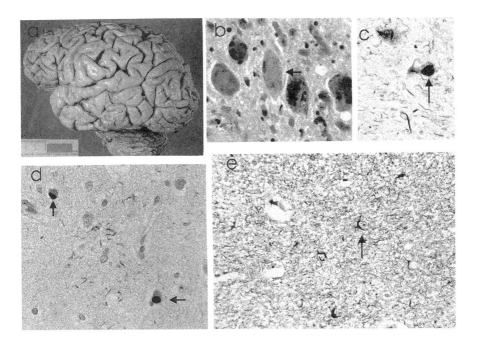

FIGURE 15.5. Corticobasal degeneration. (a) Gross atrophy restricted to the frontal lobes, in this case sparing the precentral gyrus. (b) Rounded/fibrillary inclusions (arrow) in nigral neurons (so-called corticobasal inclusions) are manifested on H&E stain by the displacement of neuromelanin. (c) The Gallyas silver stain best reveals the nigral rounded/fibrillary inclusions (black arrow), as well as a coiled body (O-I, white arrow) and numerous neuropil threads. (d) A glial plaque (A-II) in the center is associated with two rounded/fibrillary inclusions (arrows), one of which has a rounded shape reminiscent of a Pick body. Neocortex. Gallyas stain. (e) The hemispheric white matter is pervaded by a dense network of argyrophilic threads. Multiple coiled bodies (type O-I) are also seen. Gallyas stain.

ure 15.5d). However, unlike Pick bodies, the rounded neuronal inclusions in corticobasal degeneration are intensely stained by the Gallyas method. Tau immunoreactivity is demonstrated not only in all neuronal inclusions, but also in many other neurons in a diffuse pattern (DP-II type; Color Plate 3a). Conversely, there is a total absence of ubiquitin immunoreactivity (Cooper et al., 1995). The distribution of the lesions in the hippocampus is different from that in Pick body dementia, since no argyrophilic neuronal inclusions are present either in the dentate gyrus or in the pyramidal cell layer, although both of these regions show abundant argyrophilic threads. However, numerous neurons in the dentate gyrus display diffuse cytoplasmic tau immunoreactivity (DP-II). Glial plaques (astrocytic inclusions of type A-II) are the most characteristic feature of corticobasal degeneration (Figure 15.5d). They are scattered throughout the affected cerebral cortex, merging into one another in some areas and making a major contribution to the argyrophilic processes in the neuropil. Their astrocytic nature, hidden in the silver stains, is revealed in tau immunostains, which occasionally reveal a star-shaped astrocyte from which the processes emanate (Color Plate 2e). Cortical gliosis in corticobasal degeneration is maximal at the gray–white junction, where many tau-expressing astrocytes of the A-I (thorny) type can be found. The oligodendroglial inclusions are remarkable by their abundance only, being responsible for most of the argyrophilia and tau immunoreactivity in the white matter (Figure 15.5c,e).

Among subcortical structures, the substantia nigra consistently demonstrates severe neuronal loss, accompanied by occasional basophilic globose neurofibrillary tangles of NT-II type (Figure 15.5b,c). Early accounts of the condition construed these tangles as unique and referred to them as *corticobasal inclusions.* In addition, neuronal loss, gliosis, achromatic neurons, and argyrophilic inclusions in neurons and glial cells are variably present in the neostriatum, the globus pallidus, the subthalamic nucleus, the red nucleus, the periaqueductal gray, and the locus ceruleus, as well as the nucleus raphe magnus and reticular nuclei in the pons and medulla, the nucleus basalis of Meynert, inferior olive, and spinal gray matter. The amygdala is largely spared. Different parts of the thalamus may be involved, including the ventrolateral, dorsomedial, or anterior nuclei. The posterior hypothalamus is often affected. Argyrophilic threads involve the inferior olive and the cerebellar dentate nucleus, even if these nuclei show no neuronal loss (Uchihara et al., 1994).

Although the majority of the cases appear to be sporadic, there are well-documented reports of familial corticobasal degeneration in the literature (Brown et al., 1996).

Since some inclusions in neocortical—but not dentate—neurons in corticobasal degeneration are indistinguishable from Pick bodies on Bielchowsky's stain (Figure 15.5d), the traditional method used to identify these inclusions, it is not surprising to find a diagnosis of atypical Pick disease applied to these cases. However, once the diagnostic criterion for Pick body dementia becomes the presence of Pick bodies *in the fascia dentata,* and differential staining with Gallyas and immunoreactivity with ubiquitin is used to separate the lesions, the two diseases are easy to distinguish. Furthermore, the distinctive dense network of gray and white matter processes on Gallyas stain (Figure 15.5e) allows the immediate recognition of corticobasal degeneration on a single cortical section.

The relationship of corticobasal degeneration to progressive supranuclear palsy is controversial. Extension of progressive nuclear palsy pathology to the cerebral cortex, resulting in the formation of neurofibrillary tangles made up of 15-nm-wide tubules, is well documented in several case reports (Takahashi et al., 1987, 1989; Hauw et al., 1990). Cortical ballooned neurons in the parahippocampal gyrus and elsewhere are also a feature of this condition (Rebeiz et al., 1967; Mackenzie and Hudson, 1995). Although the subcortical globose neurofibrillary tangles of corticobasal degeneration and progressive supranuclear palsy appear indistinguishable, the cortical tangles in progressive supranuclear palsy are congophilic and stain with thioflavin-S (Hof et al., 1992).

Dementia with UTNNEI

This entity, defined by the presence of the characteristic inclusions, can present in at least two clinical forms. The disease was first recognized in patients in whom a progressive dementia of frontal type was followed, or rarely preceded, by amyotrophic lateral sclerosis, usually with prominent bulbar signs and symptoms. Patients, commonly 45 to 65 years of age, endure the disease for 3 years on average, with dramatic deterioration in the last 12 months of life. Pyramidal tract signs are often absent, and there is no evident degeneration of corticospinal tracts (Mitsuyama, 1984; Morita et al., 1987). Histological examination of the anterior horns shows the classical pattern of amyotrophic lateral sclerosis, with neuronal loss and gliosis, and the presence in motor neurons of Bunina bodies and ubiquitin-positive skein-like inclusions. The defining feature is the presence of crescent- or ball-shaped UTNNEI in the granule cells of the dentate gyrus, which by definition require ubiquitin immunostains to be recognized (Color Plate 2a). As few as 1% or more than half of the granule cells may be affected. The temporal and frontal cortices may show similar inclusions in small neurons located in the superficial layers (Color Plate 2b). UTNNEI are absent from the hippocampus proper, the parietal or occipital cortices, the basal ganglia, cerebellum, and brainstem (Okamoto et al., 1992).

The second group of patients demonstrating UTNNEI present with dementia of frontal lobe type not associated with clinical or pathological evidence of amyotrophic lateral sclerosis. Furthermore, approximately 25% of amyotrophic lateral sclerosis patients without documented dementia also show these inclusions (Okamoto et al., 1991), which, on the other hand, are not found in Alzheimer's disease, Pick body dementia, multiple system atrophy, or progressive supranuclear palsy. The term *dementia of motor neuron disease type* has been applied to this condition, but it seem preferable to name the entity in relation to something shared by all the patients.

In addition to the specific findings, there is mild frontal atrophy (Figure 15.6a), often accompanied by striatal atrophy (Figure 15.6b). There is prominent frontotemporal superficial linear spongiosis, perhaps due to the depletion of tertiary branches and spines of the apical dendrites of pyramidal neurons demonstrated on Golgi preparations (Horoupian et al., 1984). Dystrophic perikarya and neurites are found in all regions of the cortex in neurons expressing nitric oxide synthase, also demonstrated by their NADPH diaphorase activity. Only certain subtypes of interneurons—smooth stellate and spiny neurons—are affected (Kuljis and Schelper, 1996). Although not described in the literature, randomly oriented long, thick neurites are found scattered in the affected cortex of these patients, predominantly in the lower layers (Color Plate 3b). Tau-immunoreactive glial cells of the thorny (A-I) and oligodendroglial types can also be present.

Other features of the disease are consistent mild to severe cell loss in the substantia nigra—without Lewy bodies (Horoupian et al., 1984; Okamoto et al., 1992)—and gliosis in the subiculum, basolateral nuclei of the amygdala, and nucleus accumbens. The nucleus basalis of Meynert, locus ceruleus, and raphe nuclei are not affected (Neary et al., 1990). As in other forms of the Pick complex, cortical choline acetyltransferase activity and somatostatin levels are normal, in contrast to the decrease observed in Alzheimer's disease (Horoupian et al., 1984).

The disease is often familial, and individuals demonstrating either dementia or motor neuron disease in isolation are commonly reported in families combining the two disorders (Morita et al., 1987). For example, the mother of patient 2 of Neary (Neary et al., 1990) suffered from a dementia of frontal lobe type of 14 years' duration and never showed signs of motor neuron disease. Several siblings of patient 1 with aphasic dementia and motor neuron disease of Caselli et al. (1993) had dementia without muscle fasciculations or atrophy.

A possible third mode of presentation combining primary progressive aphasia with predominantly bulbar motor neuron disease has been reported. These patients present with language difficulties progressing to severe aphasia, along with impaired oral and reading comprehension rather than dementia. By the time they become anarthric, they show severe bulbar dysfunction but mild limb weakness and atrophy. The average age of disease onset in seven reported cases is 67 years, and death supervenes within two years of onset. In addition to the loss of lower motor neurons, the frontal and temporal cortices showed gliosis and superficial linear spongiosis in the absence of Pick bodies or ballooned neurons. The substantia nigra was mildly affected. Unfortunately, ubiquitin immunoreactivity has not yet been assessed, and thus the nosological status of this condition remain uncertain. (Caselli et al., 1993).

Basophilic Inclusion Body Disease

This rare disease, defined by the presence of a unique type of inclusion (R-III), can present as juvenile- (Nelson and Prensky, 1972; Oda et al., 1978; Matsumoto et al., 1992) or adult-onset

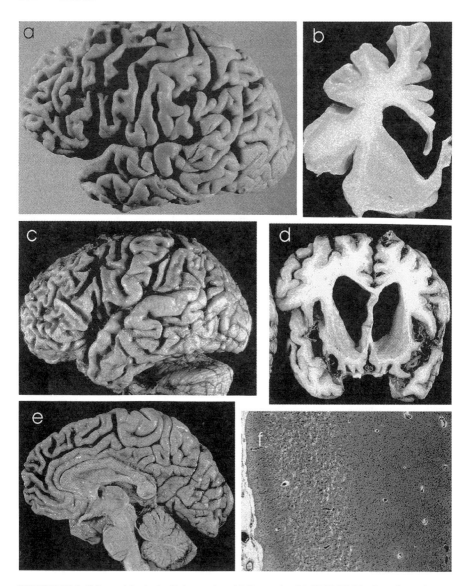

FIGURE 15.6. Other entities in the Pick complex. (a) Dementia with UTNNEI. The frontal atrophy extends caudally to involve the precentral gyrus. (b) Dementia with UTNNEI. Relatively mild caudate and cortical atrophy. (c) Basophilic inclusion body disease. The frontal lobes bear the brunt of the atrophy, which extends to involve the parietal and temporal lobes. The precentral gyrus is largely spared. (d) Severe striatal atrophy accompanies the atrophy of cortex and underlying white matter. Basophilic inclusion body disease (formerly known as *generalized form of Pick's disease*). (e) Dementia lacking distinctive histopathology. Atrophy of the mesial aspect of the frontal lobes. (f) Dementia lacking distinctive histopathology. The cerebral cortex show neuronal loss accompanied by marked superficial linear spongiosis.

(Kusaka et al., 1990, 1993) amyotrophic lateral sclerosis, a frontal lobe syndrome (Munoz-Garcia and Ludwin, 1984), or a combination of both (Hamada et al., 1995).

Patients are considerably younger than in other forms of the Pick complex: the ages of onset and death of adult patients have been 30–42 (Hamada et al., 1995); 36–45 and 52–58 (Ito et al., 1995), and 29–39 and 30–35 (Munoz-Garcia and Ludwin, 1984). As in other forms of Pick complex, patients presenting with limb or bulbar musculature weakness, atrophy, and fasciculations later develop emotional incontinence and akinetic mutism (Munoz-Garcia and Ludwin, 1984; Hamada et al., 1995). The cortical atrophy is not sharply demarcated: although more marked in frontal and temporal lobes, it extends in a less severe form to the parietal lobes (Figure 15.6c). Atrophy of the underlying white matter, caudate, putamen, amygdala, hypothalamus, and dorsomedial thalamus and depigmentation of the substantia nigra are obvious on gross inspection (Figure 15.6d). Microscopic examination reveals severe neuronal loss and gliosis, along with superficial linear spongiosis and ballooned neurons, but the specific finding is the presence of basophilic inclusion bodies (Munoz-Garcia and Ludwin, 1984) (Color Plate 2c, Figure 15.2a). The distribution of the latter in the neocortex is similar to that of Pick bodies and NT-III (corticobasal) type tangles, preferentially involving neurons in the superficial layers. However, basophilic bodies are not found in the hippocampus or dentate gyrus. They are common in several subcortical structures, including the putamen, pallidus, nucleus basalis of Meynert, subthalamus, red nucleus, periaqueductal gray, and substantia nigra. Motor neurons show neither Bunina bodies nor ubiquitinated skein-like inclusions. Another difference from amyotrophic lateral sclerosis, found even in cases with this clinical presentation, is a marked reduction in the staining of putaminal efferents to both external and internal segments of the globus pallidus, as shown by met-enkephalin and substance P immunoreactivity, respectively. This pattern had been described in striato-nigral degeneration but is unlike the normal distribution in amyotrophic lateral sclerosis (Ito et al., 1995).

Chromosome 17-Linked Dementia

This condition has also been named *disinhibition-dementia-parkinsonism-amyotrophy complex* and *primary limbic lobe sclerosis*. The terms *disinhibition* and *dementia* refer to the clinical syndrome of frontal lobe dementia, and the other two terms are self-explanatory. The familial form, transmitted in autosomal dominant form, has been linked to locus 17q21–22.

The atrophy affects the anterior portions of the frontal lobes and cingulate gyrus, the anterior and inferior temporal lobes, the substantia nigra, and in some cases the striatum. The hippocampus is spared. Microscopically, the cortex shows superficial linear spongiosis, occasional ballooned neurons, and gliosis affecting layers II, III, and IV but no argyrophilic inclusions. There is no gliosis of the subcortical white matter. Neuronal loss is severe in the amygdala, substantia nigra, ventral hypothalamus, and rostral and ventral portions of the caudate, putamen, and globus pallidus. Neurofibrillary tangles of type NT-IV are restricted to subcortical structures, including the oculomotor nucleus, periaqueductal gray, substantia nigra, subthalamic nucleus, red nucleus, globus pallidus, and ventral hypothalamus. In addition, oligodentroglial inclusions of coiled body type (O-I) are present in the white matter. The presence of prion protein has been excluded by immunohistochemistry and Western blotting (Sima et al., 1996).

Dementia Lacking Distinctive Histopathology

A major proportion of patients with lobar atrophy lack Pick bodies, the characteristic lesions of corticobasal degeneration, UTNNEI, or basophilic inclusion bodies. They may or may not show cortical ballooned neurons. The terms *frontal lobe degeneration of non-Alzheimer type* (Brun, 1987), *dementia of frontal lobe type, frontotemporal dementia,* and *dementia lacking distinctive histopathology* (Knopman et al., 1990) have been applied to this entity. Unfortunately, the first three terms invite confusion of a clinical syndrome with one of its structural substrates. Moreover, the consensus statement on clinical and neuropathological criteria for frontotemporal dementia of the Lund and Manchester groups also requires that the atrophy be mild, so that cases with severe neuronal loss and gliosis are classified as Pick's disease even in the absence of Pick bodies (The Lund and Manchester Groups, 1994). Since our proposed classification is based on histology rather than distribution of lesions, the term *dementia lacking distinctive histopathology* will be used to refer to this entity. Thus, what others have called *frontal lobe degeneration* is regarded as a variety of the distribution of dementia lacking distinctive histopathology, which can also present generalized, parietal, and mesolimbic patterns, as well as the selective frontal and temporal atrophy responsible for the syndrome of primary progressive aphasia.

The clinical presentations appear indistinguishable from those of Pick body dementia: either a frontal-type dementia or primary progressive aphasia is most commonly reported. The severity of the cortical atrophy is quite variable. It may be limited to the frontal lobe or may predominate in the temporal cortices. The parietal lobes are seldom involved (Figure 15.6e). Symmetry is the norm, although cases with preferential involvement of either hemisphere are not uncommon. In spite of considerable individual variability, it may be possible to distinguish a group in which the cerebral cortex bears the brunt of the disease and another in which the atrophy of the limbic system is combined with striatal involvement, which in addition to neostriatal structures may include the substantia nigra. These cases may also show extrapyramidal signs. This subgroup probably corresponds to the entity reported as having mesolimbocortical dementia (Torack and Morris, 1986; Verity et al., 1990). In large series, the correlation of clinical syndromes with the distribution and severity of the pathology is less than ideal (Giannakopoulos et al., 1995).

On microscopic examination, superficial linear spongiosis is a consistent feature, either limited to layer II or extending in depth to involve layer III as well (Figure 15.6f). The distribution of neuronal loss and gliosis, centered on layers II and III (Munoz-Garcia and Ludwin, 1984), is reminiscent of the location of Pick bodies or NT-III, although, of course, these lesions are absent. Pyramidal neurons seem to be preferentially lost, since the number of at least the subset of gabaergic cells expressing the calcium-binding protein parvalbumin is maintained (Arai et al., 1991). Ballooned neurons are present in many but not all cases. Sometimes they contain a condensation tantalizingly reminiscent of a Pick body. Silver stains, both Bielchowsky and Gallyas, are remarkable for the absence of findings. In most cases, tau immunohistochemistry will be similarly unrevealing. However, occasional patients demonstrate widespread neuronal perikaryal immunoreactivity for tau, as demonstrated, for example, with the antibody Alz-50 (Scheltens et al., 1994). Although no ubiquitinated neuronal inclusions are present, a recent paper describes dystrophic neurites, ubiquitin positive and vertically oriented within the region of superficial linear spongiosis in five patients with frontal lobe degeneration without associated motor neuron disease (Tolnay and Probst, 1995). However, these patients may represent cases of dementia with UTNNEI, where such dystrophic neurites are common. Synaptic loss has been proposed as a major substrate of intellectual decline in Alzheimer's disease. Measurements of the optic density of synaptophysin immunoreactivity in the molecular layer of the frontal cortex in patients with dementia lacking distinctive histopathology demonstrate a decrease comparable to that of Alzheimer's disease. In contrast, no decrease is detectable in the parietal cortex, confirming the lobar pattern of damage (Brun et al., 1995).

Dementia lacking distinctive histopathology can occur in sporadic or familial forms. In addition to the accounts of large families with frontal lobe degeneration (Passant et al., 1993), several reports of hereditary Pick's disease in fact refer to dementia lacking distinctive histopathology when current criteria are applied (Lowenberg et al., 1936; Malamud and Waggoner, 1943; Schenk, 1959; Groen and Endtz, 1982). In series comparing different forms of the Pick complex, a family history is most commonly found in this entity, even if the age of onset does not differ from that of other lobar atrophies. An autosomal dominant gene is suggested by the pattern of inheritance (Mann et al., 1993). A family history is more common among patients with presenile onset. Late-onset cases show a female predominance (Giannakopoulos et al., 1995). Recently, hereditary frontotemporal dementia has been linked to chromosome 17q21–22 in three Dutch families (some of which had been originally described as hereditary Pick's disease). Pick bodies were found "sporadically" in one brain from one of the families, an observation of great interest from the unifying perspective of the Pick complex concept (Heutink et al., 1997).

Because spongiosis—albeit superficially located—is often the most conspicuous abnormality, the question of its relationship to Jakob-Creutzfeldt's disease has been raised. There is now good evidence that dementia lacking distinctive histopathology is not related to prions. Homogenized brain samples show absence of protease-resistant prion protein on Western blots (Pollanen et al., 1993), and no staining with prion antibodies is detectable in the affected cortex (Caselli et al., 1993).

Although reports of progressive subcortical gliosis are rare, the clinical and pathological descriptions fit best with dementia lacking distinctive histopathology. There is a lobar pattern of cortical atrophy, albeit without sharp demarcation of affected and unaffected cortex, accompanied by atrophy of the striatum and substantia nigra. Although the cortical neuronal loss and gliosis are relatively mild, there is prominent superficial linear spongiosis. The absence of argyrophilic inclusions of any kind is compounded by the lack of ballooned neurons. The subiculum shows the pattern of atrophy and gliosis described in other forms of Pick complex. The white matter shows intense gliosis but minimal or no demyelination (Verity and Wechsler, 1987). Familial forms have been reported and linked to chromosome 17q21–22, the same locus as chromosome 17-linked dementia discussed above. Surprisingly, "diffuse" prion plaques in the cerebral cortex and protease-resistant fragments of prion protein were found in some subjects in the kindred. There was no mutation in the coding region of the prion gene (Petersen et al., 1995). Although these results remain controversial, they suggest that genes in chromosome 17 are involved in the metabolism of prion protein.

Lobar Atrophy with Alzheimer-Type Histopathology

A number of patients presenting with either a frontal lobe syndrome (Cooper et al., 1995) or primary progressive aphasia have been found on postmortem examination to exhibit numerous senile plaques and neurofibrillary tangles of the Alzheimer type, often but not always in association with swollen neurons. These cases have received a diagnosis of Alzheimer's disease, and indeed they fulfill published histopathological criteria for this condition. We, however, have been impressed with the discrepancy between the localized nature of the atrophy and corresponding neuronal loss and gliosis, and the disseminated distribution of Alzheimer-type lesion, unaltered in their density in the areas of atrophy. We hypothesize that these cases represent dementia lacking distinctive histopathology with superimposed Alzheimer changes. Conceptually, these cases are no different from those of combined Pick body dementia and Alzheimer's disease discussed above, but, of course, dementia lacking distinctive histopathology is not expressed in a dramatic way with Pick bodies.

CONCLUSION

Although the final elucidation of the relationship of the diverse entities comprising the Pick complex will rest on the discovery of the genetic and possibly environmental background of these disorders, the close similarities in the distribution and nature of the lesions suggest that, at a minimum, they share common pathogenic mechanisms.

REFERENCES

Alzheimer A (1911): Uber eigenartige Krankheitsfalle des spateren Alters. Z Gesamte Neurol Psychiatrie 4:356–385.

Arai H, Noguchi I, Makino Y, Kosaka K, Heizmann CW, Iizuka R (1991): Parvalbumin-immunoreactive neurons in the cortex in Pick's disease. J Neurol 238:200–202.

Arima K (1989): Involvement of subcortical nuclei and brain stem in Pick's disease: A topographical study of Pick bodies. Neuropathol Appl Neurobiol 9:105–115.

Arima K, Murayama S, Oyanagi S, Akashi T, Inose T (1992): Presenile dementia with progressive supranuclear palsy tangles and Pick bodies: An unusual degenerative disorder involving the cerebral cortex, cerebral nuclei, and brain stem nuclei. Acta Neuropathol 84:128–134.

Bergmann M, Kuchelmeister K, Schmid KW, Kretzschmar HA, Schroder R (1996): Different variants of frontotemporal dementia—a neuropathological and immunohistochemical study. Acta Neuropathol 92:170–179.

Berlin L (1949): Presenile sclerosis (Alzheimer's disease) with features resembling Pick's disease. Arch Neurol Psychiatry 61:269–383.

Braak H, Braak E (1987): Argyrophilic grains: Characteristic pathology of cerebral cortex in cases of adult onset dementia without Alzheimer changes. Neurosci Lett 76:124–127.

Braak H, Braak E (1989): Cortical and subcortical argyrophilic grains characterize a disease associated with adult onset dementia. Neuropathol Appl Neurobiol 15:13–26.

Brion S, Mikol J (1971): [Ultrastructural study of Pick's disease. Apropos of 3 cases]. Rev Neurol (Paris) 125:273–286.

Brown J, Lantos PL, Roques P, Fidani L, Rossor MN (1996): Familial dementia with swollen achromatic neurons and corticobasal inclusion bodies—a clinical and pathological study. J Neurol Sci 135:21–30.

Brun A (1987): Frontal lobe degeneration of non-Alzheimer type. I. Neuropathology. Arch Gerontol Geriatr 6:193–208.

Brun A, Liu X, Erikson C (1995); Synapse loss and gliosis in the molecular layer of the cerebral cortex in Alzheimer's disease and in frontal lobe degeneration. Neurodegeneration 4:171–177.

Cambier J, Masson M, Dairou R, Henin D (1981): [A parietal form of Pick's disease: Clinical and pathological study (author's trans)]. Rev Neurol (Paris) 137:33–38.

Caselli RJ, Windebank AJ, Petersen RC, Komori T, Parisi JE, Okazaki H, Kokmen E, Iverson R, Dinapoli RP, Graff-Radford NR, Stein SD (1993): Rapidly progressive aphasic dementia and motor neuron disease. Ann Neurol 33:200–207.

Cochran EJ, Fox JH, Mufson EJ (1994): Severe panencephalic Pick's disease with Alzheimer's disease-like neuropil threads and synaptophysin immunoreactivity. Acta Neuropathol 88:479–484.

Cole M, Wright D, Banker BQ (1979): Familial aphasia: The Pick-Alzheimer spectrum. Trans Am Neurol Assoc 104:175–179.

Constantinidis J, Richard J, Tissot R (1974): Pick's disease. Histological and clinical correlations. Eur Neurol 11:208–217.

Cooper PN, Jackson M, Lennox G, Lowe J, Mann DM (1995): Tau, ubiquitin, and alpha B-crystallin immunohistochemistry define the principal causes of degenerative frontotemporal dementia. Arch Neurol 52:1011–1015.

DeWitt DA, Richey PL, Praprotnik D, Silver J, Perry G (1994): Chondroitin sulfate proteoglycans are a common component of neuronal inclusions and astrocytic reaction in neurodegenerative diseases. Brain Res 656:205–209.

Feany MB, Mattiace LA, Dickson SW (1996): Neuropathologic overlap of progressive supranuclear palsy, Pick's disease and corticobasal degeneration. J Neuropathol Exp Neurol 55:53–67.

Ferrer I, Guionnet N, Cruz-Sanchez F, Tunon T (1990): Neuronal alterations in patients with dementia: A Golgi study on biopsy samples. Neurosci Lett 114:11–16.

Gambetti P, Parchi P, Petersen RB, Chen SG, Lugaresi E (1995): Fatal familial insomnia and familial Creutzfeldt-Jakob disease: Clinical, pathological and molecular features. Brain Pathol 5:43–51.

Giannakopoulos P, Hof PR, Bouras C (1995): Dementia lacking distinctive histopathology: Clinicopathological evaluation of 32 cases. Acta Neuropathol 89:346–355.

Gibb WR, Luthert PJ, Marsden CD (1989): Corticobasal degeneration. Brain 112:1171–1192.

Groen JJ, Endtz LJ (1982): Hereditary Pick's disease: Second re-examination of the large family and discussion of other hereditary cases, with particular reference to electroencephalography, and computerized tomography. Brain Res 105:443–459.

Hamada K, Fukazawa T, Yanagihara T, Yoshida K, Hamada T, Yoshimura N, Tashiro K (1995): Dementia with ALS features and diffuse Pick body-like inclusions (atypical Pick's disease?) Clin Neuropathol 14:1–6.

Hansen LA, DeTeresa R, Tobias H, Alford M, Terry RD (1988): Neocortical morphometry and cholinergic neurochemistry in Pick's disease. Am J Pathol 131:507–518.

Hauw JJ, Verny M, Delaere P, Cervera P, He Y, Duyckaerts C (1990): Constant neurofibrillary changes in the neocortex in progressive supranuclear palsy. Basic differences with Alzheimer's disease and aging. Neurosci Lett 119:182–186.

Heutink P, Stevens M, Rizzu P, Bakker E, Kros JM, Tibben A, Niermeijer MF, van Duijn CM, Oostra BA, van Swieten JC (1997): Hereditary frontotemporal dementia is linked to chromosome 17q21–22: A genetic and clinicopathological study of three Dutch families. Ann Neurol 41:150–159.

Hof PR, Bouras C, Perl DP, Morrison JH (1994): Quantitative neuropathologic analysis of Pick's disease cases: Cortical distribution of Pick bodies and coexistence of Alzheimer's disease. Acta Neuropathol 87:115–124.

Hof PR, Delacourte A, Bouras C (1992): Distribution of cortical neurofibrillary tangles in progressive supranuclear palsy: A quantitative analysis of six cases. Acta Neuropathol 84:45–51.

Horoupian DS, Chu PL (1994): Unusual case of corticobasal degeneration with tau/Gallyas-positive neuronal and glial tangles. Acta Neuropathol 88:592–598.

Horoupian DS, Dickson DW (1991): Striatonigral degeneration, olivopontocerebellar atrophy and "atypical" Pick disease. Acta Neuropathol 81:287–295.

Horoupian DS, Thal L, Katzman R, Terry RD, Davies P, Hirano A, DeTeresa R, Fuld PA, Petito C, Blass J, Ellis JM (1984): Dementia and motor neuron disease: Morphometric, biochemical, and Golgi studies. Ann Neurol 16:305–313.

Ikeda K, Akiyama H, Haga C, Kondo H, Arima K, Oda T (1994): Argyrophilic thread-like structure in corticobasal degeneration and supranuclear palsy. Neurosci Lett 174:157–159.

Ito H, Kusaka H, Matsumoto S, Imai T (1995): Topographic involvement of the striatal efferents in basal ganglia of patients with adult-onset motor neuron disease with basophilic inclusions. Acta Neuropathol 89:513–518.

Izumiyama Y, Ikeda K, Oyanagi S (1994): Extracellular or ghost Pick bodies and their lack of tau immunoreactivity: A histological, immunohistochemical and electron microscopic study. Acta Neuropathol 87:277–283.

Jackson M, Lowe J (1996): The new neuropathology of degenerative frontotemporal dementias. Acta Neuropathol 91:127–134.

Kalaria RN, Galloway PG, Perry G (1991): Widespread serum amyloid P immunoreactivity in cortical amyloid deposits and the neurofibrillary pathology of Alzheimer's disease and other degenerative disorders. Neuropathol Appl Neurobiol 17:189–201.

Kato S, Hirano A, Umahara T, Kato M, Herz F, Ohama E (1992): Comparative immunohistochemical study on the expression of alpha B crystallin, ubiquitin and stress-response protein 27 in ballooned neurons in various disorders. Neuropathol Appl Neurobiol 18:335–340.

Kato S, Nakamura H (1990): Presence of two different fibril subtypes in the Pick body: An immunoelectron microscopic study. Acta Neuropathol 81:125–129.

Kertesz A, Hudson L, Mackenzie IR, Munoz DG (1994): The pathology and nosology of primary progressive aphasia. Neurology 44:2065–2072.

Knopman DS, Mastri AR, Frey WH, Sung JH, Rustan T (1990): Dementia lacking distinctive histologic features: A common non-Alzheimer degenerative dementia. Neurology 40:251–256.

Kuljis RO, Schelper RL (1996): Alterations in nitrogen monoxide-synthesizing cortical neurons in amyotrophic lateral sclerosis with dementia. J Neuropathol Exp Neurol 55:25–35.

Kusaka H, Matsumoto S, Imai T (1990): An adult-onset case of sporadic motor neuron disease with basophilic inclusions. Acta Neuropathol 80:660–665.

Kusaka H, Matsumoto S, Imai T (1993): Adult-onset motor neuron disease with basophilic intraneuronal inclusion bodies. Clin Neuropathol 12:215–218.

Lippa CF, Cohen R, Smith TW, Drachman DA (1991): Primary progressive aphasia with focal neuronal achromasia. Neurology 41:882–886.

Love S, Saitoh T, Quijada S, Cole GM, Terry RD (1988): Alz-50, ubiquitin and tau immunoreactivity of neurofibrillary tangles, Pick bodies and Lewy bodies. J Neuropathol Exp Neurol 47:393–405.

Lowe J, Blanchard A, Morrell K, Lennox G, Reynolds L, Billett M, Landon M, Mayer RJ (1988): Ubiquitin is a common factor in intermediate filament inclusion bodies of diverse type in man, including those of Parkinson's disease, Pick's disease, and Alzheimer's disease, as well as Rosenthal fibres in cerebellar astrocytomas, cytoplasmic bodies in muscle, and mallory bodies in alcoholic liver disease. J Pathol 155:9–15.

Lowenberg K, Boyd DA, Salon DD (1936): Occurrence of Pick's disease in early adult years. Arch Neurol Psychiatry 41:1004–1020.

Mackenzie IR, Hudson LP (1995): Achromatic neurons in the cortex of progressive supranuclear palsy. Acta Neuropathol 90:615–619.

Malamud N, Waggoner RW (1943): Genealogic and clinicopathologic study of Pick's disease. Arch Neurol Psychiatry 50:288–303.

Mann DM, South PW, Snowden JS, Neary D (1993): Dementia of frontal lobe type: Neuropathology and immunohistochemistry. J Neurol Neurosurg Psychiatry 56:605–614.

Martinez-Lage P, Munoz DG (1996): Prevalence and disease association of argyrophilic grains of Braak. J Neuropathol Exp Neurol 56:157–164.

Masliah E, Hansen LA, Quijada S, DeTeresa R, Alford M, Kauss J, Terry R (1991): Late onset dementia with argyrophilic grains and subcortical tangles or atypical progressive supranuclear palsy? Ann Neurol 29:389–396.

Matsumoto S, Kusaka H, Murakami N, Hashizume Y, Okazaki H, Hirano A (1992): Basophilic inclusions in sporadic juvenile amyotrophic lateral sclerosis: An immunocytochemical and ultrastructural study. Acta Neuropathol 83:579–583.

Mitsuyama Y (1984): Presenile dementia with motor neuron disease in Japan: Clinico-pathological review of 26 cases. J Neurol Neurosurg Psychiatry 47:953–959.

Morita K, Kaiya H, Ikeda T, Namba M (1987): Presenile dementia combined with amyotrophy: A review of 34 Japanese cases. Arch Gerontol Geriatr 6:263–277.

Morris JC, Cole M, Banker BQ, Wright D (1984): Heredity dysphasic dementia and the Pick-Alzheimer spectrum. Ann Neurol 16:455–466.

Munoz-Garcia D, Ludwin SK (1984): Classic and generalized variants of Pick's disease: A clinicopathological, ultrastructural, and immunocytochemical comparative study. Ann Neurol 16:467–480.

Murayama S, Mori H, Ihara Y, Tomonaga M (1990); Immunocytochemical and ultrastructural studies of Pick's disease. Ann Neurol 27:394–405.

Neary D, Snowden JS, Mann DM, Northen B, Goulding PJ, MacDermott N (1990): Frontal lobe dementia and motor neuron disease. J Neurol Neurosurg Psychiatry 53:23–32.

Nelson JS, Prensky AL (1972): Sporadic juvenile amyotrophic lateral sclerosis. A clinicopathological study of a case with neuronal cytoplasmic inclusions containing RNA. Arch Neurol 27:300–306.

Oda M, Akagawa N, Tabuchi Y, Tanabe H (1978): A sporadic juvenile case of the amyotrophic lateral sclerosis with neuronal intracytoplasmic inclusions. Acta Neuropathol 44:211–216.

Okamoto K, Hirai S, Yamazaki T, Sun XY, Nakazato Y (1991): New ubiquitin-positive intraneuronal inclusions in the extra-motor cortices in patients with amyotrophic lateral sclerosis. Neurosci Lett 129:233–236.

Okamoto K, Murakami N, Kusaka H, Yoshida M, Hashizume Y, Nakazato Y, Matsubara E, Hirai S (1992): Ubiquitin-positive intraneuronal inclusions in the extramotor cortices of presenile dementia patients with motor neuron disease. J Neurol 239:426–430.

Passant U, Gustafson L, Brun A (1993): Spectrum of frontal lobe dementia in a Swedish family. Dementia 4:160–162.

Paulus W, Bancher C, Jellinger K (1993): Microglial reaction in Pick's disease. Neurosci Lett 161:89–92.

Petersen RB, Tabaton M, Chen SG, Monari L, Richardson SL, Lynches T, Manetto V, Lanska DJ, Markesbery WR, Currier RD, Autilio-Gambetti L, Wilhelmsen KC, Gambetti P (1995): Familial progressive subcortical gliosis: Presence of prions and linkage to chromosome 17. Neurology 45:1062–1067.

Pick A (1892): Ueber die Beziehungen der senile hiratrophie zur Aphasia. Prag Med Wochenschr 17:165–167.

Pollanen MS, Bergeron C, Weyer L (1993): Absence of protease-resistant prion protein in dementia characterized by neuronal loss and status spongiosus. Acta Neuropathol 86:515–517.

Prusiner SB, Hsiao KK (1994): Human prion diseases. Ann Neurol 35:385–395.

Rebeiz JJ, Kolodny EH, Richardson EPJ (1967): Corticodentatonigral degeneration with neuronal achromasia: A progressive disorder of late adult life. Trans Am Neurol Assoc 92:23–26.

Riley DE, Lang AE, Lewis A, Resch L, Ashby P, Hornykiewicz O, Black S (1990): Cortical-basal ganglionic degeneration. Neurology 40:1203–1212.

Saitoh T, Xia Y, Chen X, Masliah E, Galasko D, Shults C, Thal LJ, Hansen LA, Katzman R (1995): The CYP2D6B mutant allele is overrepresented in the Lewy body variant of Alzheimer's disease. Ann Neurol 37:110–112.

Sam M, Gutmann L, Schochet SSJ, Doshi H (1991): Pick's disease: A case clinically resembling amyotrophic lateral sclerosis. Neurology 41:1831–1833.

Sandbrink R, Hartmann T, Masters CL, Beyreuther K (1996): Genes contributing to Alzheimer's disease. Mol Psychiatry 1:27–40.

Scheltens P, Ravid R, Kamphorst W (1994): Pathologic findings in a case of primary progressive aphasia. Neurology 44:279–282.

Schenk VWD (1959): Re-examination of a family with Pick's disease. Ann Hum Genet 23:325–333.

Schochet SSJ, Lampert PW, Lindenberg R (1968): Fine structure of the Pick and Hirano bodies in a case of Pick's disease. Acta Neuropathol 11:330–337.

Shimohama S, Perry G, Richey P, Takenawa T, Whitehouse PJ, Miyoshi K, Suenaga T, Matsumoto S, Nishimura M, Kimura J (1993): Abnormal accumulation of phospholipase C-delta in filamentous inclusions of human neurodegenerative diseases. Neurosci Lett 162:183–186.

Sima AA, Defendini R, Keohane C, D'Amato C, Foster NL, Parchi P, Gambetti P, Lynch T, Wilhelmsen KC (1996): The neuropathology of chromosome 17-linked dementia. Ann Neurol 39:734–743.

Singhrao SK, Neal JW, Gasque P, Morgan BP, Newman GR (1996): Role of complement in the aetiology of Pick's disease? J Neuropathol Exp Neurol 55:578–593.

Sinha UK, Hollen KM, Miller CA (1993): Abnormal neuritic architecture identified by Di-I in Pick's disease. J Neuropathol Exp Neurol 52:411–418.

Smith TW, Lippa CF (1995): Ki-67 immunoreactivity in Alzheimer's disease and other neurodegenerative disorders. J Neuropathol Exp Neurol 54:297–303.

Sparks DL, Markesbery WR (1991): Altered serotonergic and cholinergic synaptic markers in Pick's disease. Arch Neurol 48:796–799.

Takahashi H, Oyanagi K, Takeda S, Hinokuma K, Ikuta F (1989): Occurrence of 15-nm-wide straight tubules in neocortical neurons in progressive supranuclear palsy. Acta Neuropathol 79:233–239.

Takahashi H, Takeda S, Ikuta F, Homma Y (1987): Progressive supranuclear palsy with limbic system involvement: Report of a case with ultrastructural investigation of neurofibrillary tangles in various locations. Clin Neuropathol 6:271–276.

Takauchi S, Yamauchi S, Morimura Y, Ohara K, Morita Y, Hayashi S, Miyoshi K (1995): Coexistence of Pick bodies and atypical Lewy bodies in the locus ceruleus neurons of Pick's disease. Acta Neuropathol 90:93–100.

The Lund and Manchester Groups (1994): Clinical and neuropathological criteria for frontotemporal dementia. J Neurol Neurosurg Psychiatry 57:416–418.

Tolnay M, Probst A (1995): Frontal lobe degeneration—novel ubiquitin-immunoreactive neurites within frontotemporal cortex. Neuropathol Appl Neurobiol 21:492–497.

Torack RM, Morris JC (1986): Mesolimbocortical dementia. A clinicopathologic case study of a putative disorder. Arch Neurol 43:1074–1078.

Uchihara T, Mitani K, Mori H, Kondo H, Yamada M, Ikeda K (1994): Abnormal cytoskeletal pathology peculiar to corticobasal degeneration is different from that of Alzheimer's disease or progressive supranuclear palsy. Acta Neuropathol 88:379–383.

Uchihara T, Tsuchiya K, Kosaka K (1990): Selective loss of nigral neurons in Pick's disease: A morphometric study. Acta Neuropathol 81:155–161.

Verity MA, Roitberg B, Kepes JJ (1990): Mesolimbocortical dementia: Clinico-pathological studies on two cases. J Neurol Neurosurg Psychiatry 53:492–495.

Verity MA, Wechsler AF (1987): Progressive subcortical gliosis of Neumann: A clinicopathologic study of two cases with review. Arch Gerontol Geriatr 6:245–261.

Vickers JC, Morrison JH, Friedrich VLJ, Elder GA, Perl DP, Katz RN, Lazzarini RA (1994): Age-associated and cell-type-specific neurofibrillary pathology in transgenic mice expressing the human midsized neurofilament subunit. J Neurosci 14:5603–5612.

Wakabayashi K, Oyanagi K, Makifuchi T, Ikuta F, Homma A, Homma Y, Horikawa Y, Tokiguchi S (1994): Corticobasal degeneration: Etiopathological significance of the cytoskeletal alterations. Acta Neuropathol 87:545–553.

Wechsler AF, Verity MA, Rosenschein S, Fried I, Scheibel AB (1982): Pick's disease. A clinical, computed tomographic, and histologic study with golgi impregnation observations. Arch Neurol 39:287–290.

Wisniewski HM, Coblentz JM, Terry RD (1972): Pick's disease. A clinical and ultrastructural study. Arch Neurol 26:97–108.

Wood PL, Etienne P, Lal S, Nair NP, Finlayson MH, Gauthier S, Palo J, Haltia M, Paetau A, Bird ED (1983): A post-mortem comparison of the cortical cholinergic system in Alzheimer's disease and Pick's disease. J Neurol Sci 62:211–217.

Yamada T, McGeer PL (1990): Oligodendroglial microtubular masses: An abnormality observed in some human neurodegenerative diseases. Neurosci Lett 120:163–166.

Yasuhara O, Aimi Y, McGeer EG, McGeer PL (1994a): Accumulation of amyloid precursor protein in brain lesions of patients with Pick disease. Neurosci Lett 171:63–66.

Yasuhara O, Aimi Y, McGeer EG, McGeer PL (1994b): Expression of the complement membrane attack complex and its inhibitors in Pick disease brain. Brain Res 652:346–349.

Yasuhara O, Kawamata T, Aimi Y, McGeer EG, McGeer PL (1994c): Expression of chromogranin A in lesions in the central nervous system from patients with neurological diseases. Neurosci Lett 170:13–16.

Yokoo H, Oyama T, Hirato J, Sasaki A, Nakazato Y (1994): A case of Pick's disease with unusual neuronal inclusions. Acta Neuropathol 88:267–272.

Yoshimura N (1989): Topography of Pick body distribution in Pick's disease: A contribution to understanding the relationship between Pick's and Alzheimer's disease. Clin Neuropathol 8:1–6.

CHAPTER 16

The Biochemistry of the Cytoskeleton in Pick Complex

ANDRÉ DELACOURTE, NICOLAS SERGEANT, ANNICK WATTEZ, and YVES ROBITAILLE

Unité INSERM, (A.D., N.S., A. W.), 422, 59045 Lille cedex, France and Centre de gériatrie (Y.R.), Hôpital Côte des neiges, 4565 Chemin de la Reine Marie, Montréal, H3W 1W5, Canada

INTRODUCTION

Frontotemporal dementia (FTD) is a well-defined clinical syndrome (Pasquier, 1996) associated with a primary degeneration of the frontal and anterior temporal lobes (Brun et al., 1994). Pick's disease (PiD), frontal lobe degeneration (FLD), and motor neuron disease (MND) are the most characteristic disorders demonstrating by FTD (Neary and Snowden, 1996). Focal degeneration presenting clinically as progressive aphasia has common clinical findings with FTD (Kertesz and Munoz, 1996). Other diseases can sometimes affect preferentially the frontotemporal cortices, generating clinical symptoms of FTD, such as atypical Alzheimer's disease (AD) or corticobasal degeneration (CBD) (Feany et al., 1996). Conversely, most of the patients with FLD meet the criteria for AD (McKhann et al., 1984). Therefore, the definite diagnosis of neurodegenerative disorders relies mainly on neuropathological features. However, most of them are not totally disease-specific. For instance, neurofibrillary tangles (NFT) are found in AD (Arnold et al., 1991), CBD (Mori et al., 1994; Feany et al., 1995), progressive supranuclear palsy (PSP) (Hauw et al., 1990; Hof et al., 1992a; Collins et al., 1995; Hanihara et al., 1995), postencephalitic parkinsonism (Hof et al., 1992b; Ikeda et al., 1993). This list is not exhaustive. Conversely, NFT are never found in FLD (Brun et al., 1994). Pick bodies are very characteristic inclusions that define PiD, but sometimes they are found associated with NFT (Arima et al., 1992; Hof et al., 1994). Chromatolytic neurons, also referred to as *Pick's cells, swollen neurons,* or *ballooned neurons,* are common in PiD, CBD, as well as in other varieties of Pick complex (Jendroska et al., 1995; Kertesz and Munoz, 1996). Also, the laminar spongiosis (microvacuolation), neuronal loss, gliosis, and ubiquitin stains that are used to differentiate some degenerative diseases with FTD are not, *stricto sensu,* disease-specific (Mayer et al., 1991; Cooper et al., 1995; Liu et al., 1996). Therefore, the neuropathological diagnosis of

Pick's Disease and Pick Complex, Edited by Andrew Kertesz and David G. Munoz
ISBN 0-471-17792-X   ©1998 Wiley-Liss, Inc.

FTD is impaired by the lack of precise histological markers. Actually, FLD has been described very recently by the teams of Lund and Manchester, despite the fact that this disease corresponds to the second most common cause of primary degenerative dementia (reviewed by Brun et al., 1994).

More recently, biochemical markers have been described that could help to differentiate and classify all these diseases. The most useful is certainly *tau* proteins, the basic components of many neuronal inclusions. *Tau* proteins aggregate inside neurons in different neurological disorders. Their biochemical profile is disease-specific. Indeed, the *tau* pattern distinguishes AD, PSP, CBD, PiD, FLD, and myotonic dystrophy (DM) (reviewed by Delacourte, 1994; Delacourte and Buée, 1997a). Here we will describe the information given by this outstanding biochemical marker and focus our attention on diseases that present FTD. We will also address the etiophysiopathological significance of these disease-specific *tau* biochemical signatures.

ALZHEIMER'S DISEASE

Pathological *tau* proteins (PTP) are biochemical markers of neurofibrillary degeneration coming from studies on AD. These proteins are the basic components of Paired Helical Filaments (PHF), abnormal filaments found in the cell body and neuritic extensions of degenerating neurons. *Tau* proteins belong to the family of microtubule-associated proteins. In the adult central nervous system, six human *tau* isoforms are encoded by mRNAs generated by a developmentally regulated splicing of a single gene located on chromosome 17. Exons 2, 3, and 10 are translated in adulthood. *Tau* proteins are further modified by phosphorylation. Their role is to modulate assembly of microtubules that are involved in axonal transport and neuronal plasticity (reviewed in Delacourte and Buée, 1997a).

PTP are resolved as three main bands with a molecular weight (MW) of 55, 64, and 69 kDa, as revealed by Western blot studies, using specific immunological probes such as AD2. This monoclonal antibody was originally raised against PHF. It binds to phosphorylated serines 396 and 404 on *tau* proteins (Buée-Scherrer et al., 1996a). A 74-kDa component is also present in brain extracts from AD patients with severe dementia (Figure 16.1). Other monoclonal antibodies (mAb) against phosphorylated sites are able to label specifically PTP, such as 12E8 against phosphorylated Ser 422 (Seubert et al., 1995) and AT8 against phosphorylated Ser 202 and Thr 205 (Goedert et al., 1995) (Figure 16.2A). PTP were also characterized by specific immunological probes against the polypeptidic regions encoded by exons 3 and 10, as well as with antibody 304 against exon 2 (gift from M. Goedert). With that approach, it was demonstrated that the 74-kDa band found in AD brain extracts corresponds to the longest isoform, with exons 2, 3, and 10 (Sergeant et al., 1997a) (Figure 16.2B). In AD, PTP are referred to as *PHF-tau.* They were further characterized by two-dimensional gels coupled with immunodetection by AD2. The isoelectric point (pI) of PHF-*tau* is between pH 5.92 and 6.85, while normal *tau* are above pI 7.5 (Sergeant et al., 1995; Delacourte et al., 1996; Delacourte et al., 1997b) (Figure 16.3).

Therefore, PTP seemed to be a perfect biochemical marker. In fact, in the normal autopsy-derived nervous tissue, *tau* proteins are not phosphorylated, while they are heavily phosphorylated in AD brain tissues (Buée-Scherrer et al., 1996a). This absolute difference permits precise detection and quantification of neurofibrillary degeneration using phosphorylation-dependent antibodies against *tau* (Vermersch et al., 1992, 1995b). However, in contrast, native *tau* proteins rapidly extracted and processed from normal nervous tissue are phosphorylated (Matsuo et al., 1994). The explanation is that native *tau* retrieved from autopsied brain tissues are rapidly de-

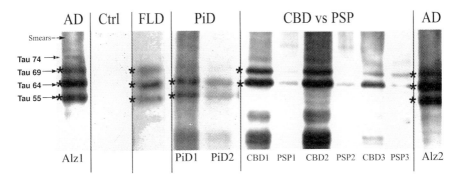

FIGURE 16.1. Comparison of the *tau* profiles observed in AD, FLD, PiD, CBD, PSP, and normal aging (Ctrl). Using a Western blot approach, the phosphorylation-dependent mAb AD2, raised against phosphorylated Ser 396 and 404 of human *tau,* was used to detect pathological *tau* proteins in brain homogenates from controls and patients with different neurodegenerative disorders. Ten microliters of brain homogenate (1 g/10 ml SDS buffer) were loaded per well. A triplet of PTP (*tau* 55, 64, 69) is detected in almost all cortical areas from AD patients (cases Alz1 and Alz2), as well as a minor 74-kDa band. These PTP are not detected in associated cortical areas from nondemented elderly individuals (Ctrl). A similar *tau* triplet is exclusively and discretely found in frontotemporal regions of patients with FLD (non-AD, non-PiD), with a characteristic absence of smears. PiD is characterized by a *tau* doublet (*tau* 55 and 64) and a minor band at 69 kDa (cases PiD 1 and 2). Another characteristic *tau* doublet (*tau* 64 and 69) is detected in CBD (cases CBD 1–3) and PSP (PSP 1–3). Immunodetection is always more prominent in CBD.

phosphorylated by postmortem endogenous phosphatase activity, while aggregated *tau* proteins that form inclusions are not (Matsuo et al., 1994; Buée-Scherrer et al., 1996a). In other words, the postmortem delay increases the differential of phosphorylation between normal and pathological (aggregated) *tau* proteins. But PHF-*tau* are different from normal native *tau* on many grounds: PHF-*tau* are highly aggregated, more acidic (Sergeant et al., 1995), and show specific phosphorylated epitopes, especially on Ser 422 (Caillet and Delacourte, 1996; Hasegawa et al., 1996). Also, other posttranslational biochemical modifications on PHF-*tau* have been reported, such as oxidation (Schweers et al., 1995), glycation (Ledesma et al., 1995), and glycosylation (Alonso et al., 1996). Altogether, these results demonstrate the concept of pathological *tau* proteins, which are markers of a pathological process (Flament et al., 1989; reviewed in Delacourte and Buée, 1997a). This concept is also demonstrated by (1) the almost perfect correlation between the presence of the marker and the density of neurofibrillary lesions at the immunohistochemical level, (2) the close relationship between the presence of the marker in the association cortex and the expression of a cognitive impairment, and (3) the fact that PTP biochemical profiles are disease-specific (see next sections).

A study of more than 60 nondemented patients versus 80 AD patients has been undertaken, with a qualitative and quantitative analysis of PHF-*tau* in more than 20 different brain regions. This study corroborates previous results (Vermersch et al., 1992, 1995b). It shows that all AD patients had the characteristic pattern of PTP (*tau* 55, 64, 69), which was found in associated brain regions, as well as in many other cortical and subcortical regions. The heterogeneity is important, particularly along the rostrocaudal axis. The frontal cortex was sometimes strongly affected, including the motor areas (Brodmann area 4). This heterogeneity explains why AD patients sometimes have clinical symptoms of FTD. Our study was combined with a bio-

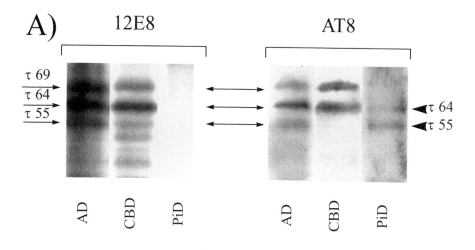

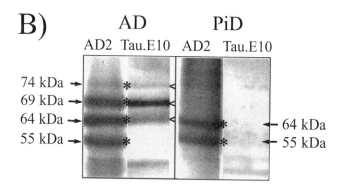

FIGURE 16.2. Analysis of the phosphorylation state and the exon 10 content of PTP from PiD versus AD and CBD. In each lane is loaded 10 μl of frontal cortex homogenate (1 g/10 ml SDS buffer). (A) Immunodetection of PTP using 12E8, an mAb against phosphorylated Ser 262. A triplet is strongly detected in AD and a major doublet in CBD (*tau* 64, 69), whereas no PTP are detected in PiD. In the same way, AT8 directed against phosphorylated Ser 202 and Thr 205 detected a triplet in AD, a doublet in CBD (*tau* 64, 69), and another doublet in PiD (*tau* 55, 64). (B) Immunodetection of the peptide sequence encoded by exon 10. Comparison with AD2 immunolabeling. In AD, PTP are strongly labeled by AD2 (*), especially the triplet *tau* 55, 64, 69, as well as the minor 74-kDa component; *tau* 74, 69, and 64 are detected by anti-*tau*-E10 (<). In PiD, a doublet (*tau* 55, 64) is mainly detected by AD2 (*), while anti-*tau*-E10 does not detect any protein.

chemical quantification of amyloid deposits, the other characteristic lesions of AD (Permanne et al., 1995). It showed that it is possible to perform a biochemical diagnosis of definite AD, since the two characteristic lesions (amyloid deposits and NFT) can be analyzed from both a qualitative and a quantitative molecular point of view (Delacourte, in preparation).

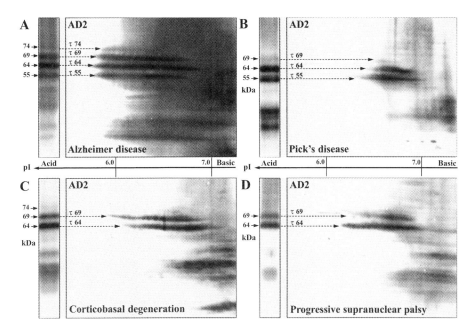

FIGURE 16.3 One- and two-dimensional Western blot analyses of PTP from patients with AD, PiD, CBD, and PSP. Molecular weights, expressed in kilodaltons, are indicated on the *x* axis, and isoelectric points (pI) are indicated on the *y* axis. PTP are immunodetected by AD2. Analysis of frontal cortex brain homogenates (1 g/10 ml SDS buffer). Loading of 10 μl for one-dimensional gels and 20 μl for two-dimensional gels. (A) AD brain PHF-*tau* components are indicated by arrows. Note the presence of four components: the characteristic triplet (*tau* 55, 64, 69) and the 74-kDa protein. (B) Profile of PiD PTP. Note the very small amount of *tau* 69 and the more basic pI of *tau* 64 and 55 versus that of AD. (C) Profile of pathological *tau* components in a representative case of CBD. Note the presence of a characteristic doublet (*tau* 64, 69) and the absence of the 55-kDa component. (D) Pathological *tau* profile of a typical PSP case. Note the presence of a doublet similar to the one of CBD, but more faintly immunodetected, the absence of *tau* 55 component, and the higher pI of *tau* 69 compared to that of CBD.

PICK'S DISEASE

PiD is a rare type of presenile dementia with clinical signs of FTD. PiD is neuropathologically confined to the prerolandic frontal convexity, orbitofrontal gyri, anteromesial temporal lobes, and occasionally parietal lobes (Pick, 1906), despite the frequently documented more diffuse forebrain atrophy with striatal involvement at postmortem examination (Constantinidis, 1985; Munoz-Garcia and Ludwin, 1986; Brion et al., 1991). The salient lesions are chromatolytic neurons and Pick bodies, with a prominent frontotemporal lobar atrophy, gliosis, and severe neuronal loss (reviewed by Hof et al., 1994). The Pick body (PB) is characteristic of PiD. Ultrastructurally, PB consist mostly of bundles of disorganized straight fibrils, which immunoreact with antisera to *tau* proteins (Kato and Nakamura, 1990; Murayama et al., 1990; Hof et al., 1994). Their immunological detection with mAb AD2 is at least two times more sensitive than that achieved with conventional silver staining (Delacourte et al., 1996).

Abnormal *tau* Proteins in PiD

At the biochemical level, PiD is characterized by a typical doublet of PTP (*tau* 55 and 64) and a minor *tau* 69 (Figures 16.1 to 16.3). This *tau* profile is characteristic of PiD because it is different from that of AD and other non-AD neurodegenerative disorders (Buée-Scherrer et al., 1996b; Delacourte et al., 1996). The characteristic pattern of pathological *tau* in PiD is well correlated with the presence of PB and a frontal-type syndrome (Delacourte et al., 1996).

The Mapping of PTP

Extensive biochemical mapping of several PiD cases was undertaken. For that purpose, we quantified PTP specifically detected by mAb AD2. The experimental protocol used was as described by Vermersch et al. (1992). A detailed analysis was carried out on 70 samples representing all Brodmann areas. Figure 16.4 shows a representative study of case 5 described in Delacourte et al. (1996). The characteristic *tau* doublet was found in almost all neocortical ar-

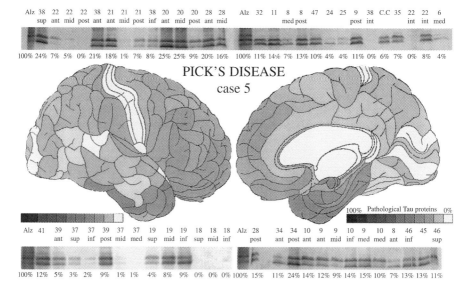

FIGURE 16.4. Cortical mapping of PTP in PiD. PTP were quantified in different brain areas from case 5 (Delacourte et al., 1996), using a Western blot approach with AD2. In each lane are loaded 10 µl of cortex homogenate (1 g/10 ml of SDS buffer). The different brain areas studied are numbered according to the classification of Brodmann. Each Brodmann area was generally subdivided for analysis (sup, inf, ant, post). Areas on the medial side are indicated (med). C.C indicates the corpus callosum. The intensity of immunodetection was quantified in comparison to the signal obtained in the temporal cortex from an AD patient. Results of quantification are presented under each analyzed brain area. The distribution of PTP was mapped with a gray scale ranging from 0 (white), corresponding to the absence of abnormal *tau*, to 100 (black), an arbitrary value given for the signal obtained from the AD brain homogenate. A triplet of PTP is observed in the AD brain extract used as a positive standard. PTP from the PiD case are characterized by a main doublet (*tau* 55 and 64) and a minor *tau* 69 in all affected Brodmann areas. PTP amounts are more important in the anterior and inferior temporal cortices and the hippocampal formation. All frontal cortex regions were affected. The sensitive primary regions (areas 1, 2, 3), the secondary visual cortex (area 18), and one gyrus of the temporal cortex (area 22 anterior and internal) were the only regions spared.

eas, limbic areas as well as subcortical nuclei. A similar pattern was found in other PiD brains, showing that the pathology affects especially the frontotemporal regions, but also many other brain regions.

The Phosphorylation State of PTP

PTP from PiD are different from those from AD, not only by their *tau* profile but also by their phosphorylation state. On two-dimensional gels, they were resolved as a large double band at 64-kDa and 55-kDa. A minor 69-kDa component was also detected. Isoelectric points of *tau* 55 and 64 were less acidic than in AD (6.4–7.00 versus 5.92–6.85), which means that *tau* from PiD are less phosphorylated than in AD (Figure 16.2A,B) (Delacourte et al., 1996). Indeed, the doublet from PiD is phosphorylated at Ser 202 and Thr 205 (the binding site of AT8; Goedert et al., 1995) and at Ser396 and 404 (binding site of AD2) (Buée-Scherrer et al., 1996a) (Figure 16.2). But interestingly, other sites are not phosphorylated, since mAb 12E8 that binds to phosphorylated Ser 262 (Seubert et al., 1995) labeled PTP from AD, PSP, and CBD but did not label those from PiD (Figure 16.2A).

The Isoform Content of Pathological *tau* Proteins from PiD

As mentioned in the section on AD, exons 2, 3 and 10 are developmentally regulated and translated only in adulthood. The regions encoded by exons 2 and 3 are on the N-terminal part of the *tau* molecule, and exon 10 is on the C-terminal part. These regions are likely those that modulate the role of *tau* proteins in adult neuronal populations. For instance, the encoded region of exon 10 corresponds to the tubulin-binding region. Its presence dramatically increases the affinity of *tau* for tubulin and therefore stabilizes the microtubule (Goode and Feinstein, 1994). We have recently developed antibodies raised against the peptidic sequence encoded by exons 3 and 10 (anti-*tau*.E3 and anti-*tau*.E10). Anti-exon 2, referred to as 304, is a gift of Dr. M. Goedert (Goedert et al., 1992). The isoform content of PTP from PiD was characterized by Western blots, using these antibodies.

As presented in Figure 16.2B, the most remarkable results were that PTP from PiD were not immunolabeled by anti-*tau*.E10. In other words, the *tau* isoforms that aggregate in PiD do not contain the protein region encoded by exon 10, unlike in AD. Anti-*tau*.E2 (304) labeled bands corresponding to *tau* 69 and 64, while anti-*tau*.E3 only detected the minor *tau* 69 band. *tau* 55 was not detected by these specific anti-exons. These results were corroborated on two-dimensional gels (Sergeant et al., 1997b).

The Etiopathogenic Significance of Specific PTP in PiD

Our results enable us to propose the following synopsis (Figure 16.5) for the correspondence between the proteins detected on Western blots and their isoform content, as well as for the number of immunodetected phosphorylation sites. Together they demonstrate that *tau* isoforms that aggregate in PiD are very different from those of AD on the basis of their primary sequence and phosphorylation sites.

These results were corroborated at the immunohistochemical level. In fact, Anti-*tau*.E2 304 strongly detected NFT from AD, as well as the PB from PiD (Figure 16.6). In parallel, on adjacent tissue sections, anti-*tau*.E10 immunodetected a large number of degenerating neurons in AD, while PB and cells were free of these epitopes (Robitaille et al., in preparation). The minor band 69 that is detected in PiD is a component of the PB. Indeed, anti-*tau*.E3 that specifically labeled *tau* 69 on Western blots of PiD brain homogenates also immunodetected PB on

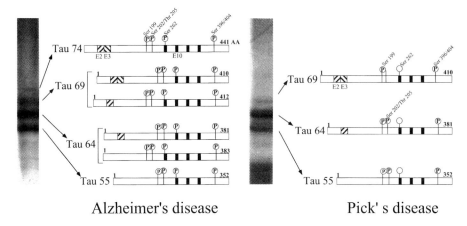

Alzheimer's disease   **Pick' s disease**

FIGURE 16.5. Synopsis of the isoforms of PTP aggregated in AD and PiD and some of their character-istic phosphorylation sites. Sites that are not phosphorylated are marked by an open circle. PTP in AD correspond to six isoforms, as described by Goedert et al. (1992) and modified by Sergeant et al. (1996). PTP from PiD, without the sequence encoded by exon 10, correspond to three isoforms. Antibodies against the peptide sequences encoded by exons 2 (304), 3 (anti-*tau*.E3), and 10 (anti-*tau*.E10) gave the corre-spondence between each electrophoretic band of PTP detected by AD2, and the *tau* isoforms (arrows). Monoclonal antibodies against different phosphorylated sites on *tau* proteins were used: AT8 for phos-phorylated Ser 202 and Thr 205, 12E8 for phosphorylated Ser 262, AD2 for Ser 396 and 404 and a poly-clonal antibody raised against phosphorylated Ser 199, namely SI99P. A difference in the phosphorylation state of PTP from PiD was noted when compared to AD: first, 12E8 did not detect PTP from PiD; second, AT8 did not detect Tau 69 from PiD.

tissue sections. Also in good agreement with biochemical findings, the labeling of PB with anti-*tau*.E3 was weaker than anti-*tau*.E2 (304), as observed on Western blots.

Neuronal populations affected in PiD are different from those affected in AD, with partic-ular involvement of granular cells of the dentate gyrus or the small neurons in layers II, III, and VI of the neocortex (Hof et al., 1994). Also, *in situ* hybridization studies showed that *tau* mRNAs with exon 10 are not expressed in granular cells from the dentate gyrus but are present in large pyramidal cells from cortical association areas (Goedert et al., 1990). From these results, one can hypothesize that neuronal populations can be distinguished by their constitutive sets of *tau* isoforms. Our data are strongly in favor of such a hypothesis. Indeed, they show that neuronal populations affected in PiD contain aggregated *tau* proteins without the encoded regions of exon 10, while neurons affected in AD express exon 10.

Therefore, we postulate that each neuronal population has a specific content of *tau* isoforms. A degenerative disorder provoking an aggregation of *tau* will generate PTP with a specific pro-file corresponding to the affected subset of neurons. Together our result emphasize at the bio-chemical level the selectivity of neurodegenerative disorders for specific neuronal populations.

FRONTAL LOBE DEGENERATION

FLD is a common but recently described disorder (Brun, 1987). It belongs, with PiD, to the group of FTD. Both diseases have a similar frontal pathology, and clinically FLD and PiD are indistinguishable. At the neuropathological level, PiD is generally easy to diagnose, especial-

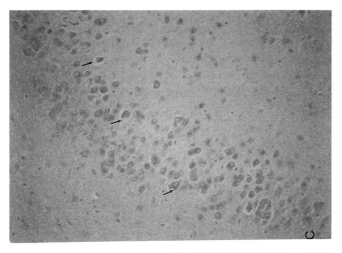

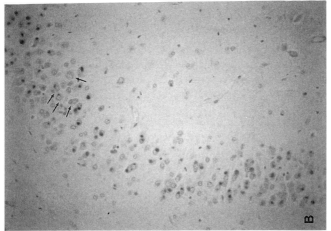

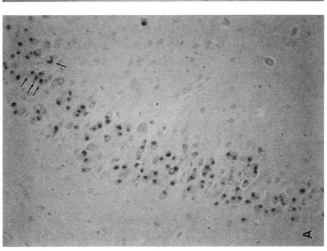

FIGURE 16.6. Dentate gyrus, PiD brain. (A) Exon 2 antibody reveals strongly immunolabeled PB within most granule cells. (B) Exon 3 shows less affinity for PB at the same dilution (1/1000), although fewer PB are marked compared with the exon 2 antibody (arrows in A and B). (C) Exon 10 displayed no PB, but rare fine intracytoplasmic elongated profiles (arrows) consistent with the neurofibrillary tangles were moderately immunolabeled (A–C × 300). Figure also appears in color section.

ly with the characteristic PB and cells immunostained with antibodies against phosphorylated *tau* proteins such as AD2 and the specific pattern of PTP (Delacourte et al., 1996). This is different for FLD, which has no specific neuropathological hallmarks. Morphological changes include neuronal cell loss, synaptic loss, spongiosis, and gliosis mainly in the superficial cortical laminae of the frontal and temporal cortices (Brun et al., 1994; Liu et al., 1996).

Vermersch et al. (1995a) reported the study of a young patient (53 years) with clinical symptoms of FTD very similar to those reported by the teams of Lund and Manchester. The neuropathology was also characteristic of FLD, non-AD, and non-Pick and was confirmed by Brun. Despite the fact that there was no neurofibrillary degeneration and therefore an absence of tangles and *tau*-positive dystrophic neurites, PTP were found in the frontotemporal region (Brodmann areas 9, 10, and 32) and the temporal pole (Brodmann area 38). The electrophoretic profile of the most affected brain regions corresponded to a *tau* triplet, as in AD, but smears of *tau* aggregates, always observed in AD, were not present in FLD. Also, the amounts of immunodetected abnormal *tau* in FLD were very low compared to those in AD. Interestingly, the hippocampus was not affected by the *tau* pathology, demonstrating that the pattern was totally different from that of AD. These results show that there is also a discrete and different *tau* pathology in FLD. It is likely that PTP assemble into small aggregates that are inaccessible to phosphatase activity generated during postmortem delay. Therefore, PTP from FLD are weakly labeled by AD2. However, these *tau* aggregates are different from those of AD, PiD, and PSP since they are not detected at the optical level. Consequently, FLD is distinguished by molecular lesions of *tau* proteins, while histological lesions of *tau* are absent. This has also been observed in a few other cases (Vermersch et al., 1995a).

These biochemical findings were also observed in a familial case of FLD (age 66 years), which was examined by Robitaille. The *tau* profile was similar to that of the previous cases reported by Vermersch et al. from a qualitative and quantitative point of view, except for discrete involvement of the hippocampal formation. The largest amounts of PTP were found in the frontal pole and represented 1% of the signal generally obtained in an AD brain. PTP were not detected in the parietal cortex. Also, in good agreement with our hypothesis on *tau* aggregation in FLD, discrete granular material was immunodetected by AD2 on tissue sections of the frontal cortex (Robitaille et al., in preparation).

However, it is clear that a study at a larger scale is necessary to determine if all FLD cases have this specific and discrete *tau* profile. From our experience, we do not exclude the possibility that some FLD cases can be without PTP (see the next section).

FTD WITHOUT PTP

As mentioned in the section "Frontal Lobe Degeneration," not all cases with FTD presented PTP. In fact, we analyzed two cases of FLD with extremely severe brain atrophy and huge gliosis. The neuropathology was therefore different from the typical FLD profile, as described by Brun et al. (1994). Our study showed that PTP were absent (Pasquier et al., in preparation). Also two cases with FTD associated with MND were investigated, which were devoid of PTP.

CORTICOBASAL DEGENERATION

CBD is a slowly progressive neurodegenerative disorder characterized by an extrapyramidal motor dysfunction (rigidity and dystonia) with asymmetrical, akinetic-rigid syndrome associated with cognitive impairment (apraxia and aphasia). Dementia usually emerges late in the course of the disease. Neuropathological examination shows neuronal loss, the presence of many chromatolytic neurons (Pick-like cells), neuritic changes, and NFT, as well as *tau*-immunoreactive glial plaques (reviewed by Feany et al., 1996). Clinically, CBD can cause symptoms similar to those of FTD. The question of the relationship between CBD, PID, and FTD was raised, and it has been suggested that CBD belongs to the Pick complex diseases (Kertesz and Munoz, 1996). Indeed, rare PB strongly immunolabeled by AD2 antibody can be readily observed in association cortex amid otherwise typical CBD lesions, such as large amounts of NFT, chromatolytic neurons, and glial plaques.

There is also an overlap, both clinically and neuropathologically, between PSP and CBD (Feany et al., 1995; Pillon et al., 1995), and it would be most helpful to distinguish these two pathologies on an immunochemical basis. PTP from PSP were characterized first by Flament et al. (1991) and Vermersch et al. (1994).

Tau Profile of PSP

This neurodegenerative disorder is characterized clinically by supranuclear ophthalmoplegia, pseudobulbar palsy, parkinsonism, and axial dystonia. Dementia is also a common feature in the later stages of the disease (Pillon et al., 1995). Using polyclonal antibodies against *tau* and anti-PHF, we demonstrated the presence of a specific profile of *tau* proteins in affected brain areas of patients with PSP (Flament et al., 1991; Vermersch et al., 1994). Their electrophoretic profile is significantly different from the one found in AD, since a characteristic doublet is revealed (*tau* 64 and *tau* 69) instead of the typical triplet found in AD. These findings have been confirmed by Schmidt et al. (1996). Also, 2-D gel analysis demonstrated that *tau* 64 and 69 had pI ranging from 6.1 to 7.2, which means that they are less acidic than the corresponding *tau* 64 and 69 of AD PHF-*tau* triplet (Delacourte et al., 1997b).

PTP in PSP are distributed in subcortical nuclei and cortical areas and are colocalized with NFT. Frontal regions are most strongly affected, especially the motor cortex. The presence of pathological *tau* 64 and 69 in frontal association brain areas suggests that the cortical pathology is likely to play a significant role in the cognitive changes observed in PSP (Vermersch et al., 1994).

Tau Profile of CBD

The profile of NFT is similar to that in PSP, as well as the *tau* electrophoretic profile (Figure 16.1) (Buée-Scherrer et al., 1996b; Feany et al., 1996). A two-dimensional gel analysis performed on samples from the frontal cortex of four CBD cases revealed that the doublet *tau* 64 and 69 was more acidic than in PSP (*tau* 69: PSP pI 6.45–7.0, CBD pI 5.95–7.0; *tau* 64: PSP pI 6.2–7.1, CBD pI 6.1–7.1) (Delacourte et al., 1997b). Furthermore, the immunoreactivity was much more intense in CBD (Figures 16.1, 16.3). Therefore, as mentioned by Feany et al. (1996), subtle changes in the *tau* profile may allow differentiation of PSP from CBD. However, this has to be corroborated in subsequent studies of more cases with clear-cut, definite diagnoses of either PSP or CBD. Nevertheless, the difference in biochemical pattern between CBD and PiD is unambiguous (Buée-Scherrer et al., 1996b; Delacourte et al., 1996).

CONCLUSION

Tau proteins are biochemical markers that are disease-specific. They are able to distinguish unambiguously nervous tissue affected by AD from normal aged tissue. This has now been verified in our laboratory on 80 AD cases versus 60 age-matched controls. Associated brain regions were always affected in AD, while they were unaffected in nondemented controls.

However, we have observed that there is an overlap of *tau* pathology in the hippocampal formation, since nondemented persons more than 75 years of age always have *tau* pathology in this brain region (Vermersch et al., 1995b).

Using the same immunochemical approach, we have typed other neurodegenerative disorders such as PSP and CBD, PiD, and myotonic dystrophy (Vermersch et al., 1996) (reviewed by Delacourte and Buée, 1997a). For that purpose, the *tau* pathology was investigated at different levels.

First, *tau* profiles on one-dimensional gels were determined using antibodies against normal *tau* and phosphorylated sites. This method is precise and accurate enough to type most of the neurodegenerative disorders. AD, Down's syndrome (Flament et al., 1990b), postencephalitic parkinsonism (Buée-Scherrer et al., 1994), and amyotrophic lateral sclerosis/parkinsonism dementia complex of Guam (Buée-Scherrer et al., 1995) are essentially characterized by a similar triplet of PTP; PSP and CBD by a *tau* doublet 64, 69 (Flament et al., 1991; Vermersch et al., 1994; Buée-Scherrer et al., 1996b; Feany et al., 1996; Schmidt et al., 1996); PiD by a major *tau* doublet 55, 64 (Delacourte et al., 1996), and myotonic dystrophy (Vermersch et al., 1996) by a major *tau* 55 band.

Second, for a given profile, it was possible to quantify the spatiotemporal extent of neurofibrillary degeneration. For instance, a strong correlation between the intensity of PTP and the number of tangles and dystrophic neurites has always been observed (Flament et al., 1991; Vermersch et al., 1992). This is not surprising, since PTP are the basic component of neurofibrillary degeneration. Also, the presence of PTP in the hippocampal formation was frequent in very old nondemented controls, while their presence in associated brain areas was always linked to a cognitive impairment. At the biochemical level, these results demonstrate that the extent of neurofibrillary degeneration explains the clinical symptoms. At last, PSP and CBD give a similar *tau* profile. But the intensity of immunodetected PTP was always stronger in CBD, and the difference was important and significant enough to distinguish both diseases.

Third, *tau* proteins were also studied on two-dimensional gels. This technique is more resolutive but also more time-consuming. It permits precise analysis of the isoelectric point of each band of PTP, as well as determination of their phosphorylation state and "exon" content. We have demonstrated that it is possible to study the charge, number, and location of each phosphorylated site if the corresponding mAb are at our disposal. At least 20 different immunological probes have been described in the literature. The most significant result presented here is that Ser 262 labeled by 12E8 (Seubert et al., 1995) is found on PTP from AD, PSP, and CBD but not on those from PiD.

We have also demonstrated that the "exon" content provides an additional possibility of typing *tau* proteins in PiD. They are characterized by isoforms that lack the region translated from exon 10, the opposite of AD.

Together our studies on PiD demonstrate that subsets of neurons can be distinguished by their specific pattern of *tau* isoforms. In fact, the specific profile of aggregated *tau* reflects diseases that affect specific neuronal populations. This result is important in understanding the etiopathogenesis of each neurodegenerative disorder.

In conclusion, PTP are helpful for the postmortem diagnosis, since some diseases with clinical and neuropathological overlap can be clearly diagnosed through this biochemical approach. Immunoprobes directed specifically against each isoform will improve diagnostic specificity and, hopefully, will also be useful for the early diagnosis of neurodegenerative disorders.

ACKNOWLEDGMENTS

Supported by INSERM and the Fonds de la Recherche en Santé du Québec network program and grants from the NIH (AG05138). Nicolas Sergeant is a recipient of a fellowship from the

France-Alzheimer Association. The authors are most grateful to Mrs. Andrée Demontigny, who provided skillful technical assistance with immunoperoxidase techniques, Mrs. Kathy Fortin, who provided expert biochemical assistance with tissue sampling and homogeneization; and Didier Lefranc for preparing anti-*tau*.E3.

Monoclonal antibody AD2 was developed through a collaboration between UMR 9921 from Montpellier University (Pr. B. Pau, Dr. C. Mourton-Gilles), Sanofi/Diagnostics Pasteur, and INSERM. 12E8, AT8, and 304 were generous gifts from Dr. D. B. Schenk (Athena Neurosciences), Dr. E. VanMechelen E (Innogenetics), and Dr. Michel Goedert (MRC, Cambridge), respectively.

REFERENCES

Alonso, AD, Grundke-Iqbal I, Iqbal K (1996): Alzheimer's disease hyperphosphorylated tau sequesters normal tau into tangles of filaments and disassembles microtubules. Nature Med 2:783–787.

Arima K, Murayama S, Oyanagi S, Akashi T, Inose T (1992): Presenile dementia with progressive supranuclear palsy tangles and Pick bodies—An unusual degenerative disorder involving the cerebral cortex, cerebral nuclei, and brain stem nuclei. Acta Neuropathol 84:128–134.

Arnold SE, Hyman BT, Flory J, Damasio AR, Van Hoesen GW (1991): The topographical and neuroanatomical distribution of neurofibrillary tangles and neuritic plaques in the cerebral cortex of patients with Alzheimer's disease. Cerebral Cortex 1:103–116.

Brion S, Plas J, Jeanneau A (1991): Pick's disease—A clinico-pathological point of view. Rev Neurol 147:693–704.

Brun A, Englund B, Gustafson L, Passant U, Mann DMA, Neary D, Snowden JS (1994): Clinical and neuropathological criteria for frontotemporal dementia. J Neurol Neurosurg Psychiatry 57:416–418.

Buée-Scherrer V, Buée L, Hof PR, Leveugle B, Gilles C, Loerzel AJ, Perl DP, Delacourte A (1995): Neurofibrillary degeneration in amyotrophic lateral sclerosis/parkinsonism-dementia complex of Guam—Immunochemical characterization of tau proteins. Am J Pathol 146:924–932.

Buée-Scherrer V, Buée L, Vermersch P, Hof PR, Leveugle B, Perl DP, Delacourte A (1994): Tau pathology in neurodegenerative disorders: Biochemical analysis. Soc Neurosci Abstr 20:1647.

Buée-Scherrer V, Condamines O, Mourton-Gilles C, Jakes R, Goedert M, Pau B, Delacourte A (1996a): AD2, a phosphorylation-dependent monoclonal antibody directed against tau proteins found in Alzheimer's disease. Mol Brain Res 39:79–88.

Buée-Scherrer V, Hof PR, Buée L, Leveugle B, Vermersch P, Perl DP, Olanow CW, Delacourte A (1996b): Hyperphosphorylated tau proteins differentiate corticobasal degeneration and Pick's disease. Acta Neuropathol 91:351–359.

Caillet-Boudin ML, Delacourte A (1996): Induction of a specific Tau Alzheimer epitope in SY-5Y neuroblastoma cells. Neuroreport 8:307–310.

Collins SJ, Ahlskog JE, Parisi JE, Maraganore DM (1995): Progressive supranuclear palsy: Neuropathologically based diagnostic clinical criteria. 58:167–173.

Constantinidis J (1985): Pick dementia: Anatomo-clinical correlations and pathophysiological considerations. In Rose FC (ed): Interdisciplinary topics in Gerontology. Modern Approaches to the Dementias. Part I: Etiology and Pathophysiology. Basel: Karger, pp 72–97.

Cooper PN, Jackson M, Lennox G, Lowe J, Mann DMA (1995): Tau, ubiquitin, and alpha beta-crystallin immunohistochemistry define the principal causes of degenerative frontotemporal dementia. Arch Neurol 52:1011–1015.

Delacourte A (1994): Pathological tau proteins of Alzheimer's disease as a biochemical marker of neurofibrillary degeneration. Biomed Pharmacother 48:287–295.

Delacourte A, Buée L (1997a): Normal and PTP as factors of microtubule assembly. Int Rev Cytol 171:67–224.

Delacourte A, Robitaille Y, Sergeant N, Buée L, Hof PR, Wattez A, Laroche-Cholette A, Mathieu J, Chagnon P, Gauvreau D (1996): Specific pathological tau protein variants characterize Pick's disease. J Neuropathol Exp Neurol 55:159–168.

Delacourte A, Sergeant N, Robitaille Y, Buée-Scherrer V, Buée L, David JP, Bussière T, Vermersch P, Hof PR, Gauvreau D, Wattez A (1997b): Pathological tau proteins are biochemical markers that differentiate several types of neurofibrillary degeneration. In Iqbal K, Winblad B, Nishimura T, Takeda M, Wisniewski H (eds): Alzheimer's Disease: Biology, Diagnosis and Therapeutics. John Wiley & Sons Ltd, pp 205–212.

Feany MB, Dickson DW (1995): Widespread cytoskeletal pathology characterizes corticobasal degeneration. Am J Pathol 146:1388–1396.

Feany MB, Ksiezak-Reding H, Liu WK, Vincent I, Yen SHC, Dickson DW (1995): Epitope expression and hyperphosphorylation of tau protein in corticobasal degeneration: Differentiation from progressive supranuclear palsy. Acta Neuropathol 90:37–43.

Feany MB, Mattiace LA, Dickson DW (1996): Neuropathologic overlap of progressive supranuclear palsy, Pick's disease and corticobasal degeneration. J Neuropathol Exp Neur 55:53–67.

Flament S, Delacourte A, Delaère P, Duyckaerts C, Hauw JJ (1990a): Correlation between microscopical changes and Tau 64 and 69 biochemical detection in senile dementia of the Alzheimer type. Acta Neuropathol 80:212–215.

Flament S, Delacourte A, Hemon B, Défossez A (1989): Characterization of two pathological Tau-protein variants in Alzheimer brain cortices. J Neurol Sci 92:133–141.

Flament S, Delacourte A, Mann DMA (1990b): Phosphorylation of tau proteins: A major event during the process of neurofibrillary degeneration. A comparative study between Alzheimer's disease and Down's syndrome. Brain Res 516:15–19.

Flament S, Delacourte A, Verny M, Hauw JJ, Javoy Agid F (1991): Abnormal tau proteins in progressive supranuclear palsy. Similarities and differences with the neurofibrillary degeneration of the Alzheimer type. Acta Neuropathol 81:591–596.

Goedert M, Jakes R, Vanmechelen E (1995): Monoclonal antibody AT8 recognises tau protein phosphorylated at both serine 202 and threonine 205. Neurosci Lett 189:167–170.

Goedert M, Spillantini MG (1990): Molecular neuropathology of Alzheimer's disease—in situ hybridization studies. Cell Mol Neurobiol 10:159–174.

Goedert M, Spillantini MG, Cairns NJ, Crowther RA (1992): Tau-proteins of Alzheimer paired helical filaments—abnormal phosphorylation of all six brain isoforms. Neuron 8:159–168.

Goode BL, Feinstein SC (1994): Identification of a novel microtubule binding and assembly domain in the developmentally regulated Inter-Repeat region of tau. J Cell Biol 124:769–782.

Hanihara T, Amano N, Takahashi T, Nagatomo H, Yagashita S (1995): Distribution of tangles and threads in the cerebral cortex in progressive supranuclear palsy. Neuropathol Appl Neurol 21:319–326.

Hasegawa M, Jakes R, Crowther RA, Lee VMY, Ihara Y, Goedert M (1996): Characterization of mAb AP422, a novel phosphorylation-dependent monoclonal antibody against tau protein. Febs Lett 384:25–30.

Hauw JJ, Verny M, Delaère P, Cervera P, He Y, Duyckaerts C (1990): Constant neurofibrillary changes in the neocortex in progressive supranuclear palsy—basic differences with Alzheimer's disease and aging. Neurosci Lett 119:182–186.

Hof PR, Bouras C, Perl DP, Morrison JH (1994): Quantitative neuropathologic analysis of Pick's disease cases—cortical distribution of Pick bodies and coexistence with Alzheimer's disease. Acta Neuropathol 87:115–124.

Hof PR, Charpiot A, Delacourte A, Buée L, Purohit D, Perl DP, Bouras C (1992b): Distribution of neurofibrillary tangles and senile plaques in the cerebral cortex in postencephalitic parkinsonism. Neurosci Lett 139:10–14.

Hof PR, Delacourte A, Bouras C (1992a): Distribution of cortical neurofibrillary tangles in progressive supranuclear palsy. A quantitative analysis of 6 cases. Acta Neuropathol 84:45–51.

Ikeda K, Akiyama H, Kondo H, Ikeda K (1993): Anti-tau-positive glial fibrillary tangles in the brain of postencephalitic parkinsonism of economo type. Neurosci Lett 162:176–178.

Jendroska K, Rossor MN, Mathias CJ, Daniel SE (1995): Morphological overlap between corticobasal degeneration and Pick's disease: A clinicopathological report. Mov Disord 10:111–114.

Kato S, Nakamura H (1990): Presence of two different fibril subtypes in the Pick body: An immunoelectron microscopic study. Acta Neuropathol 81:125–129.

Kertesz A, Munoz DG (1996): Clinical and pathological characteristics of primary progressive aphasia and frontal dementia. J Neural Trans Suppl 47:133–141.

Ledesma MD, Bonay P, Avila J (1995): Tau protein from Alzheimer's disease patients is glycated at its tubulin-binding domain. J Neurochem 65:1658–1664.

Liu XY, Erikson C, Brun A (1996): Cortical synaptic changes and gliosis in normal aging, Alzheimer's disease and frontal lobe degeneration. Dementia 7:128–134.

Matsuo ES, Shin RW, Billingsley ML, Vandevoorde A, Oconnor M, Trojanowski JQ, Lee VMY (1994): Biopsy-derived adult human brain tau is phosphorylated at many of the same sites as Alzheimer's disease paired helical filament tau. Neuron 13:989–1002.

Mayer RJ, Lowe J, Landon M (1991): Ubiquitin and the molecular pathology of chronic degenerative diseases. J Pathol 163:279–281.

McKhann GM, Drachman D, Folstein M, Katzman R, Price D, Stadlan EM (1984): Clinical diagnosis of Alzheimer's disease: Report of the NINCDS-ADRDA work group under the auspices of Department of Health and Human Services Task Force on Alzheimer's disease. Neurology 34:939–944.

Mori H, Nishimura M, Namba Y, Oda M (1994): Corticobasal degeneration: A disease with widespread appearance of abnormal tau and neurofibrillary tangles, and its relation to progressive supranuclear palsy. Acta Neuropathol 88:113–121.

Munoz-Garcia D, Ludwin SK (1986): Clinicopathological studies of some non-Alzheimer dementing diseases. Can J Neurol Sci 13:483–489.

Murayama S, Mori H, Ihara Y, Tomonaga M (1990): Immunocytochemical and ultrastructural studies of Pick's disease. Ann Neurol 27:394–405.

Neary D, Snowden J (1996): Fronto-temporal dementia: Nosology, neuropsychology, and neuropathology. Brain Cogn 31:176–187.

Pasquier F (1996): Neuropsychological features and cognitive assessment in frontotemporal dementia. In Wolters E CH, Scheltens PH (eds): Current Issues in Neurodegenerative Diseases, Vol 8. Dordrecht, the Netherlands: ICG Publications, pp 50–69.

Permanne B, Buée L, David JP, Fallet-Bianco C, Dimenza C, Delacourte A (1995): Quantitation of Alzheimer's amyloid peptide and identification of related amyloid proteins by dot-blot immunoassay. Brain Res 685:154–162.

Pick A (1906): Über einen weiteren SymptomenKomplex im Rahmen der Dementia senilis, bedingt durch umschriebene stärkere Hirnatrophie (gemischte Apraxie). Monatsschr Psychiatry Neurol 19:97–108.

Pillon B, Blin J, Vidailhet M, Deweer B, Sirigu A, Dubois B, Agid Y (1995): The neuropsychological pattern of corticobasal degeneration: Comparison with progressive supranuclear palsy and Alzheimer's disease. Neurology 45:1477–1483.

Schmidt ML, Huang R, Martin JA, Henley J, Mawaldewan M, Hurtig HI, Lee VMY, Trojanowski JQ (1996): Neurofibrillary tangles in progressive supranuclear palsy contain the same tau epitopes identified in Alzheimer's disease. PHF Tau 55:534–539.

Schweers O, Mandelkow EM, Biernat J, Mandelkow E (1995): Oxidation of cysteine-322 in the repeat domain of microtubule-associated protein tau controls the in vitro assembly of paired helical filaments. Proc Natl Acad Sci USA 92:8463–8467.

Sergeant N, Bussière T, Vermersch P, Lejeune JP, Delacourte A (1995): Isoelectric point differentiates PHF-tau from biopsy-derived human brain tau proteins. Neuroreport 6:2217–2220.

Sergeant N, David JP, Goedert M, Jakes R, Vermersch P, Buée L, Lefranc D, Wattez A, Delacourte A (1997a): Two-dimensional characterization of paired helical filament-tau from Alzheimer's disease:

Demonstration of an additional 74-kDa component and aged-related biochemical modifications. J Neurochem 69(2):834–844.

Sergeant N, David JP, Lefranc D, Vermersch P, Wattez A, Delacourte A (1997b): Different distribution of phosphorylated tau protein isoforms in Alzheimer's and Pick's diseases. FEBS Lett 412:578–582.

Seubert P, Mawaldewan M, Barbour R, Jakes R, Goedert M, Johnson GVW, Litersky JM, Schenk D, Lieberburg I, Trojanowski JQ, Lee VMY (1995): Detection of phosphorylated Ser(262) in fetal tau, adult tau, and paired helical filament tau. J Biol Chem 270:18917–18922.

Vermersch P, Bordet R, Ledoze F, Ruchoux MM, Chapon F, Thomas P, Destée A, Lechevallier B (1995a): Demonstration of a specific profile of pathological tau proteins in frontotemporal dementia cases. C R Acad Sci 318:439–445.

Vermersch P, David JP, Frigard B, Fallet-Bianco C, Wattez A, Petit H, Delacourte A (1995b): Cortical mapping of Alzheimer pathology in brains of aged non-demented subjects. Prog Neuro-psychopharmacol 19:1035–1047.

Vermersch P, Frigard B, Delacourte A (1992): Mapping of neurofibrillary degeneration in Alzheimer's disease—evaluation of heterogeneity using the quantification of abnormal tau proteins. Acta Neuropathol 85:48–54.

Vermersch P, Robitaille Y, Bernier L, Wattez A, Gauvreau D, Delacourte A (1994): Biochemical mapping of neurofibrillary degeneration in a case of progressive supranuclear palsy: Evidence for general cortical involvement. Acta Neuropathol 87:572–577.

Vermersch P, Sergeant N, Ruchoux MM, Hofmann-Radvanyi H, Wattez A, Petit H, Dewailly P, Delacourte A (1996): Specific tau variants in the brains of patients with myotonic dystrophy. Neurology 47:711–717.

CHAPTER 17

The Inflammatory Response in Pick's Disease

SIM K. SINGHRAO, JAMES W. NEAL, PHILIPPE GASQUE,
and GEOFF R. NEWMAN

Medical Electron Microscopy Unit (S.K.S., G.R.N.), Department of Medical Biochemistry
(S.K.S., P.G.), and Neuropathology Laboratory, Department of Histopathology (J.W.N.),
University of Wales College of Medicine, Heath Park, Cardiff CF4 4XN, United Kingdom

The neuropathology of Pick's disease (PiD) is characterized by a profound degree of cortical neuronal loss and spongiform change with accompanying astrocytosis restricted to the anterior parts of the temporal and frontal lobes (Constantinidis et al., 1974). Throughout the parts of the brain with severe pathological changes, the characteristic ballooned neurons are present, as well as the readily identified large intracytoplasmic inclusion, the Pick body. These inclusions contain the cytoskeletal protein tau (Murayama et al., 1987).

The central nervous system (CNS) is thought to have an immunologically privileged status due to the presence of the blood brain barrier (BBB), low levels of major histocompatibility complex (MHC), and adhesion molecules (critical for antigen presentation) and the absence of a lymphatic system (see Fabry et al., 1994, for review). On this basis, it is possible to argue that the contribution to any neurodegenerative disease, including PiD, by classic immune cells recruited from the circulation would be minor. This proposal is supported by the sparse numbers of lymphocytes and monocytes in PiD. However, there is growing evidence that resident cells play an important role in generating an inflammatory response in the CNS. It is well known that the astrocyte *in vitro* is a major source of cytokines and chemokines. Recently, it has been shown that astrocytes also express complement proteins. The synthesis of proinflammatory molecules by glial cells at the site of neuronal damage might contribute to toxicity and cell lysis.

INFLAMMATION AND COMPLEMENT IN NEURODEGENERATIVE DISEASES

A great deal of the information relating to the molecular basis of immune and inflammatory responses in the CNS has been derived from multiple sclerosis (MS) and viral encephalitis (see

Pick's Disease and Pick Complex, Edited by Andrew Kertesz and David G. Munoz
ISBN 0-471-17792-X   ©1998 Wiley-Liss, Inc.

Fabry et al., 1994; Kreutzberg, 1996; Merril and Benveniste, 1996; and Morgan and Gasque, 1996, for reviews), and both conditions have an obvious immune cell infiltrate in the form of lymphocytes and monocyte-macrophage cells. This population of cells provides a source of chemokines, cytokines (γ-interferon, tumor necrosis factor-α), and antibodies that mediates an immune and inflammatory response and induces demyelination and neuronal damage. The activation of astrocytes and microglia (the resident macrophage in the CNS) has also been associated with the inflammatory reaction in MS and encephalitis. In the neurodegenerative diseases, however, including PiD, the number of inflammatory cells is low, suggesting that perhaps glial cells are the potential mediators of an inflammatory response.

In the CNS, the complement system is an important component of the inflammatory response. The full cascade of this system has been extensively investigated in Alzheimer's disease (AD) (McGeer et al., 1989; Rogers et al., 1992; Eikelenboom et al., 1994) and in MS (Morgan, 1990, for a review), but there is little information about the potential contribution made by complement activation in PiD (Yasuhara et al., 1994).

Neurodegenerative diseases are characterized by an increase in the number of astocytes (associated with amyloid plaques) in AD and within the cortex of PiD. This is of particular interest because since 1987 a growing amount of experimental evidence has shown that astrocytes express complement and contribute to an inflammatory response in the CNS (Levi-Strauss and Mallat, 1987).

THE COMPLEMENT PATHWAY AND ITS RELEVANCE TO CNS INFLAMMATION

The expression of complement in the CNS has been reviewed elsewhere (Morgan, 1990; Morgan and Gasque, 1996, 1997). However, a brief summary of the complement system and its significance to CNS disease will be presented. The complement cascade consists of two separate sequences of functionally related proteins, the classical and alternative pathways (Figure 17.1). The classical pathway is activated at the C1 complex (containing C1q, C1r, and C1s) through binding of antigen-antibody complexes at the Fc part of the immunoglobulins (Ig). Binding of C1q to IgM or IgG produces activation of C1r, which in turn activates C1s. The next step in the sequence is the cleavage of C4 by C1s to produce C4b, which under optimum conditions becomes attached to the cell surface. C2 is the third component of the classical complement pathway, and when it binds to C4b, it results in the formation of the cleavage fragment C4b2a, which binds to C3 and creates a further complex, C4b2a3b. This complex catalyzes the cleavage of C5 and initiates the formation of the membrane attack complex (MAC). The alternative pathway differs from the classical complement pathway because the initial activation results from C3 binding to a cell membrane, which can then associate with factor B (FB) in the presence of factor D (FD) and properdin (P) to form the cleavage fragment C3bBb. The alternative pathway shares the final step with the classical pathway, with cleavage of C5 and formation of the MAC on the membrane of the target cell. The importance of the MAC complex is that it will form pores in cell membranes and induce cell lysis or cell toxicity (Figure 17.1).

Activation of either pathway also contributes to the production of an inflammatory response through a number of different effects, namely, chemotaxis (mediated by the complement anaphylatoxins C3a and C5a) and stimulation of the release of various cytokines and chemokines by myeloid cells (neutrophils and macrophages). During complement activation, target cells are opsonized (covered) with complement and complement fragments (opsonins: C1q; fragments of C3, C3b, iC3b, and C3d) to be recognized by competent macrophages (expressing receptors for complement) and removed by phagocytosis.

In view of its harmful effect, complement is closely controlled by several soluble (secreted by nucleated cells) and cell membrane-associated proteins, all named *complement regulators*.

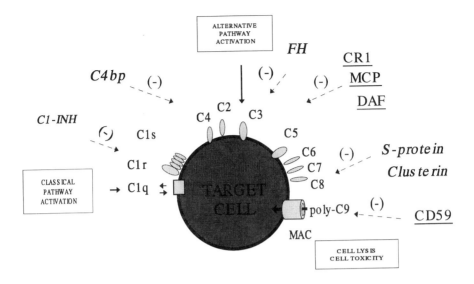

FIGURE 17.1. Complement can be activated through two different pathways. The classical pathway is activated by binding of complement C1q either to immunocomplexes (antibody-antigen, soluble or membrane bound) or to various substances (nucleic acid, myelin, amyloid fibrils etc.). The alternative pathway is activated by spontaneous binding of C3 to activating surfaces (tumour cells, virus etc.). Complement activation is tightly controlled by complement regulators expressed and secreted in the fluid phase (C1 inhibitor (C1-INH), C4b binding protein (C4bp), factor H (FH), S protein (Sp), clusterin (CLU) or regulators expressed on the membrane of nucleated cells (complement receptor type 1 (CR1), membrane cofactor protein (MCP), decay accelerating factor (DAF) and CD59.

These inhibit activation of complement at specific sites along each of the pathways (Figure 17.1). C1 inhibitor is a soluble inhibitor and blocks classical pathway activation at the C1 complex level by preventing association between C1q and C1r-C1s. The formation of C3 convertase is inhibited by C4b binding protein (C4bp), the cell surface protein DAF (decay accelerating factor, CD55), a membrane protein complement receptor type 1 (CR1, CD35), and membrane cofactor protein (MCP, CD46) (Morgan, 1990).

MAC formation is also under tight control through two membrane proteins, C8 binding protein (C8bp, HRF) and CD59 (Protectin, HRF20). Together these two proteins prevent the MAC-producing cell lysis or cell toxicity. A further protective mechanism preventing MAC formation is through two soluble regulatory proteins, S protein (Sp) and clusterin (CLU). The presence of complement regulators on a cell is good evidence for a protective mechanism preventing cell death or cell toxicity mediated by the MAC at high or sublytic doses, respectively.

EXPERIMENTAL EVIDENCE FOR COMPLEMENT EXPRESSION BY CNS CELLS

There is little information regarding the *in vivo* expression of complement in CNS diseases. Investigations have largely depended on postmortem tissue, which can be seriously altered by the effects of postmortem delay and premortem changes. For this reason, much of the initial work related to astrocyte expression of complement has been carried out *in vitro* and subsequently investigated *in situ,* using immunohistochemistry on both formalin fixed and frozen brain tissue.

Astrocytes

The astrocyte is the major glial cell and is a very important immunocompetent cell, capable (after stimulation) of expressing cytokines-chemokines, human leukocyte antigen (HLA) molecules, and adhesion molecules (Fabry et al., 1994). *In vitro* studies using human fetal astrocytes and cell lines obtained from gliomas have shown that the astrocyte is a source of all complement proteins. Cell culture studies have demonstrated that astrocytes, particularly after cytokine stimulation, synthesize complement components of the classical pathway (C1q, C1r, C1s, C4, C2, C3), of the alternative pathway (C3, FB, FD, P), and of the terminal pathway (C5, C6, C7, C9) to form a functional MAC (Gasque et al., 1992, 1993, 1995).

If astrocytes are able to express a full complement system, it seems that, at least *in vitro,* they are well protected from the undesired lytic and toxic effects of complement by expressing complement regulators. *In vitro* astrocyte cell lines express C1-INH, FH, FI, Sp, CLU, and the membrane regulators DAF, MCP, CR1, and CD59.

In vitro experiments also show that astrocytoma cell lines express a wide range of complement receptors, including CR1 together with CR2, which can bind to C3 fragments on immune complexes or on the membrane of the target cell. The anaphylatoxin C5a receptor was also recently characterized on fetal astrocytes and astrocyte cell lines, and it is believed that this receptor is implicated in cell activation and recruitment (chemotaxis) of astrocytes (Gasque et al., 1997).

Microglia

The microglia are the resident macrophages of the CNS, capable of becoming activated rapidly and of producing various cytokines (Kreutzberg, 1996). The majority of microglia remain in the adult CNS in an inactive state (ramified microglia), but when activated, notably by cytokines, they start to express high levels of HLA molecules and complement receptors (CR3 and CR4) and gain a typical amoeboid morphology.

Human microglia are very difficult to study *in vitro,* and no cell line is currently available. As a model, we have used a human macrophage cell line and have shown that *in vitro* this cell synthesizes the components of the terminal complement pathway components, C7, C8, and C9 (Gasque et al., 1995; Morgan and Gasque, 1996) together with the fluid phase regulators Sp and CLU (Gasque et al., 1995). This evidence raises the possibility that microglial cells (by analogy with macrophages) possess the capacity to synthesize complement.

Oligodendrocytes

The synthesis of complement by oligodendroglia is less well understood than that of either astrocytes or microglia. A human oligodendroglial cell line has been shown to express complement component C3, the membrane regulators CD 59, DAF, and MCP, and the fluid phase inhibitors C1 inhibitor, SP, and CLU (Gasque and Morgan, 1996).

Neurons

The majority of information relating to complement expression by neurons is derived from neuroblastoma cell lines and shows that these cells express regulatory proteins C1-INH, FH CLU, and Sp. Membrane proteins MCP and CD59 are also expressed, but not to the same degree as glial cells (Gasque et al., 1996b; Morgan and Gasque, 1996). One important feature of both oligodendroglia and neurons is that, unlike astrocytes, they are capable of activating complement spontaneously and through this are at risk of complement-mediated damage (Morgan and Gasque, 1996).

Astrocytes and microglia can express the full range of complement components and their regulators. The presence of activated astrocytes and microglial cells in the CNS capable of synthesizing complement supports the proposal that pathological changes in neurodegenerative diseases such as PiD could be mediated by local complement synthesis.

EVIDENCE FOR THE INVOLVEMENT OF COMPLEMENT IN PiD

Initial work investigating the molecular basis of the inflammatory response in neurodegenerative disease was carried out in AD (McGeer et al., 1989; Eikelenboom et al., 1994). This resulted in a great deal of information indicating the importance of the complement system as a contributory factor in the disease process. The absence of Ig and T lymphocytes in AD suggests that immune complex-mediated complement activation is not a major contributory factor. However, complement can be activated by fibrillary βA4, and it is believed that in AD, complement activation on neurons takes place after direct binding of complement C1q to amyloid fibrils present within the plaques (Rogers et al., 1992; Velazquez et al., 1997). Activation of the classical complement pathway in AD also provides an important signal to recruit microglia, and possibly astrocytes, into the vicinity of an amyloid plaque (Velazquez et al., 1997). The MAC formed on neuronal membranes will induce toxicity and cell lysis, but microglia have also been implicated in the removal of damaged neurons opsonized with complement proteins. The actual source of the complement in AD has not yet been identified.

PiD provides an excellent opportunity to study the molecular basis of inflammation in a neurodegenerative disease without the presence of numerous amyloid plaques and neurofibrillary tangles. One feature of PiD is the presence of large numbers of astrocytes, which provides an opportunity to investigate the *in vivo* expression of complement by reactive astrocytes (Figure 17.2). At present, there is little information about the contribution made by cytokines and chemokines to the disease process in PiD. The majority of the evidence used to support an inflammatory component in this disease has been obtained from investigation of the expression of a complement system in PiD brains (Singhrao et al., 1996). Immunohistochemistry results from PiD were validated by similar studies using age-matched control cases with the same postmortem time intervals as for the PiD cases. In the control cases, there was little evidence of the expression of complement components or complement activation. This suggests that postmortem autolysis does not in itself result in the activation of complement or the transfer of inflammatory cells and Ig into the brain from the systemic circulation. In the studies so far carried out, we have used both frozen and paraffin-embedded material from the same sites in the brain.

CELLULAR COMPONENTS OF INFLAMMATION IN PiD

Neurons

In PiD, evidence for activation of the classical pathway of complement was stronger than for activation of the alternative pathway, since factor B, related to the alternative pathway, was present in only two of the cases studied. The cytoplasm of neurons was strongly immunostained for antibodies to components of the classical pathway C1q, C4, C2, C3 (see Figure 17.3), C6, and C8 and weakly to C5. FB immunopositivity in two cases was present in the Pick body. The presence of membrane regulatory proteins CR1, DAF, and MCP was not detected in PiD brains. The results in this study using frozen and paraffin-embedded tissue were very similar.

Neuronal protection against complement attack in PiD is indicated by the absence of anti-MAC neo and C9 staining, together with immunopositivity for the complement inhibitors Sp, CLU, and CD59. This shows that the complement pathway does not continue to completion

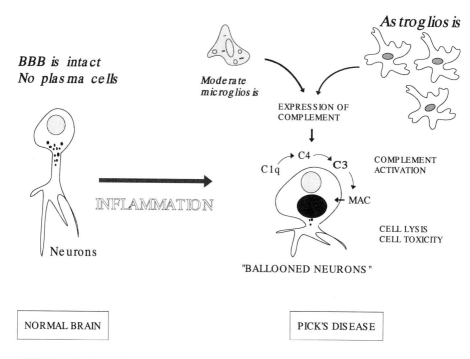

FIGURE 17.2. Expression and roles of complement in neurodegeneration: Pick's disease as a model. The complement system is not expressed or detected in normal brain. Complement can be synthesised by resident cells but at a very low level and only for some components (C1q, C3, C4). The blood brain barrier (BBB) is intact and therefore there is no transudation of plasma (source of complement) into the CNS tissue. In neurodegeneration, the astrocyte population is activated (astrogliosis) and from *in vitro* studies it is believed that astrocyte (and microglia) can synthesise a full complement system. The membrane attack complex (MAC) is cytolytic and cytotoxic to neurons but it is weakly detected in Pick's disease brain. Damaged neurons opsonised with complement fragments can, however, be specifically removed by activated phagocytes.

once activated. The intracellular localization of the complement components within Pick bodies is taken as evidence for internalization of complement-opsonized membranes that would also act as a protective mechanism, preventing continued complement activation and subsequent neuronal lysis and toxicity.

Microglia and Lymphocytes

The failure to find significant numbers of microglia stained by LN3 antibody, despite a clear inflammatory response in PiD, is surprising. LN3 is an antibody for HLA class II molecules, and our observations cannot exclude the possibility that microglia are present in PiD brains but that they are negative for HLA.

Astrocytes

Astrocytes were immunostained strongly using antibodies to C1q, C2, C3 (see Figure 17.3), C5, and C6 and weakly using antibodies to C4, C8, and anti-C9. No immunostaining was ob-

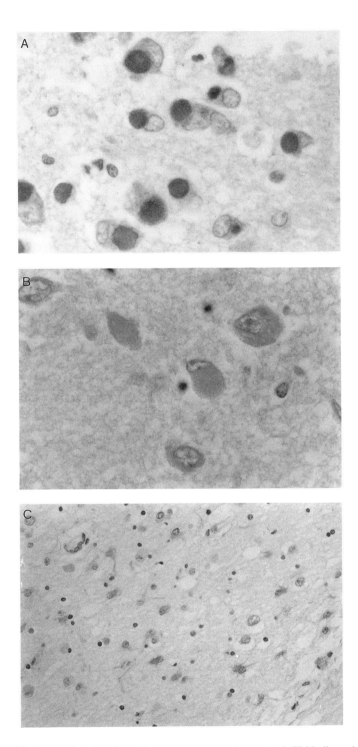

FIGURE 17.3. Immunodetection of complement on neurons and astrocytes in Pick's disease brains. Tissues sections were immunostained according to the protocol described by Singhrao et al. (1996). (A) immunostaining for tau. (B) immunostaining of ballooned neurons for complement C3. (C) staining of astrocytes for complement C3. All magnification (x1200). Parts A and B of figure also appear in color section.

tained using antibodies to MAC neo and antibodies to components of the alternative pathway. Membrane regulatory proteins were not detected, but positive immunostaining was noted for Sp and CLU. The same results were found in both frozen and paraffin-embedded, formalin-fixed tissue.

Intracellular immunopositivity for a number of complement components supports the interpretation that the astrocyte is the main source of complement in PiD, as predicted by *in vitro* experiments (Morgan and Gasque, 1996, 1997) (Figure 17.2). These findings raise the possibility that the astrocyte is an integral part of an inflammatory response and not merely a passive bystander caught up in the neuronal damage.

SIGNIFICANCE OF COMPLEMENT ACTIVATION IN PiD

The experimental evidence shows that astrocytes and microglia are capable of synthesizing a full range of complement proteins (Levi-Strauss and Mallat, 1987; Gasque et al., 1995, 1996a, b, 1997; Morgan and Gasque, 1996). The cellular basis of the inflammatory response in neurodegenerative disease is not dependent on the presence of either lymphocytes or microglia, but rather on the reactive astrocyte population. The production of complement by astrocytes could mediate neuronal lysis in neurodegenerative diseases. Variable numbers of neurons in PiD are able to survive in the presence of complement. The internalization of complement together with the presence of complement regulators (CD59, Sp, and CLU) within Pick bodies provides evidence that some neurons are capable of preventing complement-mediated damage by a number of different protective mechanisms (Singhrao et al., 1996). Unlike AD, in which there is a well-defined element in the form of fibrillary βA4 to activate complement (Rogers et al., 1992; Velazquez et al., 1997) in PiD, the mechanism responsible for complement activation has not been identified.

The potential therapeutic benefits of preventing complement activation have been exploited in several different drug trials using anti-inflammatory treatment of AD (McGeer et al., 1992; Rogers et al., 1993). The same therapeutic strategy could be applied to the treatment of PiD.

REFERENCES

Constantinidis J, Richard J, Tissot R (1974): Pick's disease histological and clinical correlations. Eur Neurol 11:208–217.

Eikelenboom P, Zhan SS, VanGool W, Allsop D (1994): Inflammatory mechanisms in Alzheimer's disease. Trends Pharmacol 15:447–450.

Fabry Z, Raine CS, Hart MN (1994): Nervous tissue as an immune compartment: The dialect of the immune response in the CNS. Immunol Today 15:218–224.

Gasque P, Chan P, Mauger C, Schouft MT, Singhrao SK, Dierich MP, Morgan BP, Fontaine M (1996a): Identification and characterization of complement C3 receptors on human astrocytes. J Immunol 156:2247–2255.

Gasque P, Fontaine M, Morgan BP (1995): Complement expression in human brain: Biosynthesis of the terminal pathway components and regulators in human glial cells and cell lines. J Immunol 154:4726–4733.

Gasque P, Ischenko A, Legoedec J, Mauger C, Schouft MT, Fontaine M (1993): Expression of the complement classical pathway by human glioma in culture. J Biol Chem 268:25068–25074.

Gasque P, Julen N, Ischenko A, Picot C, Mauger C, Chauzy C, Ripoche J, Fontaine M (1992): Expression of complement components of the alternative pathway by glioma cell lines. J Immunol 149:1381–1387.

Gasque P, Morgan BP (1996): Complement regulatory protein expression by a human oligodendrocyte cell line: Cytokine regulation and comparison with astrocytes. Immunology 89:338–347.

Gasque P, Thomas A, Fontaine M, Morgan BP (1996b): Complement activation on human neuroblastoma cell lines in vitro: Route of activation and expression of functional complement regulatory proteins. J Neuroimmunol 66:29–40.

Gasque P, Singhrao SK, Neal JW, Gotze O, Morgan BP (1997): Expression of the receptor for complement 5a (CD88) is up-regulated on reactive astrocytes, microglia, and endothelial cells in the inflamed human central nervous system. Am J Pathol 150:31–41.

Kreutzberg GW (1996): Microglia: A sensor for pathological events in the CNS. Trends Neurosci 8:312–318.

Levi-Strauss M, Mallat M (1987): Primary culture of murine astrocyte produces C3 and factor B two components of the alternative pathway of complement activation. J Immunol 139:2361–2366.

McGeer PL, Akiyama H, Itagaki S, McGeer EG (1989): Activation of the classical complement pathway in brain tissue of Alzheimer's disease patients. Neurosci Lett 107:341–346.

McGeer PL, McGeer EG (1996): Anti-inflammatory drugs in the fight against Alzheimer's disease. Ann NY Acad Sci 777:213–220.

McGeer PL, Rogers J (1992): Anti inflammatory agents as therapeutic approach to Alzheimer's disease. Neurology 42:447–449.

Merrill JE, Benveniste EN (1996): Cytokines in inflammatory brain lesions: Helpful and harmful. Trends Neurosci 19(8):331–338.

Morgan BP (1990): In Complement. Clinical Aspects and Relevance to Disease. London: Academic Press, Harcourt Brace Jovanovich. pp 141–156.

Morgan BP, Gasque P (1996): Expression of complement in the brain: Role in health and disease. Immunol Today 17(10):461–466.

Morgan BP, Gasque P (1997): Extrahepatic complement biosynthesis: Where, when and why? Clin Exp Immunol 1:1–7.

Mrak RE, Sheng JG, Griffin S (1995): Glial cytokines in Alzheimer's disease: Review and pathogenic implications. Hum Pathol 26:816–823.

Murayama S, Mori H, Ihara Y, Tomonaga M (1987): Immunocytochemical and ultrastructural studies of Pick's disease. Ann Neurol 47:393–405.

Piddlesden SJ, Morgan BP (1993): Killing of rat glial cells by complement: Deficiency of the rat analogue of CD59 is the cause of oligodendrocyte susceptibility to lysis. J Neuroimmunol 48:169–176.

Rogers J, Cooper NR, Webster S, Schulz J, McGeer PL, Stryen SD, Civin WH, Brachova L, Bradt B, Ward P, Lierburg I (1992): Complement activation by beta amyloid in Alzheimer's disease. Proc Natl Acad Sci USA 89:10016–10020.

Rogers J, Kirby LC, Hempleman SR, Berry DL, McGeer PL, Kaszniak AW, Zalinski J, Cofield M, Mansukhani L, Willson P, Kogan F (1993): Clinical trial of indomethacin in Alzheimer's disease. Neurology 43:1609–1611.

Singhrao SK, Neal JW, Gasque P, Morgan BP, Newman GR (1996): Role of complement in the aetiology of Pick's disease? J Neuropathol Exp Neurol 55:578–593.

Velazquez P, Cribbs D, Poulos T, Tenner A (1997): Aspartate residue 7 in amyloid β protein is critical for classical complement pathway activation: Implications for Alzheimer's disease pathogenesis. Nature Med 73:77–79.

Yasuhara O, Yoshinari A, McGeer EG, McGeer PL (1994): Expression of complement membrane attack complex and its inhibitors in Pick's disease. Brain Res 652:346–349.

CHAPTER 18

The Genetics of Pick Complex and Adult-Onset Dementia

LORRAINE N. CLARK and KIRK C. WILHELMSEN

Department of Neurology, University of California, San Francisco, CA 94110

INTRODUCTION

Tremendous progress in elucidating the genetics of adult-onset dementia has occurred in the last decade. The study of Alzheimer's disease (AD), the most common cause of adult-onset dementia, is perhaps one of the best examples of the advances that can be achieved by using genetics.

In addition to AD, other major causes of adult-onset dementia with a genetic etiology include frontotemporal lobar atrophy with nonspecific histology, the trinucleotide repeat disorders (TNRs), and prion disease (Table 18.1). These forms of dementia are autosomal dominant age-related disorders for which numerous risk factors, including mutations in specific genes, have been described.

Recently, several syndromes with frontotemporal lobar atrophy and nonspecific histology that are clinically related to Pick's disease (PiD) have been described (Foster et al., 1997). For the purpose of this review, we will refer to these syndromes as the *Pick complex* (Kertesz et al., 1994). These syndromes are linked to a few genetic locations, principally on chromosome 17q21–22 (Table 18.1).

This chapter will describe recent progress in our understanding of the genetics of Pick complex and adult-onset dementia in general.

ALZHEIMER'S DISEASE

Several genetic loci are associated with AD (Table 18.2). For example, one major risk factor for AD is the epsilon 4 allele at the apolipoprotein E gene (APOE) on chromosome 19q31.2 (Roses, 1996a). This allele has been found to be present in over 50% of AD patients with late-onset disease, regardless of whether or not they have a family history of dementia. Mutations

Pick's Disease and Pick Complex, Edited by Andrew Kertesz and David G. Munoz
ISBN 0-471-17792-X   ©1998 Wiley-Liss, Inc.

TABLE 18.1   Genetic Causes of Adult-Onset Dementia

Dementia	Example	Reference
Alzheimer's disease	AD1 familial	(Roses, 1996b)
CAG trinucleotide repeat disorders	Huntington's disease	(Willems, 1994)
Prion disease	Familial Creutzfeldt-Jakob disease	(Prusiner and Hsiao, 1994)
Pick complex	Disinhibition-dementia-parkinsonism-amyotrophy complex	(Foster et al., 1997)

in the presenilin 1 (PS1), presenilin 2 (PS2), and amyloid β protein precursor (APP) genes have been identified in familial Alzheimer's disease (FAD) (Chartier Harlin et al., 1991; Goate et al., 1991; Levy-Lahad et al., 1995b; Rogaev et al., 1995; Sherrington et al., 1995, 1996).

The protein product of the APP gene is a type 1 integral membrane glycoprotein. APP missense mutations associated with FAD are thought to affect precursor processing and contribute to Aβ production and to the accumulation of the amyloid deposits indicative of AD (Citron et al., 1992; Cai et al., 1993; Haass et al., 1994; Thinakaran et al., 1996).

Only a small proportion of cases of early-onset FAD are associated with missense mutations in the APP gene (Goate et al., 1991; Hendricks et al., 1992; Mullan et al., 1992). The majority of cases are linked to missense mutations (>40 missense mutations have been reported in the literature) at the PS1 gene located on chromosome 14 (St George-Hyslop et al., 1992; Alzheimer's Disease Collaborative Group, 1995; Sherrington et al., 1995). Presently, the function of the protein encoded by PS1 is unknown; however, the predicted structure deduced from its amino acid sequence is a seven-transmembrane protein that has been proposed to play a role in protein trafficking. The PS2 gene located on chromosome 1, which is associated with early-onset AD in Volga-German AD kindreds, has been proposed to have a function similar to that of PS1 based on their similar gene structures, homology of the gene products, and expression patterns in the brain (Levy-Lahad et al., 1995a; Rogaev et al., 1995; Lee et al., 1996).

Familial mutations in AD1, AD3, and AD4, when combined, account for a small percentage of the incidence of AD (Table 18.2) and have provided insight into the pathogenesis of AD. APOE alleles account for 60% of the susceptibility to AD. The APOE gene is the first gene that

TABLE 18.2   Genetic Risk Factors Associated with AD

Form of AD	Gene	Chromosome	References
AD1—familial autosomal dominant	APP	21	(Chartier Harlin et al., 1991; Goate et al., 1991)
AD2—late onset, familial, sporadic, susceptibility gene	APOE	19	(Roses, 1996a)
AD3—early onset, familial, autosomal dominant	Presenilin 1	14	(St. George Hyslop et al., 1992; Alzheimer's Disease Collaborative Group, 1995; Sherrington et al., 1995)
AD4—familial autosomal dominant	Presenilin 2	1	(Rogaev et al., 1995; Levy-Lahad et al., 1995a)

has been identified in which "normal" alleles predispose to dementia. Unlike mutations in the familial forms of AD, inheriting the E4 allele does not reliably predict whether or when a carrier will develop AD. Thus, it seems likely that more genes that predispose to AD remain to be discovered. We are gaining new insight into neurodegeneration and dementia with the identification of each new AD susceptibility gene. Whether this insight will lead to rational development of therapy cannot be predicted.

PICK COMPLEX

Several forms of non-AD dementia predominantly affecting the frontal and temporal lobes have been described. Among the most widely recognized form is PiD. Clinically, these disorders are characterized by progressive cognitive and behavioral disturbances, and they can be distinguished from AD on the basis of pathology (Brun, 1987). Until recently, the relationship of these syndromes both to each other and to PiD was unclear. Classification of these syndromes has been limited by the heterogeneity observed in both the clinical symptoms and neuropathological manifestations of patients. For example, although frontotemporal atrophy is considered diagnostic of PiD, the use of histopathological criteria, in particular the significance of the presence of Pick bodies, has differed among investigators (Constantinidis et al., 1974; Hansen and Crain, 1995). In contrast to AD, the genetics of the Pick complex is in the very early stages of research, and much remains to be elucidated. Research in this field has been hindered partly by the lack of an agreed-on classification scheme. Genetic family studies have not systematically looked at PiD with Pick bodies because it is rarely familial and because there are very few reports in the literature of PiD with Pick bodies that are described as hereditary disorders. However, the observation that approximately 50% of cases with frontotemporal dementia (FTD), a syndrome in the Pick complex, have a positive family history suggests that these syndromes may eventually be classified by molecular genetics (Neary et al., 1993; Giannakopoulos et al., 1995). The identification of two genetic loci for disorders within the Pick complex located on chromosomes 17q21–22 and 3p11.1–q11.2 suggests that such a classification scheme may soon by a reality (Wilhelmsen et al., 1994; Brown et al., 1995)

As this review focuses on the genetics of conditions in the Pick complex, the nosology that has been used in the primary literature is maintained. Syndromes that appear to be etiologically related to PiD based on linkage analysis are assumed to be part of the Pick complex. However, until the mutations that produce the syndromes in this spectrum are identified, we cannot be certain that the disorders discussed here are, in fact, etiologically related to PiD.

The frequency of Pick complex in the population is unknown. However, it has been estimated that FTD may account for as much as 20% of the cases of presenile dementia (Hulette and Crain, 1992; Giannakopoulos et al., 1995, 1996).

Chromosome 17-Linked Dementia

Disinhibition-dementia-parkinsonism-amyotrophy complex (DDPAC) is a familial adult-onset, nonspecific dementia. This syndrome was defined on the basis of a study of a family (Mo) whose members presented initially with disinhibition followed by frontal lobe dementia, parkinsonism, and amyotrophy (Lynch et al., 1994). Although this syndrome is clinically heterogeneous, the neuropathology and the linkage to chromosome 17 suggest that a mutation at a single genetic locus is responsible for this form of nonspecific dementia.

Following localization of the DDPAC locus to chromosome 17q21–22, loci for several clinically distinct disorders within the Pick complex were also mapped to the same region of chro-

TABLE 18.3   **Pick Complex Families Linked to Chromosome 17**

Kindred or Disorder	Affected Only Multipoint LOD Score	Flanking Genetic Markers	References
DDPAC, family (Mo)	>3	D17S798-D17S808	(Lynch et al., 1994)
PPND	6.8	D17S250-D17S943	(Wszolek et al., 1992)
Familial Multiple system tauopathy with presenile dementia	>3	THRA1-D17S791	
Seattle family A or DK	>3	No obligate recombinants	(Sumi et al., 1992)
FTD, Dutch family 1	>3	D17S800-D17S790	(Heutnik et al., 1997)
FTD, Duke University family 1684	>5	D17S800-D17S806	(Yamaoka et al., 1996)
HDD family 2	3.7	No obligate recombinants	(Lendon et al., submitted)
FTD, Australian family	>3	No obligate recombinants	(Hutton et al., 1996)
FTD, Dutch family 2	1.6	No obligate recombinants	(Groen and Endtz, 1982)
FTD, Dutch family 3	2.6	D17S953-D17S791	(Heutnik et al., 1996)
FTD, Karolinska family	2.7	No obligate recombinants	None
FPSG family A	1.6	No obligate recombinants	(Lansha et al., 1994; Petersen et al., 1995)
Seattle family B	1.1	No obligate recombinants	None

mosome 17. A recent report from the Chromosome 17-Related Dementia Conference (Ann Arbor, Michigan, October 1996) describes 13 families with progressive dementia linked to chromosome 17 (Table 18.3) (Foster et al., 1997). Some of the chromosome 17-linked dementias, such as FTD, clearly fall within the Pick complex. Palido–ponto–nigral degeneration (PPND) does not, suggesting that the clinical syndrome defined by Pick may be too restrictive to include all of the etiologically related syndromes that are due to mutations on 17q21–22.

All affected members of these families display prominent behavioral disturbances and parkinsonian features. The authors suggest the use of the term *frontotemporal dementia and parkinsonism linked to chromosome 17* (*FTDP-17*) until the genetic basis of these disorders is understood. Although eight families linked to the critical region of chromosome 17 were reported to have multipoint Lod scores above 3, five families did not meet the same criteria. However, families with Lod scores between 1 and 3 were considered to have a probable linkage to the critical region of chromosome 17. On the basis of the linkage data available in Table 18.3, the critical region containing the disease gene that segregates in families linked to chromosome 17q21–22 is a 2-3cM region between the genetic markers D17S800 and D17S791 (Figure 18.1).

Within this critical region numerous genes and transcribed genomic sequences have been localized (data from the human gene map at the National Center for Biotechnology Information, http://www.ncbi.nlm.nih.gov/). The functions of several genes in this region provide a list of potential candidates for mutation screening using a positional candidate gene approach (Table 18.4). Among the genes with known function (Table 18.4) located in the region implicated in the Pick complex, microtubule-associated protein tau (MAPT) has been of the most interest since aberrant forms of the MAPT protein, called tau, are associated with neurodegeneration in AD (Beyreuther and Masters, 1996). Abnormal tau pathology is also a feature of other dementias, including PiD (Buee-Scherrer et al., 1996; Delacourte et al., 1996; Jackson

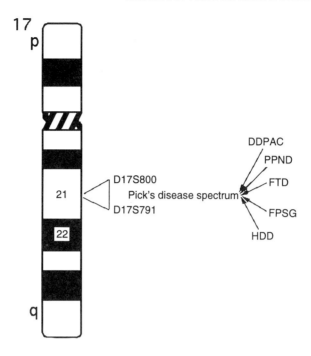

FIGURE 18.1. The FTDP-17 critical region.

and Lowe, 1996), progressive supranuclear palsy (Hauw et al., 1994; Conrad et al., 1996), parkinsonism-dementia complex of Guam (Chen, 1981; Shankar et al., 1989; Hirano, 1992; Kato et al., 1992), and FTD (Papasozomenos, 1995). For example, Vermersch et al. (1995) have detected hyperphosphorylated forms of tau with molecular weights of 55, 64, and 69 kDa in brain frontal and temporal lobes in FTD patients. We have investigated MAPT as a candidate gene for two Pick complex FTDP-17 families (DDPAC and PPND) and several sporadic cases of FTD. The MAPT gene was screened for mutations by direct sequencing of exons, and reverse transcription-polymerase chain reaction was used to check for splicing defects. Using

TABLE 18.4   Candidate Genes in the FTDP-17 Critical Region

Gene or Transcript	Function	Reference
MAPT	Cytoskeletal neuronal protein	(Kosik, 1992)
Dihydropryridine-sensitive L-type brain calcium channel β-1-B2 subunit	A subunit of a dihydropyridine-sensitive calcium channel expressed in brain (hippocampus)	(Pragnell et al., 1991; Powers et al., 1992)
Glial fibrillary acidic protein (GFAP) WI-6595	A glial specific class III intermediate filament protein GT198 mRNA, DNAJ protein homolog HSJ1; tissue-specific expression in brain neuronal layers; HSJ1 contains a DNAJ-like domain	(Brownell et al., 1991)

Data source: The human gene transcript map at http://www.ncbi.nlm.nih.gov and Clark and Wilhelmsen, unpublished data.

these approaches, we did not detect mutations in the MAPT gene that segregate with the disease in FTDP-17 families (Clark and Wilhelmsen, unpublished data, 1996). Furthermore, portions of MAPT have also been excluded as a candidate gene in an Australian (Martin et al., pers. comm.) and a Swedish (L. Lannfelt et al., pers. comm.) FTDP-17 family. There is still a possibility that mutations in MAPT regulatory sequences cause Pick complex and that some syndromes are due to mutations in MAPT.

Recently, Conrad et al. (1996) identified a polymorphic marker in MAPT that is in linkage disequilibrium with the rare late-onset neurodegenerative disorder progressive supranuclear palsy (PSP). The prevalence of PSP in the United States is estimated to be 1.39 per 100,000. The study by Conrad et al. implies that a mutation in MAPT, or at least in a gene that maps closely to MAPT, is associated with PSP. At present, it is unclear whether PSP is etiologically related to other 17q21–22-linked syndromes. Regardless of whether MAPT is responsible for Pick complex, the tau pathology in these and other neurodegenerative disorders indicates that MAPT should be investigated further.

Chromosome 3-Linked Dementia

A disease locus for familial nonspecific frontotemporal dementia located on chromosome 3p11.1–q11.2 was recently identified by linkage studies using a large pedigree from the Jutland region of Denmark. In this study, other areas of the genome known to contain dementia susceptibility loci were excluded and a locus on chromosome 3 that defines a nonspecific dementia was identified. Brown et al. (1995) propose the term *familial nonspecific dementia* because the disease is not specific in terms of the pathology of brain structures. To date, this publication is the only report of linkage of a nonspecific dementia to chromosome 3. Further studies will be necessary to determine the proportion of all cases of nonspecific dementia that are caused by a mutation at the locus on chromosome 3. However, Brown et al. (1995) propose that families with frontal lobe dementia from regions such as Denmark, southern Sweden, and northern England most likely have a common ancestry and probably share a similar etiology.

The clinical syndrome described by Pick continues to be the subject of active investigation. Clinical and pathological studies have continued to increase our understanding of the Pick complex. To date, two distinct genetic loci associated with the Pick complex have been identified. Molecular genetic studies have established that the FTDs are genetically heterogeneous and may be classified at the molecular level.

NEURODEGENERATIVE DISORDERS CAUSED BY EXPANSION OF TRINUCLEOTIDE REPEATS

Genetic loci containing expanded trinucleotide repeats have been identified for several neurodegenerative disorders, including spinal bulbar muscular atrophy (Kennedy's disease), Huntington's disease, spinocerebellar ataxia type 1 (SCA1) and type 2 (SCA2), dentatorubral-pallidoluysian atrophy (DRPLA), and Machado-Joseph disease (Willems, 1994; Warren, 1996). The incidence of Huntington's disease and SCA in the population is estimated to be approximately 4–7 per 100,000 individuals; DRPLA and Machado-Joseph disease are less prevalent than the other TNR disorders, representing 2–2.5% of all forms of spinocerebellar degeneration. These disorders have a common disease mechanism that involves unstable expansion of the trinucleotide repeat CAG (<100 CAG repeats) located in the open reading frame of a gene. These CAG repeats are translated into stretches of glutamine residues and are thought to result in a gain-of-function mutation. The age of onset of these diseases correlates with the number

TABLE 18.5   The TNR Neurodegenerative Disorders

Disorder	Chromosome Location of Expanded CAG Repeat	Reference
Kennedy's	Xq11.2–Xq12	(LA Spada et al., 1991)
Huntington's	4p16.3	(The Huntington's Disease Collaborative Research Group, 1993)
SCA1	6p23	(Orr et al., 1993)
SCA2	12q23–q24.1	(Imbert et al., 1996; Pulst et al., 1996; Sanpei et al., 1996)
DRPLA	12p13.31	(Burke et al., 1994; Koide et al., 1994)
Machado-Joseph	14q21	(Kawaguchi et al., 1994)

of repeats, and the number of repeats tends to increase in successive generations. This phenomenon, called *genetic anticipation,* is a feature observed in all of the TNR neurodegenerative disorders. Dynamic mutations of this kind may also account for other neurodegenerative disorders that display genetic anticipation and for which the disease gene has yet to be identified. The neurodegenerative disorders listed in Table 18.5 all encode proteins containing an uninterrupted stretch of glutamine residues that varies in length. For example, normal alleles of the HD gene encode 8 to 36 glutamine residues; in contrast, disease alleles result in 38 to >120 glutamine residues in the huntingtin protein (The Huntington's Disease Collaborative Research Group, 1993; MacDonald and Gusella, 1996). Although the precise mechanism of neurodegeneration involved in the TNR disorders is not understood, the presence of an expanded polyglutamine tract is neuronal proteins encoded by the TNR genes suggests a common mechanism of cell death (Burright et al., 1995; Perutz et al., 1995; Trottier et al., 1995; Ikeda et al., 1996).

Genetic anticipation has not been observed in families with Pick complex except in the Jutland pedigree with familial nonspecific frontotemporal dementia located on chromosome 3p11.1–q11.2 (Foster et al., 1997).

THE PRION DISEASES

The Prion diseases, also known as the *spongiform encephalopathies,* are a group of neurodegenerative diseases that can occur as inherited, sporadic, and transmissible forms (Prusiner and Hsiao, 1994). Four distinct human diseases comprise the prion disease group: Creutzfeldt-Jakob disease (CJD), Gerstmann-Straussler-Scheinker disease (GSS), fatal familial insomnia (FFI), and Kuru. CJD is the most common sporadic form of prion disease, while GSS and FFI represent familial forms. The exact incidence of familial prion disease is unknown, but inherited prion disease represents a small proportion of all prion diseases and is estimated to be 1–10 per 100 million individuals (Hsiao and Prusiner, 1990). GSS is inherited as an autosomal dominant Mendelian disorder by linkage to a missense mutation at codon 102 of the prion protein (PRNP) gene located on chromosome 20 (Hsiao et al., 1989). In familial forms of CJD and GSS, a group of genetic mutations consisting of missense mutations and variations in the number of octapeptide repeat elements has been identified (Owen et al., 1989; Hsiao and Prusiner, 1990; Goldfarb et al., 1991; Collinge et al., 1992; Kretzschmar et al., 1992). FFI is a rare prion disorder linked to a mutation at codon 178 of the PRNP gene and is distinguished from CJD by the presence of insomnia and thalamic involvement (Medori et al., 1992).

CONCLUSIONS

Genetic linkage analysis has led to the identification of several distinct disease loci responsible for dementia. Molecular genetic analysis has revealed significant heterogeneity among the major causes of adult-onset dementia but, more importantly, it has provided a powerful tool for classification.

The next major advance to be made in the understanding of adult-onset dementia will be to correlate the disease phenotype with the genotype. Intensive research in the fields of AD and the TNRs is already providing some clues to disease pathogenesis and has uncovered an unsuspected etiological relationship among the chromosome 17q21–22-linked Pick complex syndromes.

REFERENCES

Alzheimer's Disease Collaborative Group (1995): The structure of the presenilin 1 (S182) gene and identification of six novel mutations in early onset AD families. Nat Genet 11:219–222.

Beyreuther K, Masters CL (1996): Alzheimer's disease. Tangle disentanglement. Nature 383:476–477.

Brown J, Ashworth A, Gydesen S, Sorensen A, Rossor M, Hardy J, Collinge J (1995): Familial non-specific dementia maps to chromosome 3. Hum Mol Genet 4:1625–1628.

Brownell E, Lee AS, Pekar SK, Pravtcheva D, Ruddle FH, Bayney RM (1991): Glial fibrillary acid protein, an astrocyte-specific marker, maps to human chromosome 17. Genomics 10:1087–1089.

Brun A (1987): Frontal lobe degeneration of non-Alzheimer type. I. Neuropathology. Arch Gerontol Geriatr 6:193–208.

Buee-Scherrer V, Hof PR, Buee L, Leveugle B, Vermersch P, Perl DP, Olanow CW, Delacourte A (1996): Hyperphosphorylated tau proteins differentiate corticobasal degeneration and Pick's disease. Acta Neuropathol 91:351–359.

Burke JR, Wingfield MS, Lewis KE, Roses AD, Lee JE, Hulette C, Pericak-Vance MA, Vance JM (1994): The Haw-River syndrome: denato-rubropallidoluysian atrophy (DRPLA) in an African–American family. Nature Genet 7:521–524.

Burright EN, Clark HB, Servadio A, Matilla T, Feddersen RM, Yunis WS, Duvick LA, Zoghbi HY, Orr HT (1995): SCA1 transgenic mice: A model for neurodegeneration caused by an expanded CAG trinucleotide repeat. Cell 82:937–948.

Cai X-D, Golde TE, Younkin SG (1993): Release of excess amyloid β protein from a mutant amyloid β protein precursor. Science 259:514–516.

Chartier–Harlin MC, Crawford F, Houlden H, Warren A, Hughes D, Fidani L, Goate AM, Rossor M, Roques P, Hardy J, Mullan M (1991): Early-onset Alzheimer's disease caused by mutations at codon 717 of the β-amyloid precursor protein gene. Nature 353:844–846.

Chen L (1981): Neurofibrillary change on Guam. Arch Neurol 38:16–18.

Citron M, Oltersdorf T, Haass C, McConlogue L, Hung AY, Seubert P, Vigo-Pelfrey C, Lieberburg I, Selkoe DJ (1992): Mutation of the β-amyloid precursor protein in familial Alzheimer's disease increases β-protein production. Nature 360:672–674.

Collinge J, Brown J, Hardy J, Mullan M, Rossor MN, Baker H, Crow TJ, Lofthouse R, Poulter M, Ridley R, Owen F, Bennet C, Dunn G, Harding AE, Quinn N, Doshi B, Roberts GW, Honovar M, Janota I, Lankos PL (1992): Inherited prion disease with 144 base pair gene insertion. II. Clinical and pathological features. Brain 115:687–710.

Conrad C, Andreadis A, Trojanowski JQ, Dickson DW, Kang D, Chen X, Wiederholt W, Hansen L, Masilah E, Thal LJ, Katzman R, Xia Y, Saitoh T (1997): Genetic evidence for the involvement of tau in progressive supranuclear palsy. Ann of Neurol 41:277–281.

Constantinidis J, Richard J, Tissot R (1974): Pick's disease. Histological and clinical correlations. Eur Neurol 11:208–217.

Delacourte A, Robitaille Y, Sergeant N, Buee L, Hof PR, Wattez A, Laroche-Cholette A, Mathieu J, Chagnon P, Gauvreau D (1996): Specific pathological tau protein variants characterize Pick's disease. J Neuropathol Exp Neurol 55(2):159–168.

Foster NL, Wilhelmsen KC, Sima AAF, Jones MZ, D'Amato C, Gilman S. The Participants of the Chromosome 17-Related Dementia Conference (1997): Frontotemporal Dementia and Parkinsonism Linked to Chromosome 17: A consensus conference. Ann Neurol 41:706–715.

Giannakopoulos P, Hof PR, Bouras C (1995): Dementia lacking distinctive histopathology: Clinicopathological evaluation of 32 cases. Acta Neuropathol 89:346–355.

Giannakopoulos P, Hof PR, Savioz A, Guimon J, Antonarakis SE, Bouras C (1996): Early-onset dementias: Clinical, neuropathological and genetic characteristics. Acta Neuropathol 91:451–465.

Goate AM, Chartier Harlin MC, Mullan M, Brown J, Crawford F, Fidani L, Giuffra L, Haynes A, Irving N, James L, Mant R, Newton P, Rooke K, Roques P, Talbot C, Pericak-Vance M, Roses A, Williamson R, Rosser M, Owen M, Hardy J (1991): Segregation of a missense mutation in the amyloid precursor protein gene with familial Alzheimer's disease. Nature 349:704–706.

Goldfarb LJ, Brown P, McCombie WR, Goldgaber D, Swergold GD, Wells PR, Cervenakova L, Baron H, Gibbs CJ, Jr., Gajdusek DC (1991): Transmissible familial Creutzfeldt-Jakob disease associated with five, seven, and eight extra octapeptide coding repeats in the PRNP gene. Proc Natl Acad Sci USA 88:10926–10930.

Groen JJ, Endtz LJ (1982): Hereditary Pick's disease. Second reexamination of the large family and discussion of other hereditary cases, with particular reference to electroencephalography, a computerized tomography. Brain 105:443–459.

Haass C, Hung AY, Selkoe DJ, Teplow DB (1994): Mutations associated with a locus for familial Alzheimer's disease result in alternative processing of amyloid β-protein precursor. J Biol Chem 269:17741–17748.

Hansen LA, Crain BJ (1995): Making the diagnosis of mixed and non-Alzheimer's dementias. Arch Pathol Lab Med 119:1023–1031.

Hauw JJ, Daniel SE, Dickson D, Horoupian DS, Jellinger K, Lantos PL, McKee A, Tabaton M, Litvan I (1994): Preliminary NINDS neuropathologic criteria for Steele-Richardson-Olszewski Syndrome (progressive supranuclear palsy). Neurol 44:2015–2019.

Hendricks L, van Duijn CM, Cras P, Cruts M, Van Hul W, Van Harskamp F, Warren A, McInnes MG, Antonarakis SE, Martin JJ (1992): Presenile dementia and cerebral haemorrhage linked to a mutation at codon 692 for the b-amyloid precursor protein gene. Nat Genet 1:218–221.

Heutink P, Stevens M, Rizzu P, Bakker E, Kros JM, Tibben A, Niermeijer MF, van Duijn CM, Oostra BA, van Swieten JC (1997): Hereditary frontotemporal dementia is linked to chromosome 17q21–22: A genetic and clinicopathological study of three Dutch Families. Ann Neurol 41:150–159.

Hirano A (1992): Amyotrophic lateral sclerosis and parkinsonism-dementia complex on Guam: Immunohistochemical studies. Keio J Med 41:6–9.

Hsiao K, Baker HF, Crow TJ, Poulter M, Owen F, Terwilliger JD, Westaway D, Ott J, Prusiner SB (1989): Linkage of a prion protein missense variant to Gerstmann-Sträussler syndrome. Nature 338:342–345.

Hsiao K, Prusiner SB (1990): Inherited human prion diseases. Neurology 40:1820–1827.

Hulette CM, Crain BJ (1992): Lobar atrophy without Pick bodies. Clin Neuropathol 11:151–156.

Hutton M, Baker M, Houlden H, Crook R, Kucera S, Hardy J, Dodd P, Hayward N, Webb S, Kwok J, Schofield P, Dark F (1996): Genetic analysis of an Australian pedigree with autosomal dominant non-Alzheimer's dementia (abstract). Am J Hum Genet 1196 (59 Suppl): A 221.

Ikeda H, Yamaguchi M, Sugai S, Aze Y, Narumiya S, Kakizuka A (1996): Expanded polyglutamine in the Machado-Joseph disease protein induces cell death *in vitro* and *in vivo*. Nat Genet 13:196–202.

Imbert G, Saudou F, Yvert G, Devys D, Trottier Y, Garnier J-M, Weber C, Mandel J-L, Cancel G, Abbas N, Durr A, Didierjean O, Stevanin G, Agid Y, Brice A (1996): Cloning of the gene for spinocerebellar ataxia 2 reveals a locus with high sensitivity to expanded CAG/glutamine repeats. Nat Genet 14:285–291.

Jackson M, Lowe J (1996): The new neuropathology of degenerative frontotemporal dementias. Acta Neuropathol 91:127–134.

Kato S, Hirano A, Llena JF, Ito H, Yen SH (1992): Ultrastructural identification of neurofibrillary tangles in the spinal cords in Guamanian amyotrophic lateral sclerosis and parkinsonism-dementia complex on Guam. Acta Neuropathol 83:277–282.

Kawaguchi Y, Okamoto T, Taniwaki M, Aizawa M, Inoue M, Katayama S, Kawakami H, Nakamura S, Nishimura M, Akiguchi I (1994): CAG expansions in a novel gene for Machado-Joseph disease at chromosome 14q32.1. Nat Genet 8:221–228.

Kertesz A, Hudson L, MacKenzie IRA, Munoz DG (1994): The pathology and nosology of primary progressive aphasia. Neurology 44:2065–2072.

Koide R, Ikeuchi T, Onodera O, Tanaka H, Igarashi S, Endo K, Takahashi H, Kondo R, Ishikawa A, Hayashi T, Saito M, Tomoda A, Miike T, Naito H, Ikuta F, Tsuji A (1994): Unstable expansion of a CAG repeat in hereditary denatorubral-pallidoluysian atrophy (DRPLA). Nat Genet 6:9–12.

Kosik KS (1992): Tau protein and Neurodegeneration. Mol Neurobiol 4:171–179.

Kretzschmar HA, Kufer P, Riethmuller G, DeArmond SJ, Prusiner SB, Schiffer D (1992): Prion protein mutation at codon 102 in an Italian family with Gerstmann-Straussler-Scheinker syndrome. Neurology 42:809–810.

La Spada AR, Wilson EM, Lubahn DB, Harding AE, Fischbeck KH (1991): Androgen receptor gene mutations in X-linked spinal and bulbar muscular atrophy. Nature 352:77–79.

Lanska DJ, Currier RD, Cohen M, Gambetti P, Smith EE, Bebin J, Jackson JF, Whitehouse PJ, Markesberry WR (1994): Familial progressive subcortical gliosis. Neurology 44:1633–1643.

Lee MK, Slunt HH, Martin LJ, Thinakaran G, Kim G, Gandy SE, Seeger M, Koo E, Price DL, Sisodia SS (1996): Expression of presenilin 1 and 2 (PS1 and PS2) in human and murine tissues. J Neurosci 16(23):7513–7525.

Lendon CL, Lynch T, Norton J, Busfield F, Craddock N, Chakraverty S, Gopalakrishnan G, Shears SD, Grimmet W, Wilhelmsen KC, Hansen L, McKeel DW, Morris JC, Goate AM: Hereditary Dysphasic Disinhibition Dementia: a frontal lobe dementia linked to 17q21–22 (submitted).

Levy-Lahad E, Wasco W, Poorkaj P, Romano DM, Oshima J, Pettingell WH, Yu CE, Jondro PD, Schmidt SD, Wang K (1995a): Candidate gene for the chromosome 1 familial Alzheimer's disease locus. Science 269:973–977.

Levy-Lahad E, Wijsman EM, Nemens E, Anderson L, Goddard KA, Weber JL, Bird TD, Schellenberg GD (1995b): A familial Alzheimer's disease locus on chromosome 1. Science 269:970–973.

Lynch TS, Sano M, Marder KS, Bell KL, Foster NL, Defendini RF, Sima AAF, Keohane C, Nygaard TG, Fahn S, Mayeux R, Rowland LP, Wilhelmsen KC (1994): Clinical characteristics of a family with chromosome 17-linked disinhibition-dementia-parkinsonism-amyotrophy complex (DDPAC). Neurology 44:1878–1884.

MacDonald ME, Gusella JF (1996): Huntington's disease: Translating a CAG repeat into a pathogenic mechanism. Curr Opin Neurobiol 6(5):638–643.

Medori R, Tritschler HJ, LeBlanc A, Villare F, Manetto V, Chen HY, Xue R, Leal S, Montagna P, Cortelli P, Tinuper P, Avani P, Mochi M, Baruzzi A, Hauw JJ, Ott J, Lugaresi E, Autilio-Gambetti L, Gambetti P (1992): Fatal familial insomnia, a prion disease with a mutation at codon 178 of the prion protein gene. N Engl J Med 326(7):444–449.

Mullan M, Crawford F, Axelman K, Houlden H, Lilius L, Winblad B, Lannfelt L (1992): A pathogenic mutation for probable Alzheimer's disease in the APP gene at the N-terminus. Nat Genet 1:345–347.

Neary D, Snowden JS, Mann DM (1993): The clinical pathological correlates of lobar atrophy. A review. Dementia 4:154–159.

Orr HT, Chung M-Y, Banfi S, Kwiatkowski TJJ, Servadio A, Baudet AL, McCall AE, Duvick LA, Ranum LPW, Zoghbi HY (1993): Expansion of an unstable trinucleotide CAG repeat in spinocerebellar ataxia type I. Nat Genet 4:221–226.

Owen F, Poulter M, Lofthouse R, Collinge J, Crow TJ, Risby D, Baker HF, Ridley RM, Hsiao K, Prusiner SB (1989): Insertion in prion protein gene in familial Creutzfeldt-Jakob disease. Lancet 1:51–52.

Papasozomenos SC (1995): Nuclear tau immunoreactivity in presenile dementia with motor neuron disease: A case report. Clin Neuropathol 14:100–104.

Perutz M, Johnson T, Suzuki M, Finch JT (1995): Glutamine repeats as polar zippers: Their possible role in inherited neurodegenerative diseases. Molec Med 1(7):718–721.

Petersen RB, Tabaton M, Chen SG, Monari MD, Richardson SL, Lynch T, Manetto V, Lanska DJ, Markesbery WR, Currier RD, Autilio-Gambetti L, Wilhelmsen KC, Gambetti P (1995): Familial progressive subcortical gliosis: Presence of prions and linkage to chromosome 17. Neurology 45:1062–1067.

Powers PA, Liu S, Hogan K, Gregg RG (1992): Skeletal muscle and brain isoforms of a beta subunit of human voltage-dependent calcium channels are encoded by a single gene. J Biol Chem 267:22967–22972.

Pragnell M, Sakamoto J, Jay SD, Campbell KP (1991): Cloning and tissue-specific expression of the brain calcium channel β subunit. FEBS Lett 291:253–258.

Prusiner SB, Hsiao KK (1994): Human prion diseases. Ann Neurol 35:385–395.

Pulst S-M, Nechiporuk A, Nechiporuk T, Gispert S, Chen X-N, Lopes-Cendes I, Pearlman S, Starkman S, Orozco-Diaz G, Lunkes A, DeJong P, Rouleau G, Auburger G, Korenberg JR, Figueroa C, Sahba S (1996): Moderate expansion of a normally biallelic trinucleotide repeat in spinocerebellar ataxia type 2. Nat Genet 14:269–276.

Rogaev EI, Sherrington R, Rogaeva EA, Levesque G, Ikeda M, Liang Y, Chi H, Lin C, Holman K, Tsuda T, Mar L, Sorbi S, Nacmias B, Piacentini S, Amaducci L, Chumakov I, Cohen D, Lannfelt L, Fraser PE, Rommens JM, St George-Hyslop PH (1995): Familial Alzheimer's disease in kindreds with missense mutations in a gene on chromosome 1 related to the Alzheimer's disease type 3 gene. Nature 376:775–778.

Roses AD (1996a): Apolipoprotein E alleles as risk factors in Alzheimer disease. Ann Rev Med 47:387–400.

Roses AD (1996b): The Alzheimer diseases. Curr Opin Neurobiol 6:644–650.

Sanpei K, Takano H, Igarashi S, Sato T, Oyake M, Sasaki H, Wakisaka A, Tashiro K, Ishida Y, Ikeuchi T, Koide R, Saito M, Sato A, Tanaka T, Hanyu S, Takiyama Y, Nishizawa M, Shimizu N, Nomura Y, Segawa M, Iwabuchi K, Eguchi I, Tanaka H, Takahashi H, Tsuji S (1996): Identification of the spinocerebellar ataxia type 2 gene using a direct identification of repeat expansion and cloning technique, DIRECT. Nat Genet 14:277–284.

Shankar SK, Yanagihara R, Garruto RM, Grundke Iqbal I, Kosik KS, Gajdusek DC (1989): Immunocytochemical characterization of neurofibrillary tangles in amyotrophic lateral sclerosis and parkinsonism-dementia of Guam. Ann Neurol 25:146–151.

Sherrington R, Froelich S, Sorbi S, Campion D, Chi H, Rogaeva EA, Levesque G, Rogaev EI, Lin C, Liang Y, Ikeda M, Mar L, Brice A, Agid Y, Percy ME, Clerget-Darpoux F, Piacentini S, Marcon G, Nacimas B, Amaducci L, Frebourg T, Lannfelt L, Rommens JM, St George-Hyslop PH (1996): Alzheimer's disease associated with mutations in presenilin 2 is rare and variably penetrant. Hum Mol Genet 5(7):985–988.

Sherrington R, Rogaev EI, Liang Y, Rogaeva EA, Levesque G, Ikeda M, Chi H, Lin C, Li G, Holman K, Tsuda T, Mar L, Foncin J-F, Bruni AC, Montesi MP, Sorbi S, Rainero I, Pinessi L, Nee L, Chumakov I, Pollen D, Brookes A, Sanseau P, Polinsky RJ, Wasco W, Da Silva HAR, Haines JL, Pericak-Vance MA, Tanzi RE, Roses AD, Fraser PE, Rommens JM, St George-Hyslop PH (1995): Cloning of a gene bearing missense mutations in early-onset familial Alzheimer's disease. Nature 375:754–760.

Snowden JS, Neary D, Mann DMA (1996): Fronto-Temporal Lobar Degeneration: Fronto-Temporal Dementia, Progressive Aphasia, Semantic dementia. New York: Churchill Livingstone.

St George-Hyslop PH, Haines J, Rogaev E, Mortilla M, Vaula G, Pericak Vance M, Foncin JF, Montesi M, Bruni A, Sorbi S, et al (1992): Genetic evidence for a novel familial Alzheimer's disease locus on chromosome 14. Nat Genet 2:330–334.

Sumi SM, Bird TD, Nochlin D, Raskind MA (1992): Familial presenile dementia with psychosis associated with cortical neurofibrillary tangles and degeneration of the amygdala. Neurology 42:120–127.

The Huntington's Disease Collaborative Research Group (1993): A novel gene containing a trinucleotide repeat that is expanded and unstable on Huntington's disease chromosomes. Cell 72:971–983.

Thinakaran G, Teplow DB, Siman R, Greenberg B, Sisodia SS (1996): Metabolism of the "Swedish APP" variant in Neuro2A (N2A) cells: Evidence that cleavage at the "b-secretase" site occurs in the Golgi apparatus. J Biol Chem 271:9390–9397.

Trottier Y, Lutz Y, Stevanin G, Imbert G, Devys D, Cancel G, Saudou F, Weber C, David G, Tora L (1995): Polyglutamine expansion as a pathological epitope in Huntington's disease and four dominant cerebellar ataxias. Nature 378:403–406.

Vermersch P, Bordet R, Ledoze F, Ruchoux MM, Chapon F, Thomas P, Destée A, Lechevallier B (1995): Demonstration of a specific profile of pathological tau proteins in frontotemporal dementia cases. CR Acad Sci 318:439–445.

Warren ST (1996): The expanding world of trinucleotide repeats. Science 271:1374–1375.

Wilhelmsen KC, Lynch T, Pavlou E, Higgins M, Nygaard TG (1994): Localization of disinhibition-dementia-parkinsonism-amyotrophy complex to 17q21–22. Am J Hum Genet 55:1159–1165.

Willems PJ (1994): Dynamic mutations hit double figures. Nat Genet 8:213–215.

Wszolek ZK, Pfeiffer RF, Bhatt MH, Schelper RL, Cordes M, Snow BJ, Rodnitzky RL, Wolters EC, Arwert F, Calne DB (1992): Rapidly progressive autosomal dominant parkinsonism and dementia with pallido-ponto-nigral degeneration. Ann Neurol 32:312–320.

Yamaoka LH, Welsh-Bohmer KA, Hulette CM, Gaskell PCJ, Murray M, Rimmler JL, Helms BR, Guerra M, Roses AD, Schmechel DE, Pericak-Vance MA (1996): Linkage of frontotemporal dementia to chromosome 17: Clinical and neuropathological characterization of phenotype. Am J Hum Genet 59:1306–1312.

CHAPTER 19

Clinical and Pathological Overlap in Pick Complex

ANDREW KERTESZ and DAVID G. MUNOZ

Department of Clinical Neurological Sciences (A.K.) and Department of Pathology (D.G.M.),
University of Western Ontario, London, Ontario N6A 4V2, Canada

INTRODUCTION

Arnold Pick described progressive aphasia, apraxia, and personality changes as the major clinical syndromes of frontotemporal atrophy more than 100 years ago. Subsequent reports of extrapyramidal symptoms in Pick's disease (PiD) occurred frequently. Frontal lobe dementia (FLD) (Brun, 1987; Neary et al., 1988), primary progressive aphasia (PPA) (Mesulam, 1982), their combination with motor neuron disease (MND) (Neary et al., 1990; Caselli, 1993), and corticonigral or corticobasal degeneration (CBD) (Rebeiz et al., 1968) have recently been described as separate entities. Their clinical and pathological overlap and its extent are not widely recognized. The reason for this is mainly that longitudinal studies are rare and many autopsy reports have patchy clinical information. Series of cases exemplifying these clinical syndromes tend to emphasize the features on presentation or at the time of examination and not the evolution of the disease. Pathological diagnosis of PiD, on the other hand, is accompanied by a variety of clinical symptoms and syndromes, leading some to conclude that it is difficult to diagnose *in vivo*. Moreover, when the pathological picture lacks Pick bodies or has other distinguishing features, the relationship to PiD is not recognized or is denied even though the clinical picture is the same. We will attempt to show the extent of both clinical and pathological overlap on the basis of our own experience and the review of the literature.

In the last 15 years, we have observed 68 cases of PPA, FLD, CBD, and their various combinations in a dementia population of 365 assessed at our Cognitive Neurology Clinic. Undoubtedly, a referral bias existed since our colleagues were aware of our interest in Pick complex (Kertesz et al., 1994). We also had 15 autopsied cases. Some of these were prospectively followed, and a few (*n* = 6) were retrospectively studied when their autopsy showed Pick complex. In this study we included all patients with more than 3 years of follow-up (average, 6

Pick's Disease and Pick Complex, Edited by Andrew Kertesz and David G. Munoz
ISBN 0-471-17792-X   ©1998 Wiley-Liss, Inc.

years) if they fell into one of the following groups: FLD: patients presenting with personality and behavior disorders of the frontal lobe type ($n = 17$), PPA: progressive aphasia only as the initial feature ($n = 25$), progressive fluent aphasia (PFA) (semantic) ($n = 3$), and CBD syndrome (CBDS) ($n = 9$): presentation with unilateral parkinsonism, apraxia, and alien hand syndrome. FLD cases had behavioral symptoms compatible with the criteria of the Lund/Manchester groups (1994), and PPA cases satisfied Mesulam's (1987) criteria. Those cases that showed a nearly simultaneous presentation of progressive aphasia (PA) but were soon followed by behavioral personality changes or extra-pyramidal-apraxic syndrome were also grouped with PPA. In a few cases, it was difficult to determine from the history which symptom came first. These cases were classified by the predominant or most disabling condition.

The results of our follow-up study indicated that 20/25 PPA patients developed significant personality changes, and 11/17 patients presenting with FLD developed PA. All CBDS patients ($n = 8$) presenting with extrapyramidal or apractic features eventually developed aphasia, and five had additional behavioral or personality changes. Nine of 27 patients with PPA and 5/17 patients with FLD developed features of CBD. One patient with PPA and three patients with FLD also developed features of MND (Table 19.1).

In the FLD type, by the time the patients were seen, most of them had some logopenia or impoverished speech, but their behavioral and personality disorders were the presenting features. Four of the clinically followed patients continue to have normal speech output so far, but all those with autopsy developed a progressive nonfluent speech disorder leading to mutism that was similar to descriptions of PPA. Although FLD was originally described with emphasis on the behavioral changes and personality disturbance, the picture of nonfluent aphasia often progressing to mutism was part of the clinical description in all of the series, and it became a core symptom of what the Lund/Manchester Group called *frontotemporal degeneration*. It remains to be seen if this is different enough from the language disturbance of PPA. MND has been observed less frequently. In two of the patients, it appeared as a definite cause of shortening of the disease course. Extrapyramidal syndromes also appeared in a specific number, and subcortical (CBD) pathology was also seen. The ubiquitinated, tau-negative, non-eosinophilic inclusions (UTNNEI), that are also present in the motor neurons, were more common in FLD/MND, but they were not exclusive for this condition.

TABLE 19.1   Clinical Overlap in Pick Complex

Presentation (*n*)		Second Syndrome (*n*)		Third Syndrome (*n*)	
FLD	(17)	PA	(7)	PA	(4)
		CBDS	(3)	CBDS	(2)
		MND	(2)	MND	(1)
PPA	(27)	FLD	(16)	FLD	(4)
		CBDS	(7)	CBDS	(2)
				MND	(1)
CBDS	(8)	PA	(8)	FLD	(4)
PFA	(3)				
	(55)		(43)		(18)

Abbreviations: FLD = frontal lobe dementia (behavior and personality change is primary); PPA = primary progressive aphasia (logopenic); PA = progressive aphasia; PFA = primary fluent aphasia (some "semantic"); CBDS = corticobasal degeneration syndrome (unilateral rigidity, alien limb, or apraxia); MND = motor neuron disease.

Patients with PPA, on the other hand, often develop behavioral changes that are related to frontal lobe involvement later in their illness. This was the case in about half of our PPA patients. The extrapyramidal-apractic syndrome (CBDS) was seen in a third of PPA patients, in a few as an early feature, causing an accelerated course and early death in two. In most patients these are late developments, and PPA patients function much better than those with FLD. Both PPA and FLD patients are characteristically presenile (disease onset before 65 years of age). The duration of the illness is often 10 years or longer.

Patients with both FLD and PPA presentations may develop extrapyramidal symptoms that are often unilateral and associated with severe apraxia and the alien hand phenomenon. This can be a secondary or tertiary syndrome after the primary frontal or temporal presentation. Although CBD was originally described as a novel extrapyramidal disease, many of the typical patients with CBD develop language deficits and personality changes. Furthermore, CBD pathology is often seen without the extrapyramidal disease, with only PPA or FLD. CBD pathology resembles PiD in many respects, although the location and appearance of the inclusions are different. In addition to this is the large literature dealing with the extrapyramidal or subcortical variety of PiD.

Currently, it appears that the underlying pathology in the clinical syndromes of FLD, PPA, and CBDS can be tentatively divided into six histopathological substrates, although none of the clinical pictures predict the pathological subtype exclusively. The ubiquitin-positive variety appears to be associated with FLD and MND, but there are definite examples of this pathological picture without clinical MND in the literature. The superficial layer microvacuolation (spongiosis), neuronal loss, and gliosis appear to be common underlying features of all histological subtypes. The CBD type of pathology is far from specific for the clinical syndrome of CBDS, and it can occur with PPA and FLD without the extrapyramidal symptoms.

Our 15 autopsied cases were grouped as follows:

1. Classical PiD ($n = 4$) is defined by the presence of argyrophilic, tau-immunoreactive Pick bodies in the neurons of the dentate gyrus of the hippocampus, as well as in other hippocampal, neocortical, and subcortical sites. In addition, Pick cells are always present. There is gliosis and spongiform change in the second and third layers of the cortex. Three of these patients had PPA and one had an FLD presentation clinically (Table 19.2).

TABLE 19.2   Pick Complex: Pathological Variants and Clinical Presentation

		PPA	FLD
A SGN + Pick bodies	4	3	1
B SGN + CBD type	4	3[1]	1
C SGN only	4	2	2
SGN + UTNNEI	3	1	2[1]
Total *n*	15	9	6

Abbreviations: SGN = spongiosis, gliosis, neuronal loss; CBD = corticobasal degeneration (see text); UTNNEI = ubiquitinated tau-negative, noneosinophilic inclusions; PPA = primary progressive aphasia; FLD = frontal lobe dementia.
[1]One patient had additional ALS and faster decline in each category. ABC = Constantinidis and Tissot classification of Pick variants.

2. Corticobasal degeneration type of pathology ($n = 4$) is characterized by the combination of four findings: cortical ballooned neurons (Pick cells); argyrophilic and tau-immunoreactive clusters of astrocytic process (*glial plaques*); a dense network of argyrophilic threads in the white matter, cortex, and basal ganglia; and globose neurofibrillary tangles in the substantia nigra (*corticobasal inclusion bodies*) and other sites. Three patients had PPA and one had the FLD type of presentation. One of the FLD patients with CBD pathology also developed MND (Table 19.2).

3. Dementia of motor neuron type ($n = 3$) is characterized by the presence of ubiquitin-positive but tau-negative, noneosinophilic cytoplasmic inclusions (UTNNEI) in the granular cell layer of the dentate gyrus, and other cortical and subcortical sites. Only one of these patients developed clinical MND and had a more rapid decline. Two presented with FLD and one with PPA (Table 19.2).

4. Dementia lacking distinctive histological findings ($n = 4$), so-called because of the absence of argyrophilic or tau-immunoreactive inclusions, nevertheless consistently shows superficial linear spongiosis in the cortex, gliosis, and neuronal loss, sometimes accompanied by the presence of scattered, ballooned neurons in the deep layers. Two of the patients presented with FLD and two with PPA with this pathology. The spongiosis, gliosis, and neuronal loss (SGN) are features of all other types of pathology in the Pick complex. We do not have enough CBD presentations with pathology to suggest a definite correlation, but one patient with an almost simultaneous FLD and CBD presentation had the typical CBD type of pathology (see the description above).

Subsequent to describing all the entities included in the Pick complex, we will consider the biological significance of this concept. Some will argue that each entity represents a different biological process, and that the entities are tied together by coincidental commonality of phenotypic expression alone. The distinctions between lesions may be emphasized, and lumping of entities may be attributed to the lack of sophistication of earlier pathological studies. In contrast to this position, we postulate that the Pick complex represents a biological condition in which the different entities at least share relevant pathogenetic mechanisms and may in part represent variations of a common theme.

Several arguments can be assembled in support of this hypothesis. The lobar pattern of atrophy is the first defining feature of the group, and a more or less sharp transition from severely atrophic to normal areas sets it apart from other neurodegenerative diseases. However, the involved areas vary within each entity as much as between entities. Thus a single pathological entity, like CBD, can demonstrate at least three modes of presentation, and a single syndrome, like PPA, can have many different pathological substrata. Despite the variability, there are some common tendencies, such as the avoidance of the occipital lobes.

Examination of the neocortex at the microscopic level shows that all entities share a preferential involvement of the supragranular cortical layers accompanied by more or less prominent superficial linear spongiosis. At the level of the hippocampal formation, the preferential atrophy of the subiculum is remarkable for its consistency between entities. Involvement of the substantia nigra is severe in basophilic inclusion body disease and CBD. It is not always appreciated that it is consistently present, albeit with variable severity, in dementia with Pick bodies.

The different variety-specific inclusions bodies, namely, Pick bodies (R-I), UTNNEI (R-II), basophilic (R-III), and corticobasal-type rounded/fibrillary inclusion (R/F) all preferentially affect layer III neurons, in contrast to the involvement of layer V neurons seen in

Alzheimer's disease (AD). They all commonly adopt a spherical shape and are often girdled by a peripheral ring. The inclusions show remarkable differences in immunohistochemistry in a single case, between cases in an entity, and between entities. For example, Pick bodies with intense or absent expression of tau epitopes can be found in a single case. Only a few in any case will be stained by the Gallyas method. The Bielchowsky technique will stain some basophilic inclusions as solid masses, outline a ring in others, and leave the majority unstained. There is marked variation of chromogranin A expression in Pick bodies among apparently identical adjacent neurons in the dentate granular cell layer. The panoply of ultrastructural appearances of the filamentous component of Pick bodies is described in Chapter 15 of this volume. Rather than being rigidly defined structures with fixed antigenic phenotypes, each of the inclusion bodies shows a remarkable degree of variability, resulting in considerable overlap between the types.

Both ballooned neurons and dispersed tau immunoreactivity are neuronal lesions shared by all the entities. The accumulation of aberrantly phosphorylated tau in oligodendrocytes is also part of the common pool of lesions. The astrocytic abnormalities, on the other hand, are more akin to neuronal inclusions in their relatively specific association with a variety. However, even the robust correlation of type A-II astrocytic inclusions (glial plaques) with CBD is not absolute, since similar glial cells can be infrequently found in dementia with Pick bodies.

Differences in pathological tau protein have anchored the distinctions between the different entities first described histologically. However, biochemical studies have also brought at least a subset of dementia lacking distinctive histopathology into the fold of diseases characterized by abnormal tau proteins (see Chapter 16, this volume). The biochemical basis of the histochemical and immunohistochemical heterogeneity of the neuronal inclusions within a single case remains to be elucidated, and this precludes the exploration of overlap between entities at the molecular level. It is possible that multiple genes are involved in the diverse entities gathered under the umbrella of Pick complex. Yet, as long as diseases are defined as clinico-pathological entities, the concept of Pick complex appears to us as useful as that of AD, a malady related to at least four independent genes.

It appears FLD, PPA, frontotemporal atrophies, circumscribed parietal astrophy, CBD, hereditary dysphasic dementia, "dementia without specific pathology," and dementia with motor neuron disease may have certain similarities, both clinically and pathologically, to PiD and may all form a spectrum that may be justifiably called *Pick complex.* Others prefer to restrict the eponymic designation to the presence Pick bodies in the dentate gyrus and have renamed the clinical syndrome *frontotemporal degeneration,* claiming it has different pathologies, each representing different biological entities. Biochemical and genetic evidence of the relationship may allow less reliance on the pathological variations to provide a link. So far, chromosomes 17 and 3 have been identified as candidate sites. The incidence of FLD is considered to be 15–25% of degenerative dementia in various series (with classical PiD included). PPA represents approximately 10% of the patients seen in dementia clinics. In our clinic the incidence appears higher, but this may be related to a referral bias. Even considering that in some centers the same patient may be described as having FLD and in others as having PPA, the combined incidence of the three presentations is likely to exceed 20–25% when vascular or mixed dementias are excluded and 10–15% of all dementias in a cognitive clinic (Table 19.3). Therefore, Pick complex, including classical and atypical varieties of PiD, may be one of the largest nosological entities after AD to cause dementia, particularly in the presenile age group. This may have important implications for future research on the biology and treatment of dementias.

TABLE 19.3   Dementia Diagnosis—5 Years

			Age	
			$\bar{X}$	SD
AD	41%	222	71.0	(8.6)
Pick complex	13%	68	64.0	(9.6)
Vascular	10%	56	71.6	(8.5)
Mixed vascular/AD	9%	51	70.9	(7.2)
Depressive	10%	54	58.9	(8.5)
Subcortical	6%	30	68.5	(6.82)
Pure memory	1%	7	67.0	(11.1)
Senectophobic	1%	6	57.2	(9.5)
Others[1]	9%	46	67.1	(13.1)
Total	100%	540	68.0	(10.2)

[1]Normal pressure hydrocephalus, Creutzfeldt-Jakob, Multiple Sclerosis, Progressive supranuclear palsy, Limbic encephalopathy and contamination by language barrier, low education.

REFERENCES

Brun A (1987): Frontal lobe degeneration of non-Alzheimer type. I. Neuropathology. Arch Geront Geriatr 6:193–208.

Caselli RJ, Windebank AJ, Petersen RC, Komori R, Parisi JE, Okazake H, Kokmen E, Iverson R, Dinapol R, Graf-Radford NR (1993): Rapidly progressive aphasic dementia and motor neuron disease. Ann Neurol 33:200–207.

Kertesz A, Hudson L, Mackenzie IRA, Munoz DG (1994): The pathology and nosology of Primary Progressive Aphasia. Neurology 44:2065–2072.

Lund and Manchester Groups (1994): Clinical and neuropathological criteria for frontotemporal dementia. J Neurol Neurosurg Psychiatry 57:416–418.

Mesulam MM (1982): Slowly progressive aphasia without dementia. Ann Neurol 11:592–598.

Neary D, Snowden JS, Mann DMA, Northen B, Goulding PJ, Macdermott N (1990): Frontal lobe dementia and motor neurone disease. J Neurol Neurosurg Psychiatry 53:23–32.

Neary D, Snowden JS, Northen B, Goulding PJ (1988): Dementia of frontal lobe type. J Neurol Neurosurg Psychiatry 51:353–361.

Rebeiz JJ, Kolodny EH, Richardson EP Jr (1968): Corticodentatonigral degeneration with neuronal achromasia. Arch Neurol 18:20–33.

Index